OECD
SOCIAL POLICY STUDIES
No. 7

HEALTH CARE SYSTEMS IN TRANSITION

ORGANISATION FOR ECONOMIC CO-OPERATION AND DEVELOPMENT

Pursuant to article 1 of the Convention signed in Paris on 14th December 1960, and which came into force on 30th September 1961, the Organisation for Economic Co-operation and Development (OECD) shall promote policies designed:

– to achieve the highest sustainable economic growth and employment and a rising standard of living in Member countries, while maintaining financial stability, and thus to contribute to the development of the world economy;
– to contribute to sound economic expansion in Member as well as non-member countries in the process of economic development; and
– to contribute to the expansion of world trade on a multilateral, non-discriminatory basis in accordance with international obligations.

The original Member countries of the OECD are Austria, Belgium, Canada, Denmark, France, the Federal Republic of Germany, Greece, Iceland, Ireland, Italy, Luxembourg, the Netherlands, Norway, Portugal, Spain, Sweden, Switzerland, Turkey, the United Kingdom and the United States. The following countries became Members subsequently through accession at the dates indicated hereafter: Japan (28th April 1964), Finland (28th January 1969), Australia (7th June 1971) and New Zealand (29th May 1973).

The Socialist Federal Republic of Yugoslavia takes part in some of the work of the OECD (agreement of 28th October 1961).

Publié en français sous le titre :

LES SYSTÈMES
DE SANTÉ

A la recherche d'efficacité

This report is jointly published by the Health Care Financing Administration (HCFA), Office of Research and Demonstrations, US Department of Health and Human Services, under the title, *International Comparison of Health Care Financing and Delivery: Data and Perspectives*, Health Care Financing Review, 1989 Annual Supplement, Baltimore, Maryland.

Preface

The development of health care systems in Organisation for Economic Cooperation and Development (OECD) Member countries has been an issue of concern for a number of years now. The management of health systems has been made difficult by the conflict between budgetary constraints and the growth of health expenditures. There are growing reservations about the efficiency and effectiveness of health care services and about the wisdom of rapidly absorbing new technologies. Linked to these issues are questions about the way in which generous and open-ended provision of health insurance has altered the incentives and behavior of patients, doctors, and other health professionals. These doubts have been strengthened, on the one hand, by the lack of reliable evidence concerning the results of medical interventions and, on the other hand, by the growing evidence of wide variations that prevail in accepted medical practice.

Work at the OECD over a number of years has reflected these concerns. In addition to previous studies such as *Measuring Health Care 1960-1983* (1985) and *Financing and Delivering Health Care* (1987), OECD Ministers responsible for Social Policy, meeting in Paris in 1988, emphasized the need for continuing studies at an international level that would not only address the policy and analytical issues involved but would also provide the empirical basis for a comparative understanding of the differences and similarities between OECD countries. The result of that effort was *The Future of Social Protection* (1988).

This publication is a further step in that direction. It is particularly welcomed both because of its contents and because of the cooperation between the U.S. authorities and the OECD Secretariat and Member countries that has brought it to an early fruition and is making it available to a wide international audience.

T. J. Alexander
Director for Social Affairs, Manpower,
and Education
Organisation for Economic Cooperation
and Development

3

Also available

'OECD Social Policy Studies' Series

No. 1 — SOCIAL EXPENDITURE 1960–1990. Problems of Growth and Control (March 1985)
Out of print. Available on microfiches

No. 2 — MEASURING HEALTH CARE 1960–1983: Expenditure, Costs and Performance (November 1985)
(81 85 06 1)ISBN 92-64-12736-4 162 pages
Out of print. Available on microfiches

No. 3 — LIVING CONDITIONS IN OECD COUNTRIES. A Compendium of Social Indicators (February 1986)
(81 85 04 1)ISBN 92-64-12734-8 166 pages   £6.50   US$13.00   FF65.00 DM26

No. 4 — FINANCING AND DELIVERING HEALTH CARE. A Comparative Analysis of OECD Countries (July 1987)
(81 87 02 1)ISBN 92-64-12973-1 102 pages   £6.00   US$13.00   FF60.00 DM26

No. 5 — REFORMING PUBLIC PENSIONS (August 1988)
(81 88 04 1)ISBN 92-64-13123-X 160 pages   £15.50   US$29.00   FF130.00 DM56

No. 6 — THE FUTURE OF SOCIAL PROTECTION (December 1988)
(81 88 03 1)ISBN 92-64-13152-3 64 pages   £8.50   US$15.50   FF70.00 DM31

Prices charged at the OECD Bookshop.

*The OECD CATALOGUE OF PUBLICATIONS and supplements will be sent free of charge
on request addressed either to OECD Publications Service,
2, rue André-Pascal, 75775 PARIS CEDEX 16,
or to the OECD Distributor in your country.*

Foreword

Comparisons of the industrialized countries' health care financing and delivery systems are both a challenging and ambitious undertaking, conceived in recognition of growing global interdependence and a shared concern among industrialized countries for cost–effective, quality health care.

An examination of international differences in health care financing and delivery is possible because of an extensive data base maintained by the OECD that provides comparable statistics on Member countries.

Although there is no international health accounting framework to facilitate comparative studies, the unique OECD data bank makes a substantial contribution in this direction.

In recent decades, the growth in health care expenditures has exceeded the growth in gross domestic product across the OECD area. Despite slightly slower growth in health care outlays in more recent years relative to that experienced in the 1960s and 1970s, concern persists among Member countries because of continuing economic constraints coupled with competing pressures in the use of resources.

This concern is exacerbated by the aging of the population and its implications for more intensive and extensive use of health care resources in the future, with possible renewed acceleration in the growth of expenditures. As a result, a heightened interest in the efficiency and effectiveness of health care systems has emerged.

Although financial pressures relating to health care systems are a shared experience among Member countries, the underlying structure and delivery of health care is widely divergent from one country to another, as is the manner and extent to which different countries have been able to manage or control expenditures. It is the range of approaches and varying levels of success that make cross–national comparisons so important. The experience of each country serves as an experimental laboratory for others.

In this special issue, several analytic articles explore international differences and trends while acknowledging the inherent difficulties in making cross–national comparisons. The symposium section provides a forum for some of the best minds in the international health arena to take a wide–ranging look at many aspects of health care financing and delivery on both sides of the Atlantic with recommendations for making health care systems more manageable, efficient, and responsive.

Finally, a data compendium section is offered that features more than 60 tables from the OECD presenting comparable statistics for Member countries across a span of 28 years in the following areas: expenditure on health; health care pricing trends; social protection and public participation; utilization of medical services and available personnel resources; selected variations in common medical care practice; selected health status indicators; and demographic and general economic background data.

It is our sincere hope that the articles and the data presented represent a significant contribution to the development and use of internationally comparable statistics on health care financing and delivery and the lessons that we can learn from one another. Both should influence the state–of–the–art and the ability of researchers and policymakers to contribute to more efficient and effective health care systems and, ultimately, the improved health status of the population.

The Health Care Financing Review, which coproduces this volume with OECD, wishes to express appreciation to all contributors to this volume, not only for their unique perspectives and diversity of ideas, but also for their efforts and support in this endeavor.

Joseph R. Antos, Ph.D.
Director, Office of Research and Demonstration, Health Care Financing Administration

Contents

CONTENTS

Overview of international comparisons of health care expenditures

by George J. Schieber and Jean-Pierre Poullier

Health care expenditure and utilization trends in the 24 Organization for Economic Cooperation and Development countries are provided and analyzed in terms of trends in price, population, and volume-intensity. The United States spends more on health than other countries, both in absolute dollar terms and relative to gross domestic product. Moreover, the gap appears to have grown in recent years. Although international comparisons are difficult for a number of reasons outlined in the article, they can be useful in focusing efforts to understand what the United States is getting for its one-half trillion dollar expenditure on health services.

Introduction

This article is an overview of health care expenditure and utilization trends in the 24 Member countries of the Organization for Economic Cooperation and Development (OECD), a Paris-based international organization whose members are the Western industrialized countries. First, the basic underlying data and methodological issues in performing international comparisons are discussed. Second, trends in expenditures are analyzed. Third, increases in expenditures are analyzed in terms of price, population, and volume-intensity trends. Fourth, some concluding methodological and policy prescriptions about international comparisons are made.

Issues in international comparisons

International comparisons are difficult for a variety of reasons, including the following:

- Data are generally not comparable.
- Systems' performance cannot be easily evaluated because of our inability to measure health outcomes.
- It is difficult to measure and control for social, medical, cultural, demographic, and economic differences across countries.
- Transferability of policies across countries is problematic.

International comparisons are only as good as the basic underlying data upon which they are based. Countries produce data for administrative reporting purposes. Their data systems are based on the specific structural features of their health care financing and delivery systems. Thus, for example, if salaried hospital-based physicians are treated as part of hospital sector budgets, as is the case in the Federal Republic of Germany (hereafter called Germany), the Scandinavian countries, and the United Kingdom, then reported hospital expenditures will include these inhospital physician services. On the other hand, in countries, such as the United States and Canada, where most inhospital physician services are paid for on a fee-for-service basis, such expenditures will be reported separately as physician expenditures. Compounding this problem is the lack of internationally accepted definitions of components of health care expenditures, such as hospitals, nursing homes, and home health care.

Health care information is not presently reported in a standardized format. The data used in this article and reported in the data compendium section in this issue represent an attempt by the OECD to develop international health accounts in a manner similar to the development of national income and product accounts some 40 years ago. Although far from perfect, they represent the best attempt to date to develop comparable spending and utilization information. The spending aggregates are based on public and private health consumption and investment information reported as part of the national income and product accounts of the OECD. However, users of these data must bear in mind that individual countries are continually revising their underlying figures, often to as far back as 1960. Thus, although the orders of magnitude rarely change, analysts should not interpret these data too exactly. A brief methodological discussion is provided in the data compendium section of this issue.

A second problem in making international comparisons stems from our inability to measure the performance of health systems. This is a problem even within individual countries, where definitions, reporting conventions, etc. are relatively uniform. Although the structural characteristics of health systems differ, all countries attempt to provide access to medically appropriate and medically effective services in a cost-effective manner. Much of the difficulty in assessing how well countries meet this objective stems from the problems in defining and measuring health outcomes and access to care. Defining and measuring access involve value judgments. Measuring outcomes—beyond aggregate measures such as life expectancy, infant mortality, and cause-specific mortality—is not generally feasible. In addition to inability to measure outcomes (outputs), difficulties in measuring cost effectiveness are further compounded by our inability to allocate

Reprint requests: George J. Schieber, Health Care Financing Administration, Room 2F8, Oak Meadows Building, 6325 Security Boulevard, Baltimore, Maryland 21207.

overhead and assess efficiency in complex multiproduct firms, such as multispecialty group practices and hospitals. As a result, most comparative studies are focused on inputs such as numbers of doctors and hospital beds or intermediate outputs such as physician visits, hospital days, and number of procedures. Even this information is problematic given the lack of standard terminology, discussed earlier. The nominal expenditure information used in the following analysis is based upon relatively comparable definitions of health spending, but the health care price indexes are not. Hence, one must be extremely cautious in interpreting the results.

A third problem in international comparisons stems from comparing countries with different geographical, cultural, social, demographic, political, and economic structures. Although some factors, such as age differences and certain economic factors, can be controlled for statistically, many other factors, such as climate, attitudes about health and family, pollution, and stress levels, cannot (Organization for Economic Cooperation and Development, 1987). A related problem stems from the lack of detailed information about the structural features of different health systems. To understand the basic empirical information about a system, an understanding of the underlying structural interactions among reimbursement, benefits, cost sharing, planning, public versus private insurance, financing methods, legal systems, etc. is essential. Yet, such information is not readily available for most countries in a standardized format and in sufficient detail to provide an understanding of such interactions.

A related issue concerns the transferability of policies across countries. Despite the fact that few rigorous policy evaluations have been made at the microeconomic level, there is a great deal of rhetoric concerning transferability across countries. Yet, for a policy that has worked in one country to be successful in another requires the same set of underlying incentive structures and behavioral responses. For example, in discussing the applicability of health maintenance organizations (HMOs) to countries other than the United States, Luft (1987) points out that transferring risk from the government to the HMO or individuals may be a concept inconsistent with the welfare-state philosophy inherent in many countries; that the performance of HMOs in this country is measured against a fee-for-service system with a great deal of waste and inefficiency; and that, for HMOs to work in other countries, the same types of underlying incentives would need to be operative. Cross-national policy analyses must be based upon rigorous analytical studies and detailed information about the underlying incentive structures of the different health systems.

International trends in health expenditures

Levels and trends in both relative and absolute spending for the 24 OECD countries are analyzed for

Table 1

Total and public health expenditure as a percent of gross domestic product: Organization for Economic Cooperation and Development countries, 1975-87

Country	Total expenditure				Public expenditure			
	1975	1980	1985	1987	1975	1980	1985	1987
	Percent							
Australia	5.7	6.5	7.0	7.1	3.6	4.0	5.0	5.1
Austria	7.3	7.9	8.1	8.4	5.1	5.5	5.4	5.7
Belgium	5.8	6.6	7.2	7.2	4.6	5.4	5.5	5.5
Canada	7.3	7.4	8.4	8.6	5.6	5.6	6.4	6.5
Denmark	6.5	6.8	6.2	6.0	6.0	5.8	5.3	5.2
Finland	6.3	6.5	7.2	7.4	5.0	5.1	5.7	5.8
France	6.8	7.6	8.6	8.6	5.2	6.2	6.9	6.7
Germany	7.8	7.9	8.2	8.2	6.2	6.2	6.4	6.3
Greece	4.1	4.3	4.9	5.3	2.5	3.5	4.0	4.0
Iceland	5.9	6.4	7.3	7.8	5.3	5.7	6.4	6.9
Ireland	7.7	8.5	8.0	7.4	6.4	7.8	7.1	6.4
Italy	5.8	6.8	6.7	6.9	5.0	5.6	5.4	5.4
Japan	5.5	6.4	6.6	6.8	4.0	4.5	4.8	5.0
Luxembourg	5.7	6.8	6.7	7.5	5.2	6.3	6.0	6.9
Netherlands	7.7	8.2	8.3	8.5	5.9	6.5	6.6	6.6
New Zealand	6.4	7.2	6.6	6.9	5.4	6.0	5.6	5.7
Norway	6.7	6.6	6.4	7.5	6.4	6.5	6.1	7.4
Portugal	6.4	5.9	7.0	6.4	3.8	4.2	4.0	3.9
Spain	5.1	5.9	6.0	6.0	3.6	4.4	4.3	4.3
Sweden	8.0	9.5	9.4	9.0	7.2	8.7	8.6	8.2
Switzerland	7.0	7.3	7.7	7.7	4.8	5.0	5.2	5.2
Turkey	—	—	—	3.5	—	—	—	1.4
United Kingdom	5.5	5.8	6.0	6.1	5.0	5.2	5.2	5.3
United States	8.4	9.2	10.6	11.2	3.6	3.9	4.5	4.6
Mean	6.5	7.0	7.4	[1]7.3	5.0	5.5	5.7	[1]5.6

[1]Includes Turkey. 1987 means excluding Turkey are 7.5 percent for total expenditure and 5.8 percent for public expenditure.

SOURCE: Organization for Economic Cooperation and Development: Health Data File, 1989.

the period 1975-87. First, the shares of both total and public health spending relative to gross domestic product (GDP) are analyzed. Next, absolute levels of spending are compared.

Table 1 contains the estimated shares of both total and public health spending in GDP for the OECD countries for 1975, 1980, 1985, and 1987. In 1975, the share of total health spending in GDP (excluding Turkey) ranged from 4.1 percent in Greece to 8.0 percent in Sweden and 8.4 percent in the United States, with an OECD average of 6.5 percent. By 1980, the OECD average had increased to 7.0 percent. It has been increasing at a slower rate ever since, reaching a mean (including Turkey) of 7.3 percent in 1987. In 1987, the shares ranged from 5.3 percent in Greece (3.5 percent in Turkey) to 11.2 percent in the United States. In other analyses, the increasing share of the U.S. GDP devoted to health spending compared with the relative stability of the share in most other major industrialized countries has been documented (Schieber and Poullier, 1989).

The public share of health spending relative to GDP generally mirrors these trends. Public spending accounts for more than three-quarters of health spending, on average, in the OECD countries and accounts for more than 60 percent of spending in all countries except the United States and Turkey, where it is about 40 percent. The share of total health spending that is public has been quite stable since 1980. In 1975, public health spending ranged from 2.5 percent of GDP in Greece to 7.2 percent in Sweden, with an OECD average of 5.0. In 1987, the public share ranged from 3.9 percent of GDP in Portugal (1.4 percent in Turkey) to 8.2 percent in Sweden, with an OECD average of 5.6 percent. The ratios for the United States were 3.6 percent in 1975 and 4.6 percent in 1987, well below the OECD average. The fact that both the share of total health spending in GDP and the public share of total health spending have been relatively stable since 1980 explains the relative stability of the public health share in GDP since 1980, when it was 5.5 percent. It will be interesting to monitor future changes in this ratio in the United States, where there are competing public and private sector approaches to covering those without health insurance, as well as in other OECD countries, where some governments are focusing on more private sector involvement in the financing and delivery of health care.

Although the share of GDP devoted to health care has increased, on average, from 6.5 to 7.3 percent of GDP from 1975 to 1987, there has been some variability across countries. Table 2 contains the rates of growth in real and nominal per capita health spending relative to the rates of growth in real and nominal per capita GDP for selected OECD countries for 1975-87. These elasticities represent the percentage changes in real and nominal per capita health spending relative to the percentage changes in real and nominal per capita GDP, respectively.

The average nominal elasticity for 20 of the 24 OECD countries is 1.1, indicating that, during this

Table 2

Elasticity of per capita health expenditure relative to per capita gross domestic product (GDP): Selected countries, 1975-87

Country	Nominal	Real[1]
	Elasticity	
Australia	1.1	0.9
Austria	1.1	0.8
Belgium	1.3	1.6
Canada	1.2	0.9
Denmark	0.9	0.9
Finland	1.1	0.9
France	1.2	3.1
Germany	1.1	0.9
Greece	1.1	2.5
Iceland	1.1	1.5
Ireland	1.0	1.5
Italy	1.1	1.7
Japan	1.3	1.4
Netherlands	1.2	1.1
Norway	1.0	2.0
Spain	1.1	1.1
Sweden	1.1	1.0
Switzerland	1.2	1.0
United Kingdom	1.1	1.0
United States	1.3	1.1
Mean	1.1	1.3

[1]Health-price-deflated per capita health spending relative to GDP-deflator-adjusted per capita GDP.

SOURCE: Organization for Economic Cooperation and Development: Health Data File, 1989.

period, nominal per capita health spending grew 10 percent faster than nominal per capita GDP did. The nominal elasticities ranged from 0.9 in Denmark to 1.3 in the United States, Belgium, and Japan, indicating that in the latter countries every 10-percent increase in nominal per capita GDP was associated with a 13-percent increase in nominal per capita health spending, thus resulting in a growing share of health in GDP. In terms of the growth in real per capita health spending (health price deflated) relative to real per capita GDP (GDP deflator adjusted), the elasticities ranged from 0.8 in Austria to 3.1 in France, with a 20-country OECD average of 1.3. The U.S. real elasticity is 1.1. To a large extent, these relatively small values, on average and for most countries, reflect the time period chosen. Following the oil shocks in the mid-1970s, most countries faced a protracted period of inflation and economic stagnation. These adverse economic conditions forced many countries to constrain public spending. Elasticities for the period 1960-75, an era of strong economic growth and expansion of public programs, are substantially higher, 1.4 for the average nominal elasticity and 1.7 for the average real elasticity. In the decomposition analysis presented later in this article, these trends are further analyzed in terms of price, population, and volume-intensity changes.

Absolute health spending levels also differ significantly across countries. However, establishing absolute levels in a numeraire currency is difficult. Exchange rates reflect short-run capital flows and other confounding aspects of international capital markets. As such, they are not pure price indexes and hence will not provide real volume difference estimates when used to deflate health spending. Purchasing power parities (PPPs) are price indexes that represent the average prices in specific countries relative to the average international prices for an entire group of countries for purchasing the same market basket of goods and services (Ward, 1985). Although PPPs have been developed for health services, they are in only a preliminary stage of development and are considered less reliable than GDP PPPs.

Table 3 contains 1987 per capita health expenditures and per capita GDP denominated in U.S. dollars through the use of GDP PPPs. Per capita spending ranged from less than $400 in Turkey ($148), Greece ($337), and Portugal ($386) to more than $1,200 in Switzerland ($1,225), Sweden ($1,233), Iceland ($1,241), Canada ($1,483), and the United States ($2,051), with an OECD average of $934. Expenditures in the United States were more than double the OECD average and 38 percent higher than expenditures in Canada, the second highest country. Although the United States has the highest per capita GDP and health spending is directly related to GDP, U.S. spending exceeds the basic underlying trend relationship by more than $400 per person (Schieber and Poullier, 1989). As in the case of the health share in GDP, the United States spends more than any

other country in the world, and the gap between the United States and other countries is widening. To obtain a better understanding of these macroexpenditure trends, nominal increases in health care expenditures are disaggregated into health care price inflation, overall inflation, excess health care inflation, population, and volume-intensity changes.

Decomposition of health expenditures

Health expenditure trends across countries can also be analyzed by comparing growth in health spending, health care prices, and volume-intensity changes within individual countries based on local currencies and prices. This is done through the well-known identity stating that 1 plus the annual percentage growth in nominal health spending equals the product of 1 plus the annual percentage growth in health care prices times 1 plus the annual percentage growth in volume-intensity (utilization) times 1 plus the annual percentage growth in population. Aggregate data on volume-intensity increases do not exist, but information on nominal expenditures, prices, and population is available. Therefore, volume-intensity is calculated as a residual (Organization for Economic Cooperation and Development, 1987) in the following way. Let H = 1 + annual percentage increase in health spending, POP = 1 + annual percentage increase in population, HP = 1 + annual percentage increase in health care prices, and V = 1 + annual percentage increase in volume-intensity. Suppose that nominal health expenditures increased at a compound annual rate of 10 percent during the time period under consideration, population increased by 1 percent, and health care prices increased by 4 percent. To calculate the volume-intensity increase, the following equation is solved:

$$H = HP \times V \times POP.$$

In the example cited,

$$V = H/ (HP \times POP) =$$
$$1.10/ (1.04 \times 1.01) = 1.047.$$

In other words, volume-intensity increased at a compound annual rate of 4.7 percent over the time period in question.

Inflationary trends in the health sector relative to general inflation can be analyzed by comparing health care price increases with increases in the GDP deflator. If one makes the assumption that health sector prices should increase at the same rate as overall price increases as measured by the GDP deflator, then any excess growth in health care prices can be defined as excess health care inflation. Mechanically, this is done through the identity that 1 plus the annual percentage increase in health care prices equals 1 plus the annual percentage increase in overall prices times 1 plus the annual percentage increase in health care prices in excess of overall prices. Substituting this identity into the previous one

Table 3

Per capita health expenditure and per capita gross domestic product (GDP): Organization for Economic Cooperation and Development countries, 1987

Country	Health expenditure	GDP
	Per capita amount	
Australia	$ 939	$12,612
Austria	982	11,664
Belgium	879	11,802
Canada	1,483	17,211
Denmark	792	13,329
Finland	949	12,838
France	1,105	12,803
Germany	1,093	13,323
Greece	337	6,363
Iceland	1,241	15,508
Ireland	561	7,541
Italy	841	12,254
Japan	915	13,182
Luxembourg	1,050	14,705
Netherlands	1,041	12,252
New Zealand	733	10,680
Norway	1,149	15,405
Portugal	386	6,297
Spain	521	8,681
Sweden	1,233	13,771
Switzerland	1,225	15,842
Turkey	148	4,247
United Kingdom	758	12,340
United States	2,051	18,338
Mean	934	12,207

NOTE: Amounts are denominated in U.S. dollars through the use of GDP purchasing power parities.

SOURCE: Organization for Economic Cooperation and Development: Health Data File, 1989.

results in increases in nominal health expenditures being equal to increases in volume-intensity times increases in overall prices times increases in health prices in excess of overall prices times increases in population. Using the definitions in the earlier example and defining 1 plus the annual percentage increase in the GDP deflator as P and 1 plus the annual percentage increase in excess health care inflation as EHP:

$$EHP = HP/P,$$

$$HP = P \times EHP,$$

$$H = HP \times V \times POP = P \times EHP \times V \times POP.$$

This identity provides useful comparative information on increases in nominal health spending, health care inflation, and growth in the volume-intensity of services. However, because these relationships are based on an identity, no causality can be attributed. Moreover, because the decomposition analysis provides information only on rates of increase over some time period, it provides no information about the base levels of spending and/or the appropriateness of the base or rates of increase.

Table 4 contains a decomposition of health expenditures for the seven major OECD countries for 1975-87. Columns (1) and (9) of the table contain baseline information on the shares of GDP devoted to health care in the seven countries in 1975 and 1987. Columns (2) through (8) contain information on the annual compound rates of growth in nominal health expenditures, health care prices, GDP deflator, excess health care inflation, real health expenditures, population, and volume-intensity of services per person (i.e., real per capita expenditures). From 1975 to 1987, nominal health expenditures increased, on average, at an annual compound rate of growth of 11.8 percent; health care prices increased at a rate of 8.3 percent; real expenditures (health care price deflated), 3.3 percent; population, 0.5 percent; and volume-intensity of services per person, 2.8 percent. Health care prices, on average, increased annually 0.9 percent faster than overall inflation did.

From the perspective of individual countries, nominal annual expenditure increases ranged from 6.2 percent in Germany to 17.6 percent in Italy. Nominal expenditures in the United States increased at an annual compound rate of growth of 11.7 percent. Health care price increases ranged from 3.9 percent per year in Germany to 14.9 percent in Italy, with the U.S. increase being 8.1 percent. Excess health care inflation (the amount exceeding overall inflation) ranged from -1.1 percent in France to 2.2 percent in the United States. Increases in volume-intensity per person ranged from 1.9 percent per year in Canada and the United Kingdom to 4.9 percent in France, with the U.S. increase being 2.3 percent. As shown in other analyses for different years, U.S. and Canadian trends appear to be quite similar (Schieber and Poullier, 1989).

From a health policy perspective, the two basic endogenous factors driving health expenditures are excess health care inflation and real increases in the volume-intensity of services per person. If excess health care inflation had been eliminated in the seven countries, annual nominal expenditure growth would have been reduced by almost 1 percentage point. Reducing the annual increase in volume-intensity growth by one-third would have had about the same effect. In the United States, if the 2.2-percent annual increase in health expenditures resulting from excess health care inflation had not occurred, nominal spending during the period 1975-87 would have increased by 9.3 percent per year instead of 11.7 percent, resulting in 1987 expenditures of $390 billion instead of $500 billion. Similar analyses can be performed for other countries.

Critical to all these analyses is the validity of the price indexes employed. This is an especially difficult area for international comparisons. Health care price indexes that accurately capture the actual amounts paid per unit of quality-adjusted service are difficult to construct even in the most data-sophisticated countries. The price indexes used here are based on extant indexes in the individual countries. They are not based on standard definitions and concepts. (Refer to the data compendium section in this issue.) However, these indexes are an improvement over previous indexes used for comparative analyses in that they reflect both public and private prices, thus, to some extent, obviating the problem that public price measures are overweighted by services provided by the public sector, with the converse being true for private consumer price indexes. A second and equally serious problem is the difficulty in adjusting for productivity changes. For example, how well do most currently employed indexes that are based on charges or input costs capture the secular declines in lengths of stay and the increased sophistication in diagnostic capability witnessed recently? The negative excess health care inflation found for France may well represent an overadjustment for these factors in comparison with other countries, which do not make such adjustments. Once again, international comparisons are clearly limited by the methodological state of the art.

Conclusion

The analyses described in this article are some simple examples of the kinds of comparative studies that can be performed from existing international data bases. Unfortunately, use of such analyses for making definitive policy prescriptions is limited by both data constraints and the inherent difficulties underlying all health services research. Although some of these difficulties stem from lack of standardized definitions and data, others stem from the basic difficulties of evaluating health and other social systems. Lack of reliable outcome measures coupled with the difficulty of measuring behavioral response to policy interventions, even within individual countries,

Table 4

Decomposition of health expenditure increases into price, population, and volume-intensity increases: Selected countries, 1975-87

Country	Share of health expenditure in GDP, 1975 (1)	Nominal health expenditure growth (2)	Annual compound rate of growth, 1975-87						Share of health expenditure in GDP, 1987 (9)
			Health care price deflator (3)	Of which GDP deflator (4)	Of which excess health care inflation (5)	Real expenditure growth (6)	Of which population growth (7)	Of which per capita volume-intensity growth (8)	
			Percent						
Canada	7.3	11.8	8.6	6.5	2.0	2.9	1.0	1.9	8.6
France	6.8	13.4	7.6	8.8	-1.1	5.4	0.5	4.9	8.6
Germany	7.8	6.2	3.9	3.4	0.4	2.2	-0.1	2.3	8.2
Italy	5.8	17.6	14.9	14.1	0.7	2.3	0.3	2.0	6.9
Japan	5.5	9.1	4.1	2.9	1.2	4.8	0.8	4.0	6.8
United Kingdom	5.5	13.0	10.8	9.7	1.0	2.0	0.1	1.9	6.1
United States	8.4	11.7	8.1	5.8	2.2	3.3	1.0	2.3	11.2
Mean	6.7	11.8	8.3	7.3	0.9	3.3	0.5	2.8	8.1

NOTE: GDP is gross domestic product.

SOURCE: Organization for Economic Cooperation and Development: Health Data File, 1989.

exacerbates the problem several-fold. Even within the United States, despite detailed data and substantial resources devoted to health services research, we have little valid information about the behavioral responses of consumers, medical care providers, and third-party insurers. The debates about the costs of a Medicare drug benefit and the cost and supply response impacts of physicians to a fee schedule based on the Harvard resource-based relative value scale provide good examples of the difficulties in predicting behavioral response.

Nevertheless, several relevant facts are clear. First, the United States spends far more in absolute dollar terms and relative to GDP than any other country in the world. Second, this gap appears to have grown in recent years. Third, the higher GDP of the United States can explain only a small part of these disparities. The United States tends to have about the same physician-population ratio as the average for the OECD countries and fewer inpatient medical care beds. U.S. use rates in terms of physician visits, hospital days, and average lengths of stay are among the lowest in the OECD. Yet, the costs for medical procedures and the costs per hospital bed, day, and stay are the highest in the world by far. Americans appear to practice a much more intensive style of medicine. Nevertheless, on the basis of crude outcome measures such as infant mortality and life expectancy as well as access-to-care criteria, the achievements fall short of those in many other OECD countries (Organization for Economic Cooperation and Development, 1987).

Do Americans with good insurance coverage and access to technologically sophisticated urban tertiary care facilities really receive the best quality care in the world? Are amenities in the United States far superior to those in other countries? Is the U.S. system simply more wasteful because Americans can afford to be wasteful? The current knowledge base is not sufficient for obtaining answers to these queries. However, international comparisons can be useful in focusing our own efforts to understand what the American health care system is getting for its more than one-half trillion dollar expenditure on health services and how the system might be changed in order to promote a "kinder and gentler" America.

References

Luft, H. S.: Alternative Delivery Systems: Applicability of the United States Experience with Health Maintenance Organizations to Other Countries. Internal Working Paper. Paris. Organization for Economic Cooperation and Development, 1987

Organization for Economic Cooperation and Development: *Financing and Delivering Health Care*. Paris, 1987.

Schieber, G. J., and Poullier, J. P.: International health care expenditure trends: 1987. *Health Affairs* 8(3):169-177 Fall 1989.

Ward, M.: *Purchasing Power Parities and Real Expenditures in the OECD*. Paris. Organization for Economic Cooperation and Development, 1985.

International differences in medical care practices

by Klim McPherson

An overview of several aspects of international comparisons of medical care utilization is presented with a discussion of the usefulness of such comparisons in identifying geographic variations in utilization and in elucidating the nature of clinical decisionmaking regarding various procedures. The discussion includes the purposes of conducting international studies as well as the methodological and policy issues involved. Brief descriptions of some of the studies that have been conducted are also provided.

Introduction

Health care is consuming ever-increasing proportions of developed nations' budgets. As populations age and the ability to provide effective intervention increases, medical care inflation continues to outstrip retail price indices. The aggregate utility of these expenditures, as well as each new increment that results from new diseases such as acquired immunodeficiency syndrome, new techniques such as organ transplants, technological advances in diagnostic equipment, and more sophisticated drug therapies are being questioned by governments faced with the provision of adequate health care that requires more real funding in each year than it did in the previous one.

We are entering an age, therefore, where questioning will be axiomatic in health care provision. New techniques will no longer be universally implemented without evaluating value versus cost. Even common procedures will come under more intense scrutiny as the need for justification increases. The nature of this progression increasingly becomes a rationing process. However, to ration in medicine is to do something which is quite alien to health care provision as it has evolved. One has to be absolutely certain that real benefit is not being withheld; incontrovertible evidence of efficacy or lack of it is needed as a prerequisite for rationing.

The resolution of the health care dilemma is hindered by two factors. The first is that this era of questioning is somewhat threatening to the medical profession, which has taken, and been given, decisionmaking responsibility and power (Friedson, 1972). The second, and in the end the real hindrance, is the difficulty with which many of the important questions can actually be answered.

If limited resources are to be focused on the provision of appropriate care, one must know what appropriate care is. In health care, there is a diversity of accepted opinion on the need for and value of alternative treatments. In many situations, equally qualified physicians might disagree on which treatment is optimal. There is often no scientifically correct way to practice much of medicine. Many accepted theories concerning the treatment of illness have not been adequately assessed, and consensus based on knowledge of treatment outcomes is the exception rather than the rule.

Overall efficiency

The aggregate cost to a population of hospital health care, measured in terms of annual costs per capita, is the product of two independent components. The first is the average cost per admission. This is intensively studied and relatively easily measured, and attempts to monitor contributing factors, such as diagnostic tests, length of stay, or manpower costs, can greatly affect its magnitude. The second component, less intensively studied but often more important, is average annual admission rates per capita. This component is often assumed to reflect medical need and, as such, is not subject to questioning; to question admission itself assumes a broader concept of efficiency than is usual. However, many causes of admission are associated with large variations in their per capita rates and, therefore, can be strong determinants of per capita health expenditure.

Overall efficiency requires that the aggregate activity of the hospital service maximizes the benefit-to-cost ratio of all alternative admission and process options. This means that those patients for whom the greatest benefit is realistically expected are admitted in preference to those for whom little benefit can be expected and that, among those admitted, the therapeutic options should maximize benefit-to-cost ratios. Such criteria lead inexorably to a greater interest in measuring the outcomes associated with hospital admissions and in comparing such outcomes with those associated with alternative forms of treatment.

Measuring outcome

The crucial yardstick by which all aspects of medical care will come to be measured will inevitably be outcome and, in particular, the improvement in outcome consequent upon the particular intervention. This is the benefit. There are many problems with its measurement, not least of which is the placebo effect associated with almost all supposedly active medical intervention (Beecher and Boston, 1961).

Reprint requests: Klim McPherson, University of Oxford, Department of Community Medicine and General Practice, Oxford, OX 26 HE, United Kingdom.

Disentangling this effect from a "real" therapeutic effect is one of the major problems with its measurement.

Moreover, there are many dimensions of outcome to which different people will attach different weights (Sacket and Torrance, 1978; Llewellyn-Thomas et al., 1984). For instance, for some, the length of survival with cancer is more important than the quality of life experienced (McNeil, Weichselbaum, and Pauker, 1978). While, for others, any suffering is worth avoiding even at the cost of extended life. Such individual preferences would indicate the need for discrete sets of outcome parameters (Mulley, 1989). The probabilities of achieving these sets associated with different clinical decisions, or indeed complex sets of interwoven decisions, should be known. Only then can rational choices be made about the provision of health care and whether expenditures are justified when other possibilities are considered.

Not only are the pertinent questions often complex, but the data that are available to help answer the questions are often limited. To measure outcome, one needs followup. Routine health statistics rarely provide such information because patients are lost to the system once they are discharged. Therefore, to measure even mortality 6 months after discharge is usually impossible outside the environment of special studies, and to assess quality of life is more difficult still.

Origins of clinical uncertainty

Advances in medical knowledge have come, to an extent, from undirected basic research (Comroe and Dripps, 1977). The basic knowledge that results from research and development is then formulated into a clinically usable form, sometimes through evaluation with or without clinical trials and sometimes without evaluation. The clinical practices that emerge from this inconsistent process of diffusion may begin with a strong science base, but this base is often gradually weakened as it evolves through several stages to clinical practice (Fineberg, 1985; Bunker and Fowles, 1982). Herein lies an essential paradox in the study of medical practice. Medicine is widely held to be a science, but many medical decisions do not rely on a strong scientific foundation, simply because such a foundation has yet to be fully explored, developed, and tested.

What often happens in the medical decisionmaking process is a complicated interaction of scientific evidence, patient desire, doctor preferences, and all sorts of exogenous influences, some of which may be quite irrelevant. This tends to mean that the extent to which individual clinical decisions can actually be justified by a coherent body of scientific knowledge is likely to be variable. More importantly, it is not always obvious where, within this spectrum of variability, a particular clinical judgment might lie.

The frank recognition of the existence, or the extent, of clinical uncertainty by health professionals can be difficult, however. People, on the whole, find clinical uncertainty disconcerting both when ill and when responsible for treating illness (Ingelfinger, 1980) and there is a tendency to disguise it. Patients who are concerned with their symptoms are happier if they can believe that what is being done can be justified scientifically, and health professionals command more respect if what they do is based on professional expertise. However, to question and evaluate medical care practice fairly (so that rationing can be rational), it is necessary to recognize all important uncertainty that exists.

Detecting important uncertainty

Some insight into the variation that exists in determining medical treatment is provided by epidemiological investigation of clinical consistency. In recent years, hospital use and procedure rates have become the subject of intensive investigation in many countries with a view to describing and understanding the nature of clinical decisionmaking (Bunker, Barnes, and Mosteller, 1977; Aaron and Schwartz, 1984; Wennberg and Gittelsohn, 1982).

As early as the 1930s, differences in tonsillectomy rates were observed among school districts of Southern England (Glover, 1938). The work of Bunker (1970), Vayda (1973), and McPherson et al. (1981) have documented the extent of cross-national variation in many population-based hospital use rates and drawn attention to the generally higher rates in North America compared with the United Kingdom or other European countries for which data exist. These differences are sometimes of such magnitude that important questions are raised about the causes and consequences, such as resource cost implications, which are easily estimated (McPherson, 1988).

Small area variation studies

During the 1970s, work on variations in rates led to the study of small geographic areas. Although gross differences in morbidity, in need, or in access to health care among relatively homogeneous communities should not exist, gross differences on a per capita basis in the use of many operations or procedures were recorded. Some of this variation resulted from differences in the supply of facilities, but differences in clinical decisionmaking were also reflected. Although international differences in use rates would rarely be entirely attributable to clinical differences, such an explanation was much more difficult to avoid for small area variations. In fact, ancillary evidence from surveys of need and illness rates only served to confirm such an explanation. Moreover, the nature of the observed variation was consistent with the level of certainty involved in determining appropriate medical treatment. Those conditions, such as hip fractures, that invariably required hospitalization exhibited little variation in their rates among small areas.

Table 1

Magnitude of systematic variation (in ascending order) for selected causes of admission among 30 hospital market areas in Maine: 1980-82

Variation	Medical	Surgical
Low: 1.5 fold range	—	Inguinal hernia repair Hip repair
Moderate: 2.5 fold range	Acute myocardial infarction Gastrointestinal hemorrhage Cerebrovascular accident	Appendectomy Major bowel surgery Cholecystectomy
High: 3.5 fold range	Respiratory neoplasms Cardiac arrhythmias Angina pectoris Psychosis Depressive neurosis Medical back problems Digestive malignancy Adult diabetes	Hysterectomy Major cardiovascular operations Lens operations Major joint operations Anal operations Back and neck operations
Very high: 8.5+ fold range	Adult bronchiolitis Chest pain Transient ischemic attacks Minor skin disorders Chronic obstructive lung disease Hypertension Atherosclerosis Chemotherapy	Knee operations Transurethral operations Extraocular operations Breast biopsy Dilation and curettage Tonsillectomy Tubal interruption

SOURCE: (Wennberg, McPherson, and Caper, 1984).

Wennberg and Gittelsohn (1982) proposed that variations in procedure rates reflected supplier-induced demand. Often patterns of procedure-specific, population-based rates existed in hospital service areas that could not be explained by the characteristics of the populations served and were sustained over several years until there was a change in clinical personnel. The concept of supplier-induced demand was further supported by studies of physician feedback programs where information on rates was provided; in geographic areas where rates were found to be high, a common physician response was to reduce procedure rates (Lembcke, 1956; Dyck, 1977; Wennberg and Gittelsohn, 1973; American Medical Association, 1986). Therefore, variations in hospital use rates between communities that are similar in major determinants of health, need, or use and that are larger than could be explained by chance are likely to be a manifestation of clinical uncertainty, i.e., differences in clinical opinion (Wennberg et al., 1987). This leads to comparison of the amount of systematic variation between neighboring small areas across procedures as well as across countries or health care systems. Such comparisons require a metric for measuring variation that is robust and excludes the random component of variation (McPherson et al., 1982; Roos, Wennberg, and McPherson, 1988).

In making such comparisons, some procedures are found to exhibit much more variation than others (Table 1). If this variation is taken as a measure of clinical uncertainty among professionals, then the uncertainty attached to determining admission can be compared. Hysterectomy, for example, exhibits more variation than appendectomy. The same procedures exhibit as much relative variation in the centralized system of the United Kingdom as they do in the United States despite higher aggregate rates in

North America (McPherson et al., 1982). Therefore, the clinical uncertainty concerning the indications for these procedures and for hospitalization for medical diagnoses in general is a function of the procedure or diagnosis itself, rather than the health system through which care is provided. As shown in Table 1, there is a hierarchy of implied uncertainty. Such information is invaluable in the interpretation of international differences in rates.

For one study, 90 percent of admissions exhibited greater variation among neighboring communities than occurred for hysterectomy rates (Table 2). Such a phenomenon may indicate the level of clinical uncertainty and may encourage clinicians to question their therapeutic decisions, but it does not provide necessary information about appropriate use rates. Low rates are neither necessarily better nor worse than high rates where patient welfare is concerned.

Table 2

Percent of admissions categorized by typical diagnosis-related groups with different characteristic variation among 30 hospital market areas in Maine: 1980-82

Variation	Typical diagnosis-related group	Percent admissions	Cumulative percent
Low	Hernia	1.1	1.1
Moderate	Appendectomy	8.9	10.1
High	Hysterectomy	42.3	52.4
Very high I	Disc removal	31.7	84.1
Very high II	Tonsillectomy	15.9	100.0

NOTE: The number of admissions on which percents are based is 428,056.

SOURCE: (Wennberg, McPherson, and Caper, 1984).

Such large variations, however, can lead to acceptance of prospective clinical trials to determine the parameters of appropriate care.

Reasons for differences in rates

When comparing rates for health care practices among countries, it is important to be aware of all of the possible reasons for observed differences. Many aspects of health care differ among countries (Schieber, 1987; Poullier, 1985). The utility of any comparisons depends on the extent to which competing explanations are determined to be causative. By adopting a somewhat simplistic view of the purpose of health care, certain causes of variation can be designated as legitimate and others as artifactual.

Legitimate causes of variation

The populations being compared may have different prevailing rates of illness for which the intervention is appropriate. This alone could cause observed differences in rates. In general, comparative morbidity rates are difficult to obtain because they are measured by admission rates or consultation rates which are themselves confounded by medical practice variations.

Genuine surveys of morbidity could give insights into differences in rates, but they would be expensive to do reliably. The single exception would be cancer incidence rates (Muir, 1976) where rates of disease are uncontaminated by supply or clinical preferences. However, even these are subject to artifacts of recording, such as diagnostic ambiguities, incomplete enumeration of the population at risk, or omission of cases from private or religious hospitals. Thus, systematic differences among countries may not be entirely a manifestation of real differences in incidence (Doll and Peto, 1981).

The same difficulty exists for comparative morbidity rates that rely on cause-specific mortality rates. The designation and coding of death certificates are a function of local practices and may not reflect true epidemiological differences. However, large differences in genuine incidence of disease may exist, particularly between the developing and developed world.

Different age and sex characteristics of populations also have an impact. Diseases are usually more common with increasing age and more prevalent in one gender than the other. If a population consists of a higher proportion of elderly females (as in Sweden), then this could explain differences in rates. Therefore, comparisons among countries should be standardized for the age and sex distribution of the populations, when possible. This way, any residual differences are unlikely to be a consequence of different demography. However, among the countries of the Organization for Economic Cooperation and Development (OECD), demography should not be a major determinant of large variations in rates.

Artifactual reasons for variations

When comparing rates, it is vital to exclude all artifactual reasons for differences. For example, high rates of intervention in previous years may give rise to low rates for current time periods. For relevant comparisons to be made, the rates need to be related to the estimated population at risk (Gittelsohn and Wennberg, 1976).

Hospital use statistics may underestimate the real population because of the systematic exclusion of some hospital admissions, for example in private or religious facilities. Also, patients who are discharged on the same day as admission (day cases) will often not appear in hospital statistics (Nicholl, Beeby, and Williams, 1988). A low rate in a community for hernia repair may indicate a larger proportion of day cases and a preference for day surgery rather than reflect any other practice variation. If one must be careful that population estimates provide the proper denominators for the calculation of rates, it is equally important to account for cross-boundary flow to ensure that numerators are not inflated by people not at risk of admission in the geographic area (Wennberg and Gittelsohn, 1973).

In addition to the completeness of recording all admissions and accurate and reliable population estimates, there may be other coding artifacts that require careful scrutiny. For example, some health information systems record up to three procedures per admission while others record only one. An incidental appendectomy that would be included in the former would be excluded in the latter. Also, the nomenclature used to record operations may differ, for example, "cholecystectomy" versus "operations on the gallbladder" (McPherson et al., 1981).

Such considerations imply the need for great care in interpreting rates, particularly among countries where significant distinctions exist in the mode of care and data collection activities. In comparing rates among countries, one has to be certain that an important part of the observed variation is not attributable to any of these factors. However, known epidemiology gives insights into plausible differences in illness rates and their relationship to age and gender, and limits on likely variation can be set. The observed variations outside these limits that are not artifactual are taken to be manifestations of practice variation (and in large part, the level of professional uncertainty concerning appropriate treatment) until demonstrated to be attributable to something else.

Clinical judgment

Clinicians may differ in making diagnoses, but even assuming the same diagnosis, they may have different opinions about the relative merits of various treatment options for a given condition, in the absence of biological certainty. Their beliefs are based on their respective educations, understanding of the literature, and personal experiences in practice. Whatever the basis for these beliefs, medical evidence is open to interpretation and may later be proven wrong. Such evidence may nonetheless appear convincing. When clouded by financial and professional considerations, such beliefs are more difficult to evaluate.

The greater concern is that strongly held beliefs can prohibit randomized comparison, which provides the most reliable information on the relative efficacy of competing treatments (Hill, 1962; Cochrane, 1971). It is the lack of this reliable information, which in turn contributes to the level of uncertainty, that ultimately impacts on the variation found in medical practice. Unfortunately, the determination of medical efficacy, in all its dimensions of outcome, is often extremely difficult. The consequence of doing one rather than another intervention for a given disease state is, in such circumstances, imprecisely understood by anyone, so clinicians must rely on their own best judgments and some medical consensus where it exists.

Prevailing custom

Some communities might eschew certain kinds of medical intervention more than others, notwithstanding availability or recommendation. This may be the result of prevailing medical opinion or of patient preferences by long-standing custom or tradition. Such things might affect the dominant case mix of admission procedures.

Supply and availability of resources

The availability of resources inevitably affects clinical decisions. Either some decisions are prohibited because the necessary resources are not available at the right time or some rationing occurs when priorities are set for the use of available resources.

Annual health budgets within countries affect availability. For those nations where per capita outlay is minimal, almost nothing is provided to the majority of the population. Yet there are some where the average expenditure might be several hundred dollars, and still others where health resources are consumed at even higher rates (Maxwell, 1981; Organization for Economic Cooperation and Development, 1989).

The method of payment for medical services also has an impact on availability. Fee-for-service systems tend to provide high levels of availability for acute services for patients with adequate medical insurance and low levels for patients without such coverage, in particular for chronic diseases. On the other hand, prepayment systems tend to under provide services because of incentives to minimize expenditures. For these reasons, the payment method is confounded by both availability and clinical judgment. As George Bernard Shaw (1971) said in 1906, "Nobody supposes that doctors are less virtuous than judges; but a judge whose salary and reputation depended on whether the verdict was for the plaintiff or the defendant, prosecutor or prisoner, would be as little trusted as a general in the pay of the enemy."

Another important consideration is the way in which patients are admitted to the hospital. In an exclusively referral system, all decisions to hospitalize are the outcome of several screening processes. For example, in the United Kingdom patients have to decide to obtain advice from their general practitioners, who in turn have to decide to refer out their patients, at which point other decisions will have to be made about the need for hospital admission. Since the decisions made at each point in this process are constrained by different exogenous influences, the outcomes could be systematically different from those that could occur when patients seek advice directly from specialists. Specialists can be expected to be enthusiasts for their specialties and have a less detached view of the need for their services. Second opinion programs in the United States have shown that hospitalization rates are reduced when an opinion is sought from an independent consultant (McCarthy, Finkel, and Ruchlin, 1982). Where such programs are a normal part of medical care, use rates for uncertain indications could be expected to be lower; where they are not, they may well be higher. In either case, the rates are not necessarily appropriate; however, the former will cost less to current budgets.

The effect of the distribution of specialists should not be underestimated. Stevens (1977) has argued that the evolution of specialist guilds in different countries gives rise to quite different influences on the referral process. Primary care is more dominant in some countries than in others. In constrained health systems, patients may be discouraged from seeking services if they suspect that a wait or a delay is involved. In this way, the availability of resources operates as a direct restraint by precluding certain actions, but it also indirectly affects both patients' readiness to seek advice and clinical decisions about priorities. By the same token, a higher level of availability may directly encourage use by patients whose perceived benefit may be marginal, but this indirectly mitigates the need for rationing.

All of these factors contribute to observed variations; the purpose in studying variations in use rates is to understand the dominant causes and to identify fruitful areas of research and evaluation. International comparisons could invoke sensible models for incorporating data from each country to measure indices of these parameters. Unfortunately, many countries still cannot provide utilization data.

Variations in admission rates

Many studies have documented large variations among countries in hospital admission rates for surgical and medical causes. The literature on variations in utilization rates among countries was recently reviewed by Sanders, Coulter, and McPherson (1989), and useful bibliographies are provided in Sanders (1988) and Ham (1988). As shown in Table 3, variations in admission rates were evident for the populations at risk for selected

Table 3

Reported admission rates for selected procedures: Selected countries for which data were reported, 1980

Country	Procedure								
	Tonsill-ectomy	Coronary bypass	Cholecyst-ectomy	Inguinal hernia repair	Exploratory laparotomy	Prostat-ectomy	Hyster-ectomy	Operation on lens	Append-ectomy
	Number of admissions per 1,000 population								
Australia	115	32	145	202	99	183	405	101	340
Canada	89	26	219	224	105	229	479	139	143
Denmark	229	—	21	—	—	234	255	118	248
Ireland	256	4	91	100	52	124	123	64	245
Japan	61	1	2	67	—	—	90	35	244
Netherlands	421	5	131	175	—	116	381	68	149
New Zealand	102	2	99	211	110	191	431	95	169
Norway	45	13	30	78	—	238	—	71	64
Sweden	65	—	140	206	111	48	145	—	168
Switzerland	51	—	49	116	68	—	—	22	74
United Kingdom	26	6	78	154	116	144	250	98	131
United States	205	61	203	238	41	308	557	294	130

NOTES: These figures are not age standardized and assume equal proportions of men and women. Some are likely to be incomparable for artifactual reasons.

SOURCE: Organization for Economic Cooperation and Development: Health Data File, 1989.

procedures around 1980 in those OECD countries that reported such data.

The first international study was by Pearson et al. (1968), and striking differences were noted in the frequency of operations in Liverpool, England, the Uppsala hospital region in Sweden, and the New England region of the United States. The Liverpool region discharged fewer patients than the other two regions, despite having more discharges of adults than any other hospital region in the United Kingdom. Tonsillectomy and adenoidectomy were performed more than twice as often in New England as in Liverpool and four times as often as in Uppsala. Although Uppsala and Liverpool had similar surgical rates, Uppsala had significantly more gallbladder and gynecological operations than Liverpool.

Comparing operations and surgeons in the United States with those in the United Kingdom, Bunker (1970) found that there were twice as many surgeons in proportion to the population in the United States as in the United Kingdom and that the population underwent twice as many operations. Comparing specific operations, Bunker reported that tonsillectomy and adenoidectomy operations as well as hernia repair operations were performed almost twice as often in the United States, and cholecystectomy operations were performed almost three times as often.

Vayda (1973) compared surgical rates in Canada with those in the United Kingdom and standardized the rates for age and sex. Comparisons showed that surgical rates in Canada in 1968 were 1.8 times greater for men and 1.6 times greater for women than in the United Kingdom. The standardized rates for diverse elective and discretionary operations such as tonsillectomy, hemorrhoidectomy, and hernia repair operations were two or more times higher in Canada than in the United Kingdom.

Both Bunker and Vayda commented that the disparity resulted from sources other than the incidence and prevalence of disease, relating it particularly to the supply of services and number of surgeons. Subsequently, Vayda, Mindell, and Rutkow (1982) compared surgical rates in Canada, the United Kingdom, and the United States between 1966 and 1976, and again reported that overall surgical rates in the United States were twice those of the United Kingdom, while the rates for Canada were 1½ times the rates for the United Kingdom. Kohn and White (1976) examined hospital utilization rates in 12 areas of 7 countries and found that standardized hospitalization rates varied more than two-fold among areas. The availability of short-term beds was found to account for most of the variation.

McPherson et al. (1981) studied the use of common surgical procedures among the United Kingdom, Canada, and the United States, and reported that rates of surgical utilization, standardized by age and sex, varied up to seven-fold among the countries. Appendectomy was the only operation carried out at similar levels in these countries. Large variations were also found among regions of the countries. Although supply and cultural variables might account for the international differences, the variation within countries was only somewhat attributable to indices of supply, but much variation remained unexplained.

As an example of the magnitude of differences in cross-national rates for a specific procedure in the mid-1970s, McPherson (1988) reported an age-standardized rate for hysterectomy of 700 per 100,000 in the United States, approximately 600 in Canada, 450 in Australia, 250 in the United Kingdom, and 110 in Norway. Coulter, McPherson, and Vessey (1988) reported more recent rates for hysterectomy of 130 per 100,000 in Sweden, in contrast to 360 in neighboring Denmark. Several possible explanations for these differences have been discussed at length in McPherson et al. (1981). The method of payment, supply of resources, availability of manpower, and reimbursement and referral patterns may all play a part. The definitive causes of these differences remain, in most cases, unknown, and the outcome differences associated with these variations as well as whether the benefits are commensurate with the costs also remain unresolved without explicit further study.

The role that demand for medical and surgical services might play in the observed variations in hospitalization rates has received considerable attention. Bunker and Brown (1974) demonstrated that the wives of men in different professions did have significantly different rates for hysterectomy and for several other discretionary surgical procedures. Of special interest was the observation that the wives of physicians reported operation rates as high, or higher, than those for the other professional groups. Whether this was demand-led or a manifestation of more available (and less expensive) supply is difficult to tell. Bloor (1976), in an extensive study of childhood tonsillectomy, has failed to discern a demand component in the decisionmaking process, and a study by Coulter and McPherson (1985) found little social class difference in the probability of discretionary surgery in the Oxford region of the United Kingdom, or any support for the notion of an effect of differential consumer demand.

Bridgman (1979) presented an international study on hospital utilization in nine regions of eight countries. One of the significant outcomes of the study was to show the correlation between the pattern of hospital utilization and the level of socioeconomic development of the countries. The rates of hysterectomy were much lower in Norway than in either Denmark or the State of Massachusetts in the United States (Anderson and Kamper-Jorgensen, 1984); the strikingly low rate of hysterectomy in Norway was noted by McPherson et al. (1982). Women in Italy were much more likely to have a hysterectomy than those in France (Van Keep, Wildemeersh, and Leher, 1983).

Caesarean section rates similarly show large variations among countries. National rates varied four-fold from less than 5 percent of all deliveries in the Netherlands and Fiji to nearly 20 percent in Singapore, Canada, and the United States (Chalmers, 1985). Notzon, Placek, and Taffel (1987) studied caesarean rates in 19 industrialized countries of Europe, North America, and the Pacific, and there were sharp differences in rates per 100 hospital deliveries in 1981, ranging from a low of 5 in Czechoslovakia to a high of 18 in the United States. The percentage of mothers who had a vaginal birth after a previous caesarean section was only 5 in the United States, compared with 43 in Norway. Women in the United States had a significantly higher rate of caesarean section for dystocia or abnormal labor than women in Ireland (Sheehan, 1987).

Ulcer disease accounted for 35 percent more bed-days per 100,000 population in Denmark than in Sweden, with the main source of the difference being accounted for by admissions for duodenal ulcer (Joensson and Silverberg, 1982). The higher consumption of hospital care in Denmark was largely explained by the fact that more medical cases were treated as in-patients in Denmark than in Sweden. The appendectomy rate in the Federal Republic of Germany was two to three times higher than that of other comparable European countries (Lichtner and Pflanz, 1971).

Plant et al. (1973) compared the number of gallbladder operations in 1961 and 1971 in three similar towns in Canada, France, and the United Kingdom and concluded that the incidence of gallbladder disease was six times higher in North America than in Western Europe, because of the much higher rate of cholecystectomy in the United States. However, evidence from morbidity surveys using necropsy studies of the prevalence of gallstones indicated a lower, rather than higher, prevalence in North America (McPherson et al., 1985).

Within the United Kingdom, morbidity differences did correlate positively with cholecystectomy rates in a study of six English towns (Barker et al., 1979). It is interesting to note that the original studies of international variations showed Canada with a higher rate than anywhere else, and this high rate was most marked among middle-aged females (McPherson, 1988). As shown in the OECD data compendium section of this issue, cholecystectomy rates among females in Canada are approaching the rates in the United States. In the early 1970s, however, the Canadian rate was twice as high as the American rate. This would strongly suggest that, at that point in time, 50 percent of the women receiving cholecystectomies in Canada would not have received them in the United States. By the same token, based on the latest OECD data, two-thirds of the women receiving cholecystectomies in the United States (where the rate is 200 per 100,000 population) might not receive the operation in the United Kingdom (where the rate is 68 per 100,000 population).

In 1982, the number of cardiac operations in the United Kingdom, with 107 operations per one million population, was significantly lower than in other countries such as Australia, with 410 operations per one million, or the United States, with 750 operations per one million (English et al., 1984). Japan has a corresponding rate of around 10 operations per one million population, which must reflect the low incidence of coronary heart disease in that country (Tunstall-Pedoe, Smith, and Crombie, 1986). Unfortunately, other countries with apparently low coronary heart disease incidence or mortality, such as France, Spain, Greece, and Switzerland, do not yet produce procedure rates.

In the book, *The Painful Prescription: Rationing Hospital Care*, Aaron and Schwartz (1984) provide an illuminating analysis of the provision of 10 medical procedures in the United States and the United Kingdom. Most services were provided at lower levels in the United Kingdom than in the United States: for example, the rate of coronary artery bypass surgery in the United Kingdom was only 10 percent of that in the United States. The overall rate of treatment for chronic renal failure in the United Kingdom was less than half that in the United States. The low rate of treatment for patients with kidney failure in the United Kingdom compared with other countries has also been commented on by Wing (1983). Three procedures—bone marrow transplants, radiotherapy for cancer, and treatment for hemophilia—were provided at essentially the same levels in both countries.

Issues for the future

Just as it is difficult to provide mass screening services without clear evidence of the benefits received, it is also difficult to provide appropriate health services without clear evidence of the relative efficacy of various treatment approaches. In the face of uncertainty, however, therapy, in contrast to screening, is difficult to withhold. Therefore, health services are provided, and implicitly rationed, but the variations shown in the OECD data compendium would indicate that all are not provided rationally. Since the information base for judging appropriateness is often inadequate, research protocols must efficiently address the important uncertainties.

Rational rationing

In comparing rates among nations, low rates are often taken implicitly to be a manifestation of under-supply. In contrast, since feedback on high rates usually results in rate reduction, high rates are taken as an indication of over-supply. These are examples of glib assumptions about the nature of the relationship between process and outcome (Donabedian, 1966), without empirical validation.

Until recently, almost all evidence of under-supply was considered detrimental to the health of the community, and indeed, in some circles (Lowry, 1988), it still is. Low rates reflected the inefficient use of resources, low productivity, and unmet need, whereas high rates reflected too much specialist enthusiasm, over-provision of resources, and unnecessary intervention. Such crude analysis pushes countries towards an average which has no rationale. It pretends that the appropriate intervention rate is known, when it is not, and indeed assumes that there is such a thing.

The policy implications of observed variations depend on knowledge about their causes and consequent outcomes, not on the magnitude of the variation alone, and certainly not on an average. If variations in rates occur because of legitimate reasons, then the policy implications are negligible. Aspects of culture and demand, when commensurate with explicit social policy and budgets, can give rise to large

international variations in use rates that are wholly unproblematic.

Procedures with low variation

When combined with knowledge about small area variation and the epidemiology of relevant diseases, observed differences among countries can be interpreted with greater precision. Large differences among countries for a procedure that is relatively invariant among small areas might well point to differences in morbidity as the first, most plausible, explanation. If the variation observed is out of proportion to feasible morbidity differences, then the influence of culture, education, or availability on clinical decisions would be the next most obvious explanation.

Examples of such procedures are cholecystectomy and appendectomy. Although these procedures vary little among neighboring small areas within countries, there appear to be four- to five-fold variations among the countries themselves. The search for systematic differences in morbidity rates has proved inadequate to justify these international differences, as has the search for artifactual explanations. The evidence suggests that there may be strong national consensus on the nature of what constitutes sufficient indications, but that this consensus appears to be quite different in different countries, and in some it may be changing.

Presumably, the within-country consensus represents a view or teaching about the correct use of an operation. As such, it is not explicitly recognized as being uncertain within a country. However, by inspecting international differences, it becomes quite clear that wholly different policies are invoked in different countries for sufficient indications to perform an operation. On the one hand, aspects of prudent prophylaxis are possibly being used where, on the other hand, only the most urgent need is being admitted. Such differences have enormous financial implications for any health sector, particularly when multiplied by other similar procedures.

The next step in evaluation is assiduous decision analysis based on the most reliable data in the literature and data from longitudinal studies (e.g., Wasson et al., 1985). For this, one requires estimates of outcome associated with various treatment options. From the literature, this would come from randomized trials and case series. Information from data bases should come from several countries where the rates are different and where the evidence for an artifactual or morbidity explanation is lacking. The application of other health information to approximate randomized comparison is possible (McPherson and Bunker, 1989). Claims data have been successfully used (Wennberg et al., 1987), as have record-linkage studies (Roos et al., 1989). It is possible to compare mortality and readmission rates at various followup times between treatment options, and such comparisons may not be seriously confounded by unmeasured indices of prognosis.

If one country has a rate twice that of another for a procedure, and if this can be attributed to practice style, it is reasonable to assume that 50 percent of the most seriously ill patients in the latter country will be receiving the procedure. In some circumstances, it might be possible to identify, from primary health care consultations, the remaining 50 percent of patients who are not admitted. It could then be argued that the combination of these two patient groups represents a cohort that is comparable to the treated cohort in the high-rate country. The advantage to using these alternative techniques is that randomized controlled comparisons could be by-passed in circumstances where they are unethical, and hence impossible, because the clinicians have few doubts. To identify all patients presenting with symptoms but not being recommended for surgery might well be to identify a cohort that could legitimately comprise a control group in a randomized study. The comparison would have to be between all those treated in the high-rate area with all those identified (both treated and not) in the low-rate area that had comparable symptoms, in essence, a comparison between a policy of intervention and a policy of conservative management.

The advantages of such studies are legion. The actual practice variations among countries can be quite enormous and, since these are often for common interventions, the sample sizes obtainable from such natural experiments can be huge. Most importantly, comparisons can be made between different treatment policies that already exist, ones that could not otherwise be duplicated in an ethical environment for the sake of experimentation. Large differences in management policy can be compared where there may be few case-mix comparability problems (Coronary Drug Project Research Group, 1980). With such potentially large data bases, it may be possible to examine the effect of policy among subgroups and even for long followup periods.

Procedures with high variation

Some discretionary procedures, such as tonsillectomy, prostatectomy, and hysterectomy, vary a great deal among small areas. Hysterectomy is variable both within and among countries. This must reflect massive uncertainty about the appropriate indication for this operation. There may well be few "correct" indications, and each decision may be an individual matter concerned with finely balanced assessments of anticipated benefits and losses (Coulter, McPherson, and Vessey, 1988). If this is the case, then such decisions ought to be made with an eye on the foregone opportunities associated with each marginal hysterectomy. It is difficult to justify marginal operations when there are any genuine unmet needs elsewhere in the health sector, which there are most likely to be. No epidemiological evidence suggests that hysterectomy rates are, to any important extent, determined by demand from

consumers. However, many opportunities exist for outcome studies and for the types of studies previously discussed to evaluate the relative benefit of interventionist versus conservative policies and to examine the detailed determinants of these varying rates.

In almost all cases for which we have data, highly variable procedures among small areas are also highly variable among countries. Moreover, countries with fee-for-service systems and/or high expenditures tend to have the higher rates (Schieber and Poullier, 1988). Health care provision which, at the margin, may provide relatively little net benefit may be provided because, in unconstrained systems where uncertainty exists, it is tempting to over-emphasize the benefit and under-emphasize the cost. It is precisely for these types of procedures that guidelines and publicly discussed policies are required so that health care budgets can be monitored in a way that is consistent with national policy. Countries could then decide which operations with marginal indications are more important, and then might end up with higher rates than in other countries as a matter of public policy.

At the moment, these policies happen in ignorance of their own determinants. They are formulated without knowing outcome, because longitudinal studies are not done, and without knowing the rates in other countries, because the data are incomplete. It is important to collect these data because many hypotheses about the determinants of health care practice, such as cultural considerations, availability of manpower and resources, and method of payment could be tested with complete data. In particular, the role of method of payment on health care practice remains impossible to disentangle from other systematic differences among countries. If these data were made available, observational information to complement the RAND Corporation's (Brook et al., 1983) randomized studies in a single country would be extremely useful.

Such policies also happen in the face of observational evidence which refuses to show a sensible association between the amount of health care provided and outcome (Cochrane, Leger, and Moore, 1978). They happen largely in ignorance of patient preferences as well, because people are unaware that such international and intranational variations exist and are, therefore, apt to view their physicians' decisions to hospitalize them as above their own preferences and inclinations. In many circumstances, patient preferences should be the ultimate determinants of these decisions (Barry et al., 1988). However, patient participation requires that information about health care practices be broadened and deepened and that the knowledge that is gained about what determines different practice styles be widely disseminated. Such knowledge can also help determine research priorities. Now that the need for answers is becoming so critical, the difficulties inherent in assessing these things can no longer be allowed too much dominance (Ellwood, 1988).

Acknowledgments

The author is grateful to colleagues and friends, particularly Angela Coulter and Diana Sanders for ideas and stimulation. A long-standing collaboration with Professors Jack Wennberg and John Bunker has been essential and also extremely fruitful. Professors Martin Vessey and, lately, David Skegg oversee a convivial working environment with lots to do and talk about. Finally, Mrs. Isobel Pairman has greatly helped with data reduction and preparation.

References

Aaron, H. J., and Schwartz, W. B.: *The Painful Prescription: Rationing Hospital Care*. Washington, D.C. The Brookings Institute, 1984.

American Medical Association: *Confronting Regional Variations: The Maine Approach*. Chicago, Ill. 1986.

Anderson, T. F., and Kamper-Jorgensen, F.: Variation in surgical rates and the organisation of health care. *Institute of Social Medicine*. Denmark. University of Copenhagen, 1984.

Barker, D. J. P., Gardner, M. J., Power, C., and Hutt, M. S. R.: Prevalence of gallstones at necropsy in nine British towns. *British Medical Journal* 2:1389-1392, 1979.

Barry, M. J., Mulley, A. G., Fowler, F. J., et al.: Watchful waiting vs. immediate transurethral resection for symptomatic prostatism: The importance of patients' preferences. *Journal of the American Medical Association* 259(20):3010-3017, 1988.

Beecher, H. K., and Boston, M. D.: Surgery as a placebo. *Journal of the American Medical Association* 231:1102-1107, 1961.

Bloor, M.: Bishop Berkeley and the adenotonsillectomy enigma: An exploration of variation in the social construction of medical disposals. *Sociology* 10:44-61, 1976.

Bridgman, R. F.: *Hospital Utilisation: An International Study*. Oxford, England. Oxford University Press, 1979.

Brook, R. H., Ware, J. E., Rogers, W. H., et al.: Does free care improve adults' health: Results from a randomized controlled trial. *New England Journal of Medicine* 309(23):1426-1434, 1983.

Bunker, J. P.: Surgical manpower: A comparison of operations and surgeons in the United States and in England and Wales. *New England Journal of Medicine* 282:135-144, 1970.

Bunker, J. P., Barnes, B., and Mosteller, F.: *Costs, Risks and Benefits of Surgery*. New York. Oxford University Press, 1977.

Bunker, J. P., and Brown, B.: The physician as an informed consumer of surgical services. *New England Journal of Medicine* 290:1051-1055, 1974.

Bunker, J. P., and Fowles, J.: Between the laboratory and the patient. *Nature* 298: 405-406, 1982.

Chalmers, I.: Trends and variations in the use of caesarean section. In Clinch, J., and Mathews, T., eds. *Perinatal Medicine*. Lancaster, England. MTP Press, 1985.

Cochrane, A. L.: *Effectiveness and Efficiency: Random Reflections on Health Services*. London. Nuffield Provincial Hospital Trust, 1971.

Cochrane, A. L., Leger, A. S., and Moore, F.: Health service 'input' and mortality 'output' in developed countries. *Journal of Epidemiologic Community Health* 32:200-205, 1978.

Comroe, J. H., and Dripps, R. D.: *The Top Ten Clinical Advances in Cardiopulmonary Medicine and Surgery, 1945-1975*. DHEW Pub. No. 78-1521. Department of Health, Education, and Welfare. Washington. U.S. Government Printing Office, 1977.

Coronary Drug Project Research Group: Influence of adherence to treatment and response of cholesterol on mortality in the Coronary Drug Project. *New England Journal of Medicine* 303:1038-1041, 1980.

Coulter, A., and McPherson, K.: Socioeconomic variations in the use of common surgical operations. *British Medical Journal* 291:183-187, 1985.

Coulter, A., McPherson, K., and Vessey, M. P.: Do British women undergo too many or too few hysterectomies? *Social Science and Medicine* 27(9):987-994, 1988.

Doll, R., and Peto, R.: *The Causes of Cancer*. Oxford, England. Oxford University Press,1981.

Donabedian, A.: Evaluating the quality of medical care. *Milbank Memorial Fund Quarterly* Suppl. 44:166-178, 1966.

Dyck, F. J., Murphy, F. A., Murphy, J. K., et al.: Effects of surveillance on the number of hysterectomies in the province of Saskatchewan. *New England Journal of Medicine* 296:1326-1329, 1977.

Ellwood, P. M.: Shattuck lecture. Outcome management: A technology of patient experience. *New England Journal of Medicine* 318(23):1549-1556, 1988.

English, T. A. H., Bailey, A. R., Dark, J. F., et al.: The UK cardiac surgical register, 1977-82. *British Medical Journal* 298:1205-1208, 1984.

Fineberg, H. V.: Effects of clinical evaluation on the diffusion of medical technology. Chap. 4. *Assessing Medical Technologies*. Committee for Evaluating Medical Technologies in Clinical Use, Institute of Medicine. Washington, D.C. National Associated Press, 1985.

Friedson, E.: *Profession of Medicine*. New York. Dodd-Mead, 1972.

Gittelsohn, A., and Wennberg, J. E.: On the risk of organ loss. *Journal of Chronic Diseases*. 29:527-535, 1976.

Glover, J. A.: The incidence of tonsillectomy in school children. *Proceedings of the Royal Society of Medicine* 31:1219-1236, 1938.

Ham, C.: *Health Care Variations: Assessing the Evidence*. London. Kings Fund Institute, 1988.

Hill, A. B.: *Statistical Methods in Clinical and Preventive Medicine*. Edinburgh, Scotland. Livingston, 1962.

Ingelfinger, F. J.: Arrogance. *New England Journal of Medicine* 303:1507-1511, 1980.

Joensson, B., and Silverberg,R.: Variations between and within countries in hospital care for peptic ulcer: A comparison between Denmark and Sweden. *Scandinavian Journal of Social Medicine* 10:63-70, 1982.

Kohn, P., and White, K. L.: *An International Study*. Oxford, England. Oxford University Press, 1976.

Lembcke, P. A.: Medical audit by scientific methods: Illustrated by major female pelvic surgery. *Journal of the American Medical Association* 162:646-651, 1956.

Lichtner, S., and Pflanz, M.: Appendectomy in the Federal Republic of Germany: Epidemiology and medical care patterns. *Medical Care* 9:311-317, 1971.

Llewellyn-Thomas, H., Sutherland, H. J., Tibshirani, R., et al.: Methodological issues in obtaining values for health states. *Medical Care* 24:113-118, 1984.

Lowry, S.: Focus on performance indicators. *British Medical Journal* 296:992-994, 1988.

Maxwell, R. A.: *Health and Wealth. An International Study of Health Care Spending.* Lexington, Mass. Lexington Books, 1981.

McCarthy, E. G., Finkel, M. L., and Ruchlin, H. S.: Current status of surgical second opinion programs. *Surgical Clinics of North America* 62(4):705-719, 1982.

McNeil, B. L.,Weichselbaum, R., and Pauker, S. G.: Fallacy of five-year survival in lung cancer. *New England Journal of Medicine* 299:1397-1400, 1978.

McPherson, K: *Variations in Hospitalization Rates: Why and How to Study Them.* London. Kings Fund Institute, 1988.

McPherson, K., and Bunker, J. P.: Application of health information to health services. In Holland, W. W., Knox, G., and Detels, R., eds. *Oxford Text Book of Public Health.* Oxford, England. Oxford University Press, 1989.

McPherson, K., Strong, P. M., Epstein, A., et al.: Regional variation in the use of common surgical procedures within and between England and Wales, Canada and the United States of America. *Social Science Medicine* 15A:273-288, 1981.

McPherson, K., Strong, P. M., Jones, L., et al.: Do cholecystectomy rates correlate with geographic variations in the prevalence of gallstones? *Journal of Epidemiologic and Community Health* 39:179-182, 1985.

McPherson, K., Wennberg, J. W., Hovind, O., et al.: Small area variations in the use of common surgical procedures: An international comparison of New England, England and Norway. *New England Journal of Medicine* 307:1310;-1314, 1982.

Muir, C. S.: Classification. In Doll, R., Muir, C., and Waterhouse, J., eds. *Cancer in Five Continents.* 3rd Edition. International Agency for Research in Cancer, 1976.

Mulley, A. G.: Assessing patients' utilities: Can the ends justify the means? *Medical Care* 27(3):269-281, 1989.

Nicholl, J. P., Beeby, N. R., and Williams, B. T.: Role of the private sector in elective surgery in England and Wales. *British Medical Journal* 298:243-247, 1988.

Notzon, P. A., Placek, P. J., and Taffel, S. M.: Comparisons of national cesarian section rates. *New England Journal of Medicine* 316(7):386-389, 1987.

Organization for Economic Cooperation and Development: Health Data File. Paris. Directorate for Social Affairs, Manpower, and Education, 1989.

Pearson, R. J. C., Smedby, B., Berfenstam, R., et al.: Hospital case loads in Liverpool, New England and Uppsala: An international comparison. *Lancet* 2:559-566, 1968.

Plant, J. C. D., Percy, I., Bates, T., et al.: Incidence of gallbladder disease in Canada, England and France. *Lancet* 2:249-251, 1973.

Poullier, J. P.: *Measuring Health Care, 1960-1983. Expenditures, Costs and Performance.* Social Policy Studies No. 2. Paris. Organization for Economic Cooperation and Development, 1985.

Roos, N. P., Wennberg, J. E., Malenka, D. J., et al.: Mortality and reoperation following open and transurethral resection of the prostate for benign prostatic hyperplasia.*New England Journal of Medicine* 320(17):1120-1124, Apr. 27, 1989.

Roos, N. P., Wennberg, J. E., and McPherson, K.: Using diagnosis-related groups for studying variations in hospital admissions. *Health Care Financing Review.* Vol. 9, No. 4. HCFA Pub. No. 03265. Office of Research and Demonstrations, Health Care Financing Administration, Washington. U.S. Government Printing Office, July 1988.

Sacket, D. L., and Torrance, G. W.: The utility of different disease states as perceived by the general public. *Journal of Chronic Disease* 7:347-351, 1978.

Sanders, D.: *Bibliography on Geographic Variations in Hospital Admission Rates.* Department of Community Medicine. Oxford, England. Radcliffe Infirmary, 1988.

Sanders, D., Coulter, A., and McPherson, K.: *Variations in Hospital Admission Rates: A Review of the Literature.* London. Kings Fund Institute, 1989.

Schieber, G. J.: *Financing and Delivering Health Care. A Comparative Analysis of OECD Countries.* Social Policy Studies No 4. Paris. Organization for Economic Cooperation and Development, 1987.

Schieber, G. J., and Poullier, J. P.: International health spending and utilization trends. *Health Affairs* 7(4):105-122, Fall 1988.

Shaw, G. B.: Preface on doctors. *The Doctor's Dilemma.* London. The Bodley Head, 1971.

Sheehan, K. H.: Caesarian section for dystocia: A comparison of practices in two countries. *Lancet* 1:548-51, 1987.

Stevens, R.: The evolution of health care systems in the United States and the United Kingdom: Similarities and differences. *Priorities for the Use of Resources in Medicine.* Fogarty International Centre Proceedings. Washington, D.C. U.S. Department of Health, Education, and Welfare, 1977.

Tunstall-Pedoe, H., Smith, W. C. S., and Crombie, I. K.: Level and trends of coronary health disease mortality in Scotland compared with other countries. Scottish Home and Health Department. *Health Bulletin* 44(3):153-61, 1986.

Van Keep, P. A., Wildemeersh, D., and Leher, P.: Hysterectomy in six European countries. *Maturitas* 5:69-75, 1983.

Vayda, E.: A comparison of surgical rates in Canada and in England and Wales. *New England Journal of Medicine* 289:1224-1229, 1973.

Vayda, E., Mindell, W. R., and Rutkow, I. M.: A decade of surgery in Canada, England and Wales and the United States. *Archives of Surgery* 117:846-853, 1982.

Wasson, H. H., Sox, H. C., Neff, R. K., et al.: Clinical prediction rules: Application and methodological standards. *New England Journal of Medicine* 313:793-799, 1985.

Wennberg, J. E., and Gittelsohn, A.: Small area variations in health care delivery: A population based health information system can guide planning and regulatory decision making. *Science* 182:1102-1109, 1973.

Wennberg, J. E., and Gittelsohn, A.: Variation in medical care among small areas. *Scientific American* 246:100-112, 1982.

Wennberg, J. E., McPherson, K., and Caper, P.: Will payment based on diagnosis-related groups control hospitalcosts? *New England Journal of Medicine* 311(5):295-300, Aug. 1984.

Wennberg, J. E., Roos, N. P., Sola, L., et al.: Use of claims data systems to evaluate health care outcomes: Mortality and reoperation following prostatectomy. *Journal of the American Medical Association* 257:933-936, 1987.

Wing, A. J.: Why don't the British treat more patients with kidney failure? *British Medical Journal* 287:1157-1158, 1983.

Cost containment in Europe

by A. J. Culyer

Health care cost containment is not in itself a sensible policy objective, because any assessment of the appropriateness of health care expenditure in aggregate, as of that on specific programs, requires a balancing of costs and benefits at the margin. International data on expenditures can, however, provide indications of the likely impact on costs and expenditures of structural features of health care systems. Data from the Organization for Economic Cooperation and Development for both European countries and a wider set are reviewed, and some current policies in Europe that are directed at controlling health care costs are outlined.

Introduction

Questions of cost containment resolve into two distinct sorts of question. One sort is normative: For example, what are the right level and growth rate of health care costs? This question in welfare economics is appropriately discussed in terms of the value of the beneficial outcomes that health services produce in relation to the value of what is necessarily forgone. The other sort is positive: For example, given the available technology, what resources are necessary in order to produce any given level of outcome? These questions can be tackled at either the microeconomic or the aggregate level. In microeconomic analysis, the focus is on cost effectiveness, cost utility, and cost-benefit analysis (Drummond, Stoddart, and Torrance, 1987). The aim is to make cross-program comparisons of marginal costs and benefits in order to determine both the optimal mix of programs and the payoff to increased spending (or the marginal lost benefits of reduced spending). A dense jungle must be hacked through here, and, although the methodology that ought to be used seems clear, its empirical implementation is underdeveloped. (A pioneering study is Williams, 1985.) In aggregate analysis, the emphasis is on total spending, its share in gross domestic product (GDP) and its principal components, the determinants of this total and its components, and the value-judgmental element involved in assessing the marginal payoff of the aggregate and its marginal opportunity cost.

A cost cannot be held too high or too low in relation either to itself or to costs elsewhere. This is true at a microeconomic level. For instance, the capital and recurrent costs of a new imaging procedure in diagnosis or treatment are worth incurring only if the expected benefit is deemed high enough. (I do not imply a narrow financial notion of benefit.) It is also true at the macroeconomic level: The overall expenditure (public and private) on health care is worthwhile only for what it enables the system to accomplish, bearing in mind that benefits at the margin from extra health spending have as their real costs the nonhealth benefits that could have been had, but were not, because less is being spent on other sources of human welfare. (These are opportunity costs.) Such comparisons are, of course, intrinsically difficult to make, because they involve approximations and judgments about what is worth while, but they are necessary. The only rational and humane way in which to make such comparisons, however imperfectly, is in terms of benefits gained and forgone. (I insist on this latter assertion without seeking to justify it.)

Expenditure is not synonymous with opportunity cost. Much of the concern commonly expressed about cost containment is more accurately represented as a concern about overall expenditure levels and, in particular, a concern about the share of health care expenditures in either public expenditure or GDP. A part of this concern may relate to a belief that existing levels or shares are too high in the sense that, at existing levels of expenditure, marginal benefits are less than marginal costs. Another part relates to a concern that levels and shares are too high because the same benefit could be had at a lower level of expenditure. (This is particularly true in Britain.) Yet a third may be a more global concern on political or macroeconomic policy grounds to reduce public expenditure (or at least its growth rate), with the implication that health services must take their share along with other parts of public spending.

The focus in this article is mainly on the aggregate approach and, within that, on the aggregate determinants and broad policy instruments available that may affect the total. At the aggregate level, there is no satisfactory measure either of the aggregate outcome of health care expenditures (let alone their value) or of the aggregate health production function either in Europe or elsewhere. Nonetheless, an aggregate analysis can help to identify some of the factors on which policy to control expenditure might be targeted and also identify areas where further more detailed inquiry is needed. The next section is a review of the expenditure patterns observed in Europe. Some theories as to why these patterns are observed are then discussed and the evidence for them reviewed. Finally, some other institutional and environmental factors, not included in these theories of aggregate expenditure, are identified and their impact on health care costs assessed.

Reprint requests: A. J. Culyer, Department of Economics and Related Studies, University of York, Heslington, York Y01 5DD England.

Table 1
Health care expenditure (HCE) and gross domestic product (GDP) per capita: Selected countries, 1970 and 1987

Country	1970			1987			Annual compound rate of change	
	HCE	GDP	HCE/GDP	HCE	GDP	HCE/GDP	HCE	GDP
							Percent	
Austria	$163	$3,056	.053	$988	$11,710	.084	11.2	8.2
Belgium	147	3,652	.040	881	12,183	.072	11.1	7.3
Denmark	252	4,147	.061	784	13,129	.060	6.9	7.0
Finland	183	3,280	.056	970	13,061	.074	10.3	8.5
France	223	3,685	.061	1,117	12,849	.087	9.9	7.6
Germany	220	3,993	.055	1,072	13,308	.081	9.8	7.3
Greece	70	1,756	.040	337	6,410	.053	9.7	7.9
Iceland	288	3,382	.085	1,205	15,566	.077	8.8	9.4
Ireland	122	2,196	.056	553	7,446	.074	9.3	7.4
Italy	171	3,093	.055	837	12,190	.069	9.8	8.4
Netherlands	232	3,881	.060	1,041	12,263	.085	9.2	7.0
Norway	191	3,083	.062	1,149	15,495	.074	11.1	10.0
Spain	102	2,473	.041	521	8,676	.060	10.1	7.7
Sweden	359	4,976	.072	1,233	13,770	.090	7.5	6.2
United Kingdom	161	3,563	.045	763	12,414	.061	9.6	7.6
Mean (unweighted)	192	3,347	.057	896	12,031	.073	9.6	7.8

NOTE: U.S. dollars at GDP purchasing power parities and current prices are used.

SOURCES: (Organization for Economic Cooperation and Development, 1987, Table 20); Organization for Economic Cooperation and Development: Health Data File, 1989.

European expenditure patterns and growth

In this section, an aggregated statistical picture is drawn for those countries for which data from the Organization for Economic Cooperation and Development (OECD) are available.

Expenditure and income

The overall levels of expenditure and GDP (current prices) in 1970 and 1987 are shown in Table 1 for 15 European countries. In 1970, health care expenditures per capita, valued at OECD purchasing power parities, averaged (unweighted) $192; they rose to $896 in 1987, an annual nominal growth rate of 9.6 percent. GDP per capita during the same period rose from $3,347 to $12,031, an annual nominal growth rate of 7.8 percent. The average share of health care expenditures in GDP rose from 5.7 percent to 7.3 percent. In all countries, save Denmark and Iceland, the share of health care expenditures in GDP rose. Countries with a below average nominal rate of growth of health care expenditures were Denmark, Iceland, Ireland, Netherlands, and Sweden. The fastest growth rates of health care spending (>10 percent) were in Austria, Belgium, Finland, Norway, and Spain. Of these, only Belgium and Spain experienced a growth of GDP below the European average.

The elasticity of real health care expenditure with respect to GDP has been calculated for several OECD countries (Organization for Economic Cooperation and Development, 1987) for the pre- and post-1975 periods in order to compare the responses before and after the oil shock. These elasticities, shown in Table 2, are based on constant price data for each country using the country's own price deflators for the health care sector and the GDP deflators for GDP. The average elasticities exceed 1 for both periods (a point discussed later). Real health spending increased 70 percent faster than GDP in the period 1960-75, before the oil price shock, and 30 percent faster after it. In Belgium, France, Italy, and Spain, the elasticity after the oil shock was, however, higher than the pre-shock elasticity. In fact, in the early 1980s, the rate of growth of real health care expenditures, both absolutely and relative to GDP, slowed. Recent OECD unpublished estimates of elasticities for the period 1970-87 suggest, however,

Table 2
Real gross domestic product elasticities of health care expenditures: Selected countries, 1960-75 and 1975-84

Country	1960-75	1975-84
Austria	0.7	0.7
Belgium	1.3	1.5
Denmark	1.9	1.4
Finland	2.0	0.9
France	1.6	2.6
Germany	1.2	0.9
Greece	1.8	1.8
Ireland	2.3	0.9
Italy	0.9	1.3
Netherlands	1.5	0.5
Norway	1.7	1.5
Spain	1.7	2.1
Sweden	2.4	1.6
United Kingdom	2.1	1.0
Mean (unweighted)	1.7	1.3

SOURCE: (Organization for Economic Cooperation and Development, 1987, Table 21).

that the elasticity has risen substantially in more recent years in some countries, especially in Austria, Belgium, France, the Federal Republic of Germany (hereafter called Germany), and Italy (Organization for Economic Cooperation and Development, 1989).

Regressions

A close association between income and spending on health care has been highlighted, particularly by Newhouse (1975 and 1977). For 13 countries in the early 1970s, he found a linear relationship between per capita health care expenditures (HCE) and per capita gross national product (GNP). (When t values for the constant term are reported in these studies, they indicate that it is not significantly different from zero.) Working in U.S. dollars calculated at annual average exchange rates, he obtained the following results (t values are shown in parentheses):

$$HCE = -60 + 0.079 \text{ GNP}$$
$$(11.47) \qquad R^2 = 0.92$$

The coefficient on GNP is the same as that Kleiman (1974) had found earlier. My own exploration of a more complete set of OECD data (Culyer, 1988) using GDP for 20 countries produces similar results:

$$HCE = -67 + 0.083 \text{ GDP}$$
$$(12.45) \qquad R^2 = 0.91$$

Using OECD's purchasing power parity rates rather than average exchange rates in order to obtain a more consistent measure of dollar command over resources, the results are:

$$HCE = -95 + 0.085 \text{ GDP}$$
$$(8.32) \qquad R^2 = 0.81$$

Parkin, McGuire, and Yule (1987), also using OECD data, found values for 1980 of

$$HCE = -134.4 + 0.086 \text{ GDP}$$
$$(11.79) \qquad R^2 = 0.87$$

using exchange rates and

$$HCE = (+)80.6 + 0.092 \text{ GDP}$$
$$(4.94) \qquad R^2 = 0.60$$

for a subset of countries for which purchasing power parities were available.

The implied income elasticity of 1971 health care expenditures per capita with respect to GDP per capita was +1.35, the same result as that obtained by Newhouse (1975 and 1977), that reported by Leviatan (1964) for Israel in the early 1960s, and that reported by the Organization for Economic Cooperation and Development (1985) for the period 1960-82. Parkin, McGuire, and Yule (1987) found income elasticities of +1.18 for their exchange rate equation but only +0.90 using purchasing power parity. In more recent analysis of OECD data for 1983, however, higher elasticities, +1.47, were found using purchasing power parities (Gerdtham et al., 1988).

The income elasticity of health care expenditure is defined as the percentage change in per capita health care expenditure divided by the percentage change in per capita income (GDP) that induced it. Thus, the results imply that, in 1971, a $100-increase in GDP

per capita could have been expected to increase health care expenditure by $8, or that a 10-percent increase in GDP could have been expected to increase health care expenditures by about 13 percent. It is this high income elasticity that gives rise to the view that health care is a luxury good, for it is conventional to classify goods with income elasticities that exceed unity as luxuries.

Interpreting the regression results

A number of points need to be borne in mind when interpreting results of this kind. First, some elements that must be held constant in the microeconomic concept of income elasticity are not held constant in macroeconomic relationships such as these. If, for example, income elasticity is not the same for all income groups, the distribution of income within countries will distort the pure relationship. In particular, if the income elasticity rises with income and if the more unequal countries are also the richer (within the relatively high-income group of the OECD countries), then the slope of the graph will be artificially high.

Second, health care is not homogeneous. Both Germany and the United States are richer countries per capita than the United Kingdom is. Using purchasing power parities, the index of GDP per capita in 1983 was: United States = 100, Germany = 82, and United Kingdom = 71. Thus, the United States was, on average, 40 percent richer and Germany 15 percent richer than the United Kingdom. Homogeneity might be taken to imply that the United States would have about 40 percent more and Germany 15 percent more real health service inputs. In fact, in 1983, the United States had 60 percent more doctors per capita than the United Kingdom had, but 27 percent fewer hospital beds and 30 percent fewer nurses! (Organization for Economic Cooperation and Development, 1985 and 1988). The claim sometimes heard that higher health expenditures go primarily into caring rather than curing (e.g., Newhouse, 1977) is not supported by this evidence. On the other hand, Germany had 40 percent more beds and 85 percent more physicians, but 59 percent fewer nurses! Clearly, once one looks beyond the aggregated expenditure picture, it can be seen that the things people are buying for their health care dollars vary greatly from country to country, and not in any way that is universally systematic with their ability to pay. The relationship between income and inputs within countries is not simple either. After 1960, the stock of beds steadily fell in the United States and the United Kingdom. In Germany, however, it rose until 1975 and only thereafter began to fall. In all three countries, the stock of doctors rose. In all three, the stock of nurses also rose, although it peaked in Germany in 1982. Clearly, more factors are at work than merely the ability to pay. Such factors include the ways in which professionals are paid and the extent to which they earn monopoly rents or the state uses its monopsony power.

Third, there is no reason to expect individual preferences for health care to remain homogeneous within countries, let alone in cross-sectional comparisons. The tastes of individuals (partially conditioned, no doubt, by established custom and the medical culture) for styles of care (e.g., generalist versus specialist community-based physicians; long versus short inpatient stays) vary. Moreover, they are likely to vary both intrinsically and in response to incentive structures, such as insurance benefits when off work sick, that are not endogenous to the model explaining overall levels of expenditure in relation to income.

Fourth, administrative costs are more a function of the organization of finance than of income. The U.S. systems of health insurance are costly (compared, say, with a country such as Canada that has public health insurance). The European systems that rely on social insurance are also relatively costly compared with countries, like the United Kingdom, that rely on taxation.

Finally, in several of the studies reported here, it was found that the intercept of a linear expenditure function was not significantly different from zero. If it were actually zero, then, of course, the income elasticity is constrained to be unity. With a significant positive slope and a significant negative intercept, the elasticity will always exceed unity. With both slope and intercept positive, the elasticity will always lie between zero and unity. This leads to a curiosity in the interpretation of Newhouse's results, as pointed out by Parkin, McGuire, and Yule (1987), that (given a negative intercept), as GDP increases, the income elasticity decreases, implying not only that health care is always a luxury but also that the higher is GDP, the less of a luxury health care becomes!

An iron law?

Because of the typically high R^2 values that have been found, some have suggested that HCE is not really a policy variable. For example, in the exchange rate equations reported earlier, from 87 percent to 92 percent of the variation in expenditure per capita was statistically explicable by variations in income per capita. The danger is that the income relationship easily becomes interpreted as a kind of iron law of health care expenditures. If income explains so much, there is nothing left for other determinants to explain: "[T]he negative inference may be drawn that other factors hypothesized to affect medical-care spending are not of quantitative significance" (Newhouse, 1977). Newhouse was careful not to claim that factors other than income, such as the form of organization and the finance of health care, bore no relationship to total expenditure. In fact, he suggested that there might be an association between the organizational forms of health care and total health care spending. Socialization (or at least centralized control of or influence over budgets) is itself a response to low income and a desire to control costs. The mode of organization is endogenous. Low per

capita income, according to his argument, leads to both controls and low per capita expenditure. That argument would seem more plausible had concern over rising health care expenditures been less universal than it has been, had their composition been more homogeneous, and had the United States been less active in developing cost-control mechanisms (albeit largely within a fairly decentralized system).

One is therefore tempted to conclude that the inexorable nature of the relationship is beyond the reach of policy. But this, it turns out, is not the case, for relevant variables are plainly omitted from estimating equations. Although the omitted variables may be hard to measure for econometric purposes or may not actually have varied over the period used for estimating relationships or across the sample used in a cross-sectional analysis, some of them may correlate with GDP per capita.

Price, population, and utilization effects

The well-known identity relating $\% \triangle$ HCE to the $\% \triangle P_H$, $\% \triangle POP$, and $\% \triangle (Q_H/POP)$ is a useful way of identifying three components in the rate of change of health care expenditures ($\% \triangle$ HCE): price changes ($\% \triangle P_H$), population changes ($\% \triangle POP$), and changes in the utilization of health care ($\% \triangle (Q_H/POP)$), as shown in the Schieber and Poullier article in this issue. The last of these terms is not directly measurable and is a residual after the effect of the other two has been taken into account. It will depend on changes in demographic structure (for example, aging populations), changes in technology, and changes in the style of medical practice insofar as they can be separated from changes in technology.

The results of such an exercise for the period 1960-84 are shown in Table 3. It can easily be seen that the population component of the growth rate is typically small, 0.7 percent (save insofar as it is reflected in utilization rates). The principal components of HCE nominal growth are health care input price inflation and utilization. Although HCE price inflation is the major part (on average, 9.6 percent, compared with an average rate of increase in utilization of 5.7 percent), it should be remembered that general inflation was also high. For the 16 countries shown, general inflation was 9.0 percent. Therefore, on average, excess health care inflation contributed 0.6 percent per year to the growth of HCE. In some countries, however, the inflation differential between the health sector and the general economy was above average, notably Austria (3.2 percent differential), Iceland (2.8 percent), Netherlands (2.2 percent), Switzerland (1.7 percent), Norway (1.3 percent), and Germany (1.3 percent). In six countries, the differential was negative, notably in Sweden (− 1.3 percent) and Greece (− 1.0 percent). Because general inflation is largely exogenous to health care inflation, the conclusion is hard to resist that the main endogenous health care factor contributing to rising HCE in Europe has been utilization. More information can be

Table 3

Annual compound rate of change in health care expenditure (HCE), by component, and gross domestic product deflator: Selected countries, 1960-84

Country	Annual compound rate of change				
	HCE growth				
	Total	Health care prices	Population	Utilization	GDP deflator
	Percent				
Austria	11.3	8.3	0.3	2.7	5.1
Belgium	11.8	6.3	0.3	5.2	5.4
Denmark	14.1	8.2	0.5	5.4	8.2
Finland	15.4	8.1	0.4	6.9	8.8
France	15.3	6.9	0.8	7.6	7.5
Germany	10.1	5.6	0.4	4.1	4.3
Greece	18.3	9.3	0.7	8.3	10.3
Iceland	34.8	30.2	1.3	3.3	27.4
Ireland	18.2	10.0	0.9	7.3	10.3
Italy	17.6	10.5	0.5	6.6	10.5
Netherlands	13.7	8.4	1.0	4.3	6.2
Norway	14.5	8.4	0.6	5.5	7.1
Spain	21.8	13.0	1.0	7.8	12.1
Sweden	13.7	6.0	0.5	7.2	7.3
Switzerland	12.1	6.7	0.9	4.5	5.0
United Kingdom	13.1	8.3	0.3	4.5	8.7
Mean (unweighted)	16.0	9.6	0.7	5.7	9.0

SOURCE: Calculated from (Organization for Economic Cooperation and Development, 1987, Table 22).

found in (Organization for Economic Cooperation and Development, 1987.)

This conclusion should, however, be seen as tentative, because it depends crucially on the adequacy of the OECD deflators for HCE. These are intended to be consumer price indexes and are therefore weighted by shares of consumer out-of-pocket expenditure in total consumer expenditure. However, shares of out-of-pocket expenditures are inappropriate weights for measures of total health care expenditure inflation. For example, hospital prices are typically heavily subsidized and have a small weight in consumers' expenditure but take up the bulk of total health care expenditure. There are also other snags. For example, an element of the hospital price index may be based on per diem costs of care rather than cost per case. If so, falling lengths of stay (indicating, all things being equal, a falling cost per case and increasing productivity) will not be picked up by the price index. In fact, a perverse price rise may be signaled if the patients not experiencing a falling length of stay are sicker, more costly cases on average and if the bed stock and occupancy rates remain roughly constant.

Composition of health care expenditures

In Table 4, public health expenditures are grouped into the four categories used by OECD. No consistent data are available for breakdowns of total health care expenditures. Even the data that are available are fraught with problems, and overinterpretation must be

avoided. Percentages do not add to 100 because the data, even for single countries, do not relate invariably to the same year. For some countries (e.g., Belgium) it is difficult to assign physician incomes between the institutional and ambulatory sectors. The balance between outpatient care provided by institutions and that provided by community-based physicians varies. For example, in Germany, virtually no outpatient care is provided by hospitals; in Sweden, 5 percent of physician visits are to doctors working in hospital outpatient departments. The use of outpatient diagnostic services in hospitals compared with diagnostic procedures in doctors' clinics and offices is variable. The remarkable growth in ambulatory care in the Netherlands is probably an artifact of the data.

In general, however, it is clear that hospital care is the largest component of health care expenditure. The most variable component is pharmaceuticals, and this element has also had the greatest variation in its growth rate. This is, in large part, the result of different methods of paying for drugs. Patient out-of-pocket shares vary greatly, thus affecting the public share.

Systematic comparisons must await greater harmonization of the data. A breakdown of

Table 4

Composition of public health care expenditure: Selected countries, selected years

Country and year	Institutional	Ambulatory	Pharmaceutical	Other
	Percent			
Austria, 1983	25.3	20.3	9.9	44.7
	(1.2)	(−1.4)	(−2.6)	(1.5)
Belgium, 1981	21.0	37.7	11.8	29.5
	(2.0)	(−0.3)	(−3.4)	(1.8)
Denmark, 1984	73.9	22.0	4.8	—
	(1.0)	(−1.2)	(0.3)	(—)
Finland, 1983	55.2	28.1	5.9	10.7
	(−1.0)	(5.0)	(0.1)	(−1.6)
France, 1984	59.5	22.9	13.1	7.9
	(2.1)	(−1.2)	(−2.6)	(—)
Germany, 1983	43.0	25.5	19.2	12.3
	(0.3)	(−1.6)	(0.4)	(4.1)
Greece, 1982	49.5	13.4	14.8	22.3
	(2.0)	(−1.9)	(−1.9)	(−0.4)
Ireland, 1983	73.4	11.5	7.0	9.7
	(—)	(—)	(15.9)	(—)
Italy, 1984	55.3	27.8	13.0	4.6
	(0.5)	(−1.1)	(−1.3)	(—)
Netherlands, 1984	69.3	23.2	7.2	3.7
	(1.7)	(31.3)	(0.6)	(−8.0)
Norway, 1981	69.9	15.3	7.2	7.6
	(−0.5)	(−2.0)	(−1.3)	(—)
Portugal, 1983	46.3	20.7	20.3	12.7
	(—)	(−1.7)	(2.3)	(1.0)
Spain, 1981	42.5	16.7	15.8	25.7
	(—)	(−0.1)	(−5.2)	(—)
Sweden, 1983	72.6	10.2	4.9	12.3
	(0.3)	(3.7)	(0.2)	(−2.7)
United Kingdom, 1979	59.7	11.2	10.3	20.0
	(0.7)	(−1.6)	(0.3)	(0.0)
Mean (unweighted)	54.4	20.4	11.0	14.9

NOTE: Annual compound rates of growth from 1970 to the 1980s are given in parentheses.

SOURCE: (Organization for Economic Cooperation and Development, 1987, Table 24).

expenditure for doctors, nurses, pharmaceuticals, other supplies, and other hospital expenses, which would ideally be by type of hospital, is not available.

The data in this section can be used to gain only a broad indication of European patterns, and one that cannot be held to be particularly accurate. It is nonetheless useful to pursue an aggregate analysis by investigating the determinants of the more reliable elements in these data, particularly total health care expenditures.

Public choice view[1]

One way of trying to build a more complex narrative is the public choice approach of Buchanan (1965) and Leu (1986). Such work is not narrative in any historical sense—Buchanan's self-confessedly so—but is an attempt to provide a systematic explanation for the international differences that are observed.

Buchanan thesis

The thesis of Buchanan (1965) was prompted by the 1965 crisis in Britain's National Health Service (NHS). Many members of the medical profession were poised to withdraw from the NHS, and problems of waiting lists and medical emigration were seen, each of which was much exaggerated into a failure of the NHS.

At the time, economists' standard objection to the provision of health care at zero price to the patient was that doing so encouraged overuse. Excess demand, they had predicted, would inexorably draw too many resources into the health sector ("too many" in the sense that the cost of the additional resources would exceed any reasonable assessment of their value in health care). After 17 years of socialized medicine, however, it was all too clear that this oversupply had not materialized. Buchanan proposed an alternative theory: Political decisions about the supply of services are made independently of demand, so inefficiency (failure) manifested itself not as oversupply but as reduced quality in the form of more congestion, longer waits, less qualified immigrant nurses and doctors, and so on.

This theory is derived from consideration of the nature of the decision each member of the community confronts as a demander of publicly provided health care and as a taxpayer. As a demander of what is, to all intents and purposes, a private good (or so it was assumed), each has an incentive to extend his or her demand (malingering) as long as additional service has value, no matter how small. As a taxpayer, however, each recognizes that the health care benefits to be had per tax dollar directly compete with the other publicly provided goods that tax dollars can buy (education, social security, and so on) and that tax-supported health care benefits must be shared with other beneficiaries. In other words, in the supply-side decision, the taxpayer both confronts the costs of providing the service (which he or she does not do on

the demand side, there being no price) and has the potential personal benefit reduced by virtue of having to share access with others. It follows that supply will not be sufficient to meet the excess demand and queues will develop. The result is that the individual as taxpayer gets the same chance in the queue as anyone else rather than the direct ability to purchase personal service.

For present purposes, the significance of Buchanan's analysis does not lie in the accuracy of his predictions about the NHS. Many of these have proved factually wrong, as seen in (Bosanquet, 1986), demonstrating that theory without history can be as misleading as evidence without theory. The significance lies rather in his recognition that the financing of collectivized health care is itself subject to decisions. Financing is not automatic, as it would be under a full market system in which price both brought supply and demand into equilibrium and provided the funding via the care supplied.

Of course, the same may be argued of health care financed by private insurance, which also severs the intimate links among demand, supply, and finance. However, the public element in the finance of health care is special in that decisions about spending are quintessentially political. It is beside the point whether voters behave as Buchanan suggested (refusing to will the financial means, but, in their other role as patients, inflating demand and driving it still further apart from supply) or whether they only appear to behave like that thanks to the accurate interpretation of their supply-side wishes by democratic politicians. In either case, the political process and the way in which health care is financed and provided have a prima facie claim to our attention. We have an expectation that expenditure will be related to these factors in some way.

Leu thesis

The analysis of Leu (1986) is founded on a useful identification of three types of actors and decisionmakers in the system. Real health care expenditures depend on the behavior of patients, of health care providers, and of health care financiers. The last group is especially significant to health care because, in all developed countries, direct, out-of-pocket charges to consumers are not the typical method by which the providers acquire their revenue. Instead, they get it from government, from insurance agencies, or from charitable gifts.

In this model, public finance of health care will raise the level of spending on health care so long as the user price to the consumer falls (but fees to providers do not) and providers have an incentive to respond to the increase in demand by increasing supply (rather than, for example, letting queues develop). Given these circumstances, we expect a correlation between total spending on health care and the share of public finance in that spending.

Leu therefore postulated that total expenditure on health care increases as the share of public finance in

_____
[1]This section is largely drawn from Culyer (1988).

the total increases. This proposition can be seen to depend on two conditions: that the public finance increases demand (by reducing the user price to the consumer) and that it increases supply (by maintaining or increasing, as necessary, the price paid to suppliers). Both must be present; having either without the other implies no correlation at all between total expenditure on health care and health care's share of public finance. Both—in particular, the second—imply willingness on the part of the taxpayer (or insurance-premium payer) to finance whatever supply is determined.

Notice that the argument just described concerned public finance, not public ownership: Paying for health benefits with tax dollars raises spending even if suppliers remain in the private sector. Leu also argued, however, that public ownership affects total expenditure. Drawing on the general property-right literature and a scattering of specific studies of hospitals, he argued that the lack of competition for the ownership of publicly owned institutions leads to a reduced incentive for management to minimize costs at each rate of activity. Therefore, other things being equal, publicly owned hospitals are costlier per unit of activity than privately owned hospitals are. In addition, nonprofit institutions in both the public and private sectors have bureaucracies whose behavior seems to be that of budget maximizers. So, said Leu, the public sector is likely to evince not only oversupply but oversupply at inflated cost.

Again, then, a public variable—this time, the share of public provision in total provision—is expected to correlate with total expenditure: The higher the public share, the greater the total expenditure. Notice that this argument, like the previous one, depends on particular assumptions, especially the assumption that the supply of finance is perfectly responsive to whatever level of provision bureaucratic decisionmakers prefer.

Leu recognized the theoretical significance of the financing constraint and included it as a variable additional to the shares of public finance and public provision. The variable he used to capture it was the centralization of political decisions about the size of the health care budget (centralization that he held to exist only in New Zealand and the United Kingdom). He also used a nontheoretical public variable to represent direct, as distinct from representative, democracies. He held that public expenditures are smaller in direct democracies (the Swiss effect). In addition, two demographic variables were included: proportion of the population under 15 years and degree of urbanization.

Leu's public choice model thus contained six explanatory variables in addition to GDP per capita:

- PF, share of public finance in total health care expenditures.
- PP, share of public provision in total provision (of hospital beds).
- CB, a dummy variable for the two countries having a centralized health care budget.
- DD, a dummy variable for direct democracy (Switzerland).
- POPU15, proportion of the population under 15 years of age.
- URB, percentage of population living in cities of more than 100,000 inhabitants.

He then ran a cross-sectional multiple regression on 1974 data for the OECD countries (excluding Luxembourg, Iceland, Japan, Portugal, and Turkey) and obtained the elasticities shown in Table 5. One estimating equation (column 1) included PF, one used PP (column 2), and one had both PF and PP (column 3); all three included CB and DD.

The income elasticities of +1.18 to +1.36 were similar to those reported earlier. (In fact, these seem to be robust results that vary little from study to study.)

According to equation (1), a 10-percent increase in the share of public and nonprofit beds was associated with a 9-percent increase in expenditure per capita. The presence of centralized budgetary control was associated with a much more substantial fall in expenditure, 21 percent. Direct democracy was associated with a dramatic fall of 31 percent.

According to equation (2), in which PP is replaced by PF, a 10-percent increase in the share of public finance was associated with a 3-percent increase in health expenditure per capita. The impact of centralized budget control rose, reducing per capita expenditure by 24 percent. The effect of the direct democracy variable was smaller and insignificant.

In equation (3), which includes both public-share variables, the effect of public provision appears to be smaller, and the impact of public finance has fallen dramatically, ceasing to be significantly different from zero. Centralized budget control was significant, and so was the Swiss effect.

Table 5

Elasticities of per capita health care expenditures: Selected countries, 1974

Item	Equation		
	(1)	(2)	(3)
GDP per capita	1.18	1.36	1.21
PF	—	0.34	*0.16
PP	0.90	—	0.85
CB	−0.21	−0.24	−0.23
DD	−0.31	*−0.20	−0.29
POPU15	0.56	1.10	0.69
URB	*0.11	0.28	—
Intercept	−12.41	−9.65	−10.06
R^2	0.97	0.96	0.97

*Elasticities were not significant at the 5-percent level.

NOTES: GDP is gross domestic product. PF is public finance share of total health care expenditures. PP is public provision share of total hospital beds. CB is a dummy variable for the 2 countries having a centralized health care budget. DD is a dummy variable for direct democracy (Switzerland only). POPU15 is proportion of population under 15 years of age. URB is percentage of population living in cities of more than 100,000 population. Equation (1) included PP but not PF; equation (2) included PF but not PP; equation (3) included both. All equations included CB and DD.

SOURCE: (Leu, 1986).

Is public provision inefficient?

Detailed microeconomic evidence casts serious doubts on the empirical validity of the claim that public provision is relatively X-inefficient. Explicit comparisons have been made between investor-owned for-profit hospitals and voluntary nonprofit hospitals. Such comparisons are relevant for Europe, which has been experiencing some growth in the market share of for-profit organizations. Care must be taken, however, to determine those differences that reflect the inherent qualities of the for-profit and nonprofit hospitals as distinct from those that are reflections of particular features in the system of financing and organizing health care delivery in the United States. Great care must also be taken to ensure that like is compared with like. Bays (1977), studying the United States, and Butler (1984), studying Australia, both found that for-profit hospitals specialized in the less complicated case mixes, concentrating on routine and non-urgent surgery. Stoddart and Labelle (1985), in a review of the entire field, concluded that evidence "does not substantiate (indeed it refutes) claims that privately owned for-profit hospitals operate more efficiently (i.e., at lower costs of production) than do non-profit hospitals." The case for privatization as a method of cost control or an agent for the promotion of efficiency is thus uneasy.

The absence of an unambiguous effect of ownership on overall spending should not come as a surprise. It is not self-evident that private sector bureaucracies are better controlled than public sector ones; that costs in the service market are higher in the public sector than in the presence of competition (a claim that standard theory does not imply, given the presence of advertising and other selling costs); or that market pressures are more reliable than professional ethics and regulation as a means of ensuring high quality. Of course, case mix varies greatly between the two sectors.

The pioneering econometric work by Newhouse and Leu continues to be followed up by others, and the definitive story remains to be unraveled. Most recently, Gerdtham et al. (1988) made a careful econometric analysis of the public choice issue. Their results differed from Leu's in that some of the variables changed signs and all had reduced *t* values.

The model preferred by Gerdtham et al., after extensive econometric testing of alternatives, was a linear in logarithms specification in which HCE per capita was a function of GDP per capita, the proportion of the population under 15 years of age, the share of public financing, and the proportion of public finance for inpatient care. Pooled OECD data for 1974 and 1983 were used. The income elasticity was highly significant and relatively high, +1.52. (The intercept term was negative and statistically significant.) The young population variable had a small elasticity (-0.085) of the opposite sign to Leu's finding, apparently denying the assumption that the young, like the elderly, are relatively high utilizers of health care (in value terms). The PF variable also changed signs, becoming negative, possibly suggesting less rather than more X-inefficiency under public than private financing and probably also reflecting heavier transaction costs. (The elasticity was -0.515.)

The foregoing suggests some lessons for those seeking effective leverage on overall expenditures:

- The wealthier (per capita) a country is, the more it spends on health care per capita and the greater the proportion of its total income spent on health.
- Centralized control of health care budgets seems to result in lower spending levels than otherwise would be expected.
- The effect of both public finance and public provision or ownership is ambiguous, but the former probably lowers expenditure.

Aggregate expenditures: Determinants and controls

In addition to centralized budgetary controls, other general institutional arrangements may be conducive to both cost control and greater efficiency. Although these do not emerge as candidates from aggregate analysis of the sort discussed in the previous section, there are either a priori or empirical reasons (sometimes both) for regarding them as policy instruments worth exploring.

Competition among hospitals

It has been frequently observed that, in most European countries, there is a large variance in cost per case (adjusted for diagnostic mix) among hospitals in both private and public sectors. In Britain, the evolution-survivor approach to industry theory (Alchian, 1950) has been espoused. This has led to the official policy idea that no a priori view of the inherent superiority of one form of ownership over another need be taken. It is better to create instead market conditions under which the more efficient providers (whatever their ownership) will tend to thrive and the relatively costly or inefficient will tend to be driven out via contestable markets and open competition among supplying agencies for the custom of publicly financed health authorities (with predetermined budgets).

This proposal for hospital financing (United Kingdom Department of Health, 1989a) has two main features. Both features rest on an important distinction of principle: that the principal public bodies responsible for ensuring the availability of health care to client populations (the District Health Authorities, or DHAs) need not be directly responsible for the provision of the care as distinct from its purchase. This separation of function is clearest in the case of the proposals for self-governing hospital trusts (SGHTs) run by boards of directors (based on ideas by Enthoven, 1985a and 1985b). SGHTs and private sector hospitals will compete for the business of DHAs. (They also will compete for the business of private patients and that of large practices of general practitioners, as discussed later.) Contracts between SGHTs and DHAs will specify workloads, quality assurance procedures, etc. The intention is to liberate managerial enterprise in those hospitals that are sufficiently geared up with internal information and management systems, to widen choice, and to provide market-type incentives for cost effectiveness. The responsibility of DHAs will remain to ensure adequate provision at the time of need for their clients. Even for hospitals that do not successfully apply to become SGHTs and remain under the direct control of DHAs, explicit management budgets will embody clear targets for quantity and quality with formal performance assessment.

Group practices of general practitioners (GPs) that serve more than 11,000 patients are also to be given the opportunity to receive practice budgets. Out of these budgets, they may purchase outpatient services, a defined set of elective surgical procedures, and diagnostic kits, such as X-ray and pathology services, directly from DHA hospitals and SGHTs (United Kingdom Department of Health, 1989a, b, c, and d).

Prospective payment for hospitals

Hospital-based care accounts for the lion's share of health costs. Countries that achieve relatively short lengths of stay and short turnover intervals will tend to have lower costs per case and, if they also achieve a low rate of hospitalization, will have lower overall costs. The pattern in Europe is extremely variable. In some countries, such as Germany, an above average rate of admissions, a higher than average bed stock, and long lengths of stay seem to raise health care expenditures substantially. Of the European countries, Finland has the most hospital-intensive style of medical practice, reflected in its admission rate and its bed stock. It is also among those with the longest lengths of stay. The United Kingdom, in contrast, is below average in all respects and offers a relatively cost-effective service.

The determinants of these differences are complex. One is plainly financial. German hospitals, for example, are reimbursed on a per diem basis, whereas United Kingdom hospitals have annual prospective budgets. Because most profit is to be made out of days that are not treatment intensive, long lengths of inpatient stay are profitable for hospitals paid per diem. However, other factors must be at work, too. It seems clear that clinical practice in Europe is not uniformly guided by the results of clinical trials and cost-effectiveness inquiries into the optimal length of stay, use of day-case surgery, and so on.

Clearly, any system that uses open-ended retrospective reimbursement for hospitals is likely to see a higher overall level of expenditure per capita and possibly a faster rate of health care cost inflation. Almost any form of prospective payment is likely to limit these tendencies by relating rewards to planned workload and encouraging awareness of cost per case. Costs could be reduced by improving efficiency; for example, by substituting less expensive inputs for costlier ones or reducing the number of unnecessary hospital stays or tests. Minimizing costs might, however, also be achieved by cutting corners and providing a lower quality of care. It thus becomes important to audit quality under this system. Another way acute care hospitals can reduce costs is to shift the burden of care to other providers, such as GPs. For example, early discharge from hospital increases the use of long-stay facilities, community services, GP visits, and so on.

The authors of the aggregate studies to date do not effectively identify a distinction between open-ended and closed-ended systems of finance, and it is clear that Leu's centralization variable is a poor proxy for closed-endedness (Culyer, 1988). Prepaid group practices such as health maintenance organizations are, for example, closed-ended systems without budget centralization; public health insurance, by contrast, may be centralized and governmentally operated but open ended. Systems that are closed ended lend themselves, on the face of it, more readily to expenditure control (Hurst, 1985), but they confront starkly the difficult issue of determining what the prospective budgets of health care suppliers should be. This task is made the more difficult by the nearly total ignorance of decisionmakers about the marginal costs and benefits of additional health care. It is also made the more politically daunting because of decisionmakers' vulnerability to charges (which may not be valid) that essential care is not being (or will not be) provided. Systems that are open ended seem to avoid this political charge, only to run into another: that costs are out of control. Moreover, ignorance of the marginal costs and benefits is not less under open-ended systems. Yet only when this ignorance has been substantially removed is it possible accurately, or even approximately, to assess which of these two approaches is more likely to produce an approximation to the optimal rate of expenditure.

Throughout Europe, there has been much discussion of the potential for using methods related to the U.S. system of diagnosis-related groups (DRGs) for prospective funding of hospitals (though not for billing purposes). DRGs are used to classify acute inpatients in groups using routine medical records data. The inventors of DRGs at Yale University claim that the groups are clinically meaningful and homogeneous in resource use (Fetter et al., 1980). The use of DRGs to pay hospitals creates, however, new patterns of penalty and reward. A limitation of DRGs in the United States is that they do not extend to outpatients and day cases, which therefore remain funded at cost. This provides an incentive for shifting costs from inpatient budgets to outpatients or day care. Such shifts could be achieved by genuinely efficient substitution or, less happily, at the expense of proper patient care. As a consequence, researchers at Yale have been developing ways of extending the DRG system to cover ambulatory categories. Like any classification system, the DRG system still contains a considerable range of costs per case. This encourages hospitals to select cheaper cases. Moreover, DRGs are based on the recorded primary diagnosis, comorbidities, and complications, which are based on clinicians' judgments, some of which may not be firmly based. Clinicians who are aware of the financial consequences for their hospitals of differing reporting conventions will be under pressure to adopt those that maximize income. (This medical form of creative accounting has been termed "DRG creep.")

Evidence on the consequences of prospective payments in the hospital sector is limited to the early U.S. experience with the Medicare prospective payment system. It should be interpreted with caution not only because experience is based on a fairly limited period but also because there would be major difficulties in transferring the results to Europe, with its different cultures, traditions of medical practice, and general levels of funding. U.S. hospitals financed by the DRG system were found to have reduced costs per day by 9.8 percent and costs per admission by 14.1 percent. Average length of stay in a hospital was shortened by 6.5 percent under the DRG program. (A review is contained in Culyer, Brazier, and O'Donnell, 1988.) The effect on total costs was, however, largely offset by an 11.7-percent rise in admissions with the DRG program. The net savings with the DRG program was, as a result, only 2.4 percent at a maximum.

The early U.S. experience with DRGs is still inconclusive. Although it would appear that length of stay has been significantly reduced, it cannot be determined whether this has been brought about by cost shifting among agencies and budgets, a rise in readmission rates, or a reduction in the quality of care and a deterioration of outcome. Evidence on the consequences of DRGs for throughput is conflicting. In general, total expenditure continues to rise. There has been a dearth of analyses of effects on patient outcomes. The potential for cost savings via this route would, of course, vary in Europe.

Medical remuneration

Because reimbursement methods can affect behavior, they can also affect economic rents and opportunity costs. Although there is some controversy about the ways in which doctors alter workload in response to changes in their methods of payment, it seems fairly clear that fee-for-service methods result in both more active treatment and higher incomes for doctors. Evans (1974) originated the theory of supplier-induced demand (SID). The idea here is that physicians have a target income; under a fee-for-service system of paying doctors, they will adjust workload in response to changes in the environment. The concept of SID seems to have grown out of the empirical observation in the United States that regional utilization of health care is positively associated with the regional stock of doctors, holding price and other variables constant. The hypothesis is that physicians will induce patients to use more services in order to maintain income. A positive association has also sometimes been found between physician stock and prices, although this

result is even more disputed than the fundamental utilization effect is. There are a number of econometric and empirical problems in testing for SID, but Rice's claim (Rice, 1983; Gabel and Rice, 1985) that experimental rather than routine data strongly support an inverse relationship between reimbursement rates and use of services seems persuasive. (A review can be found in Culyer, Donaldson, and Gerard, 1988.)

The evidence from the United States seems to be borne out by Canadian experience. Extra billing was banned in Ontario in 1986; the fee-for-service profession expanded billable items of service substantially (by about 18 percent) in subsequent years. In Quebec, a doubling of fees for home visits was followed by rapid increases in the number of home visits: 14.6 percent in 1977, 25.2 percent in 1978, and 28.4 percent in 1979 (Poullier, 1987), despite a general decline in home visits by community-based doctors generally.

No evidence for Europe exists that is comparable to that for North America. However, the relative remuneration of doctors seems to correlate with the method of payment. Although most countries adopt a mixture of systems of remuneration that differ between hospital-based and community-based doctors, those that use a predominantly fee-for-service method (Belgium, France, Germany, and Switzerland) have relatively high earnings for the profession. Slightly less than one-half of Germany's doctors are community based, are paid on a fee-for-service basis, and have complete freedom as to choice of practice location, and there is no effective control on the numbers entering the profession. Senior hospital doctors in private practice are also on a fee-for-service basis. Gross earnings for private doctors and some specialists (e.g., radiologists) are twice or three times those of salaried hospital doctors. Physician expenditures in Germany amount to about 25 percent of total HCE, the highest share in Europe. It is striking that the four countries that do not use fee for service as the principal means of payment (Denmark, Italy, Sweden, and the United Kingdom) have the four lowest ratios of average doctor income to GDP per capita (Organization for Economic Cooperation and Development, 1985 and 1988).

A related factor affecting expenditure for physicians' services is entry into the profession. The outputs of medical schools in European countries vary considerably, as does the proportion of doctors trained outside Europe. The highest rate of admission to medical school seems to be in Belgium, where entry is unrestricted (33 per 100,000 population), but the wastage rate is also high (only one-half graduate). In Germany, the rates are 19 admitted and 11 graduated. In the Netherlands, the rates are 13 and 10, and in the United Kingdom, 7 and 6, but the United Kingdom has the highest proportion of foreign medical graduates, 26 percent (Schroeder, 1984). In each of these countries save the United Kingdom, there has been a recognized oversupply of doctors and, in particular, of specialists.

Direct price and quantity controls

There has been no study in Europe in which the effect of the exercise of the state's monopsony power on the remuneration of personnel or the prices and quantities of medical supplies has been quantified. However, it is widely believed that the effect has been substantial in some countries, especially in those, like Britain, that have centralized pay negotiating machinery. The potential efficiency losses of the exercise of monopsony power have not been estimated.

One of the most regulated parts of the health care industry in Europe has typically been the pharmaceutical industry. Because of this regulation, countries with a substantial local pharmaceutical industry have experienced a tradeoff between the desires for low-cost modern medicines and for having a dynamic, high-technology, exporting (but oligopolistic) industry. In addition, most European countries subsidize drug consumption, but they have widely differing consumer copayments. In Europe, the highest expenditure per capita on drugs was in Germany ($194 in 1983, which was nearly five times that of Denmark). The variability derives not only from price regulation but also from quantity controls. For example, several European countries have limited lists from which physicians must select their prescriptions, and some allow pharmacists to substitute generic drugs for branded products. The United Kingdom is about to introduce cash-limited budgets for general practitioners' prescribing (United Kingdom Department of Health, 1989e). Perhaps surprisingly, no correlation has been found between the number of physicians or pharmacists per capita and the expenditure per capita on drugs (Organization for Economic Cooperation and Development, 1987). If adequate statistical controls could be placed on the other factors affecting drug expenditures, such a relationship might emerge. The variability in spending per capita strongly suggests that this component of HCE (on average about 10 percent of the total in the early 1980s) is rather sensitive to policy variables.

It may be possible to argue that the exercise of monopsony power; use of prospective cash-limited health care budgets; a preference for capitation and salary over fee for service; and price, quantity, and prescribing regulation in pharmaceuticals are all endogenous elements from the perspective of some overarching model of public choice and are therefore more likely to be chosen by countries with a relatively low GDP per capita. They nonetheless remain options for selection in any country wishing to exercise greater control over the growth of health care expenditures. The idea of harnessing competitive forces in a relatively poor OECD country like the United Kingdom seems, however, to be an entirely new option, neither obviously predicted by public choice theory nor, as yet, subjected to empirical test.

Conclusions

Aggregate international comparisons cannot be used to indicate what health care spending ought to be, nor can they be used to prescribe its optimal growth rate. Such issues require patient and fairly detailed cost-benefit analysis of specific health care programs. Aggregate comparisons can, however, be used to test theories of the determinants of spending. The principal conclusion to be drawn from such analyses is that in Europe, as elsewhere, income per capita is the main determinant. Income is also, however, likely to be related to particular policies adopted to control HCE. Therefore, the existing cross-sectional regression analyses do not permit any independent measure of the impact of such policies other than the general conclusions that centralized cash-limited budgets have a significant negative impact on the total and that public finance also reduces total expenditures. Microeconomic, as distinct from aggregate, comparisons suggest that private for-profit ownership of hospitals tends to raise costs.

The large variations in the composition of HCE in Europe are, in turn, the product of the great variety in forms of finance, provision, and regulation that exist. Detailed investigation of the causes of this variety remains to be done. Meanwhile, it is hard to resist the conclusion that the selective use of instruments that appear to bear on these components currently offers the best way forward: promoting competition among suppliers, use of closed-ended prospective systems for paying suppliers, controlling entry to the major professional groups, use of salary and capitation rather than fee for service in medical remuneration, and various direct price and volume controls. None is a panacea and none is without its own cost. Moreover, it should always be borne in mind that cost containment in itself is not a sensible objective. The ultimate objective of any system of health care is to promote the health and welfare of its clients. More precisely, the objective is to maximize health and welfare subject to the resources available and to adjust these resources so that, at the margin, they are neither more nor less valuable in the health care sector than elsewhere. The practical difficulties entailed in making these judgments, whether one depends on markets or planning mechanisms, should never serve as an excuse for mere cost cutting, regardless of its consequences.

Acknowledgments

My thanks for helpful comments from Jeremy Hurst, Bengt Jönsson, David Parkin, Jean-Pierre Poullier, and an anonymous Health Care Financing Administration reviewer. I have not taken all the advice given, sometimes because I stubbornly persisted in an original position and sometimes because space did not permit further elaboration. Therefore, most and probably all of any remaining faults are entirely my own.

References

Alchian, A. A.: Uncertainty, evolution and economic theory. *Journal of Political Economy* 58(3):211-221, June 1950.

Bays, C. W.: Case-mix differences between non-profit and for-profit hospitals. *Inquiry* 14(1):17-21, Mar. 1977.

Bosanquet, N.: Inconsistencies of the NHS: Buchanan revisited. In Culyer, A. J., and Jönsson, B., eds. *Public and Private Health Services: Complementarities and Conflicts.* Oxford, England. Basil Blackwell, 1986.

Buchanan, J. M.: *The Inconsistencies of the National Health Service.* London. Institute of Economic Affairs, 1965.

Butler, J.: On the relative efficiency of public and private hospitals. In Tatchell, P. M., ed. *Economics and Health 1983, Proceedings of the Fifth Australian Conference of Health Economics.* Canberra. Health Economics Research Unit, Australian National University, 1984.

Culyer, A. J.: *Health Care Expenditures in Canada: Myth and Reality; Past and Future.* Canadian Tax Paper No. 82. Canadian Tax Foundation. Toronto, Canada. 1988.

Culyer, A. J., Brazier, J. E., and O'Donnell, O.: *Organising Health Service Provision: Drawing on Experience.* London. Institute of Health Services Management, 1988.

Culyer, A. J., Donaldson, C., and Gerard, K.: *Financial Aspects of Health Services: Drawing on Experience.* London. Institute of Health Services Management, 1988.

Drummond, M. F., Stoddart, G. L., and Torrance, G. W.: *Methods for the Economic Evaluation of Health Care Programmes.* Oxford, England. Oxford University Press, 1987.

Enthoven, A. C.: *Reflections on the Management of the NHS: An American Looks at Incentives to Efficiency in Health Services Management in the UK.* London. Nuffield Provincial Hospitals Trust, 1985a.

Enthoven, A. C.: National Health Service—Some reforms that might be politically feasible. *The Economist* 61-64, June 1985b.

Evans, R. G.: Supplier-induced demand: Some empirical evidence and implications. In Perlman, M., ed. *The Economics of Health and Medical Care.* London. Macmillan, 1974.

Fetter, R. B., Shen, Y., Freeman, J. L., et al.: Case mix definition by diagnosis-related groups. *Medical Care* 18(Supp.), 1980.

Gabel, J. R., and Rice, T. H.: Reducing public expenditures for physician services: The price of paying less. *Journal of Health Politics, Policy and Law* 10(4):595-609, Winter 1985.

Gerdtham, U., Anderson, F., Sogaard, J., and Jönsson, B.: Economic analysis of health care expenditures: A cross-sectional study of the OECD countries. *CMT Rapport 1988:9.* Linköping, Sweden. Centre for Medical Technology Assessment, 1988.

Hurst, J.: *Financing Health Services in the United States, Canada, and Britain.* London. King Edward's Hospital Fund for London, 1985.

Kleiman, E.: The determinants of national outlay on health. In Perlman, M., ed. *The Economics of Health and Medical Care.* London. Macmillan, 1974.

Leu, R. R.: The public-private mix and international health care costs. In Culyer, A. J., and Jönsson, B., eds. *Public and Private Health Services: Complementarities and Conflicts.* Oxford, England. Basil Blackwell, 1986.

Leviatan, L. I.: *Consumption Patterns in Israel.* Jerusalem, Israel. Falk Project for Economic Research in Israel, 1964.

Newhouse, J. P.: Development and allocation of medical care resources: Medico-economic approach. In *Development and Allocation of Medical Care Resources.* Proceedings of the 29th World Medical Assembly. Tokyo. Japan Medical Association, 1975.

Newhouse, J. P.: Medical care expenditure: A cross-national survey. *Journal of Human Resources* 12(1):115-125, Winter 1977.

Organization for Economic Cooperation and Development: *Measuring Health Care 1960-1983, Expenditure, Costs and Performance.* Paris, 1985.

Organization for Economic Cooperation and Development: *Financing and Delivering Health Care: A Comparative Analysis of OECD Countries.* Paris, 1987.

Organization for Economic Cooperation and Development: Measuring Health Care. Draft Report MAS/WP1(88)07. Paris, 1988.

Organization for Economic Cooperation and Development: Health Data File. Paris. Directorate for Social Affairs, Manpower, and Education, 1989.

Parkin, D., McGuire, A., and Yule, B.: Aggregate health care expenditures and national income: Is health care a luxury good? *Journal of Health Economics* 6(2):109-128, June 1987.

Poullier, J. P.: From the Kaiserliche Botshafts Rede to Kremsmuenster: Has Montesquieu's Paradox Evolved? Paper presented at a symposium of the European Institute of Social Security, Present and Future Structural Problems of Social Security. Oct. 1-3, 1987.

Rice, T. H.: The impact of changing Medicare reimbursement rates on physician induced demand. *Medical Care* 21(8):803-815, Aug. 1983.

Schroeder, S. A.: Western European responses to physician oversupply. *Journal of the American Medical Association* 252(3):373-384, July 20, 1984.

Stoddart, G. L., and Labelle, R. J.: *Privatisation in the Canadian Health Care System.* Ottawa, Canada. Ministry of Supply and Services, 1985.

United Kingdom Department of Health: *Working for Patients.* Command No. CM555. London. Her Majesty's Stationery Office, 1989a.

United Kingdom Department of Health: Self-Governing Hospitals. Working Paper 1. London. Her Majesty's Stationery Office, 1989b.

United Kingdom Department of Health: Funding and Contracts for Hospital Services. Working Paper 2. London. Her Majesty's Stationery Office, 1989c.

United Kingdom Department of Health: Practice Budgets for General Medical Practitioners. Working Paper 3. London. Her Majesty's Stationery Office, 1989d.

United Kingdom Department of Health: Indicative Prescribing Budgets for General Medical Practitioners. Working Paper 4. London. Her Majesty's Stationery Office, 1989e.

Williams, A.: Economics of coronary artery bypass grafting. *British Medical Journal* 291(6491):326-329, Aug. 3, 1985.

Health services utilization and physician income trends

by Simone Sandier

Statistics from several Organization for Economic Cooperation and Development countries on consumption and cost of health care services, physician workload, and physician earnings are presented. Data are analyzed according to type of physician payment used: fee for service, per case, capitation, or salary. Incentives theoretically embodied in each payment method are often offset by other factors—scale of charges, patient out-of-pocket payment, and patient access or physician activity restrictions. Moreover, the impact of payment method on use appears to be weaker than the impact of such factors as population morbidity, national health insurance, professional ethics, and medical technology.

Introduction

This article is a presentation of a set of statistics gathered to describe the behavior of patients and doctors, the consumption and cost of health care services, and physician earnings in a number of Organization for Economic Cooperation and Development (OECD) countries. The countries concerned are Canada, Denmark, France, the Federal Republic of Germany (hereafter called Germany), Italy, Japan, the Netherlands, the United Kingdom, and the United States. (In Canada, health care systems differ somewhat from province to province. Quebec's system is studied in more detail here because some aspects of its system of remuneration for physicians are unique.) The data are studied in relation to the methods used in the different countries to compensate physicians. First, the scope and comparability of the data available across the countries as well as analysis of the possible impact of the remuneration methods on the behavior of patients and their doctors are discussed.

Methodological remarks

The aggregate statistical data used in this article were derived from a variety of different sources. In some cases, various primary data were combined so as to get as comparable estimates as possible. In the "Technical note," the sources and computations used for each parameter are listed. It must be stressed that the concepts and definitions used in the different countries—and sometimes inside the same country—vary. Therefore, the parameters used to describe the operation of the health care system in general and the activity or income of physicians in particular are not identical even though the term used may be the same.

Depending on the method of data collection—surveys of households, surveys of physicians, use of

The main ideas for this article were put together during 1988, which the author spent at the Organization for Economic Cooperation and Development on sabbatical from the Centre de Recherche, d'Etude et de Documentation en Economie de la Santé (Sandier, 1989). More detailed work is expected to be published in due course.

Reprint requests: Simone Sandier, CREDES, Association Loi de 1901, 1 rue Paul Cezanne, 75008 Paris, France.

health insurance records, or use of national accounts—the data cover a different scope of population, practitioners, and expenses. The discrepancies are sometimes real, but sometimes they are only apparent. For example, using data from the National Ambulatory Medical Care Survey of the National Center for Health Statistics (NCHS), one could quote the figure of 2.7 physician contacts per person per year in the United States during 1985. On the other hand, using 1985 NCHS data from the National Health Interview Survey, one could quote the figure of 5.3 physician visits per person per year. The explanation of the apparent difference lies in the fact that the first estimate refers only to office visits. In other countries, the scope of the data reported by national health insurance funds is generally more restricted than that of data reported in patient interviews. In most cases, the explanations of the differences can be found by careful reading of the detailed methodological appendixes of publications. The data selected for this study are as comparable across countries as possible. However, some bias might be introduced in the intercountry comparisons by the fact that data are not available for all countries on a yearly basis.

The influence of a particular method of payment on the functioning of a health system should, strictly speaking, be assessed in terms of the outcome of the incentive or disincentive effects of each of its dimensions, e.g., basis of remuneration, scale of charges, and type of health coverage provided by the health insurance agency or agencies. However, the methods of payment for medical services can influence the behavior of both those seeking health care and physicians (who are providers in their own right and also prescribers of services supplied by other members of the profession). Therefore, problems arise from the interaction of various other factors when one tries to isolate the impact of methods of remuneration on the functioning of the health care system or to determine the incentive effect of a particular aspect of remuneration.

Patient factors that influence the demand for health care include sociodemographic and cultural characteristics, geographic environment, and self-perception of their state of health. It is difficult to separate the effects of these factors from the effects of economic factors in general and the methods of paying for care in particular.

To some extent, physicians behave like other suppliers: The way they are paid will have some effect on their assessment of the patient's state of health and their consequent decisions regarding the therapy required. Such effects are difficult to isolate from the effects of other factors, such as their professional knowledge, code of ethics, and the medical-technical environment (the possibility to refer patients to hospital consultants, detection and screening services, etc.).

Moreover, each of these factors, depending on how it is applied, has an influence not only on its own account but also because it is coupled with others in a given set of conditions. In practice, the observable variants are not simply random combinations. On the contrary, it would seem that, in most countries, the adoption of particular methods of remuneration has been aimed at achieving compatibility between the different aspects of these methods of payment and their acceptability by the profession. Accordingly, the incentive effects of one feature of physician remuneration are often offset by those inherent in another of its features. Consequently, it might be unrealistic to attribute a separate incentive or disincentive effect to each individual characteristic of a particular method of payment.

From the statistical standpoint, a number of warnings should be given with regard to the conclusions to be drawn from international comparisons. In order to assess the impact of a particular factor, one needs to be able to measure the deviation it causes from a normal situation. However, in the health care area, more than elsewhere, no stable reference values exist. The pace of technological progress is such that the norms as regards numbers and concentration of personnel or equipment are constantly being revised, as is the level of needs. In assessing the values for a particular parameter in the different countries, without knowing whether these are unduly high or unduly low, it is tempting to take as the norm the average derived from a sample of countries. However, such values cannot be used as standards. On the one hand, they are obtained by aggregating highly different situations; on the other hand, it is impossible to say whether they represent an optimum.

How are physicians compensated?

In the different countries considered, there are four main basic ways of remunerating physicians: fee-for-service payment, payment per case, capitation payment, and payment of a salary. These remuneration methods are not mutually exclusive. The full description and analysis of how physicians are paid in different countries can be found elsewhere: Chadwick (1987); Contandriopoulos, Lemay, and Tessier (1987); Glaser (1970); Hogarth (1963); and Reinhardt, Sandier, and Schneider (1986). To avoid repetition, only some comments on the

incentives built into each method are provided in this article.

Different points derived from the observation of various countries should be stressed:

• In practice, each method of remuneration is applied in a number of ways across countries, depending on the conditions under which it operates. For example, payment to the physician of a fee agreed upon at the time of treatment, as is often the case in the United States, bears only a remote resemblance to the fee-for-service system operated in Germany. Under Germany's statutory health insurance scheme, neither the patient nor the doctor knows at the time of treatment the exact amount the doctor will be paid. The patient, moreover, will never know. The doctor will receive payment later through his professional association on the basis of an agreed-upon nomenclature of services and in accordance with a scale of fees worked out on the basis of the forecast overall budget agreed on by the Health Insurance Funds and apportioned among the physicians within a region in relation to their workload.

• Most countries have adopted a combination of methods for remunerating different categories of physicians on the basis of their specialty or where they practice, remunerating the same doctor when he or she performs different activities, or paying for treatment given to a particular category of patient. A physician may be paid by one or more different methods, depending on the type of patients treated. In the Netherlands, for example, the statutory health insurance scheme fixes an earnings target for general practitioners and calculates the capitation payment in such a way that it will provide 70 percent of these earnings, on the assumption that the remaining 30 percent will be derived from private practice, for which payment is on a fee-for-service basis. In the United States, a combination of payment methods is the general rule. Each payment method is represented, ranging from no patient out-of-pocket payment in the case of Medicaid, full or partial direct payments in the case of private insurance schemes, and full or partial reimbursement of the patient's expenditure to full payment with no refund for uninsured patients or for expenditure below a certain level for patients under some insurance arrangements. In some countries, the system of remuneration for specialists differs from that for general practitioners, and in some different systems of payment are used for hospital and ambulatory care.

• Each method of payment has a particular sphere of application. Fee-for-service payment applies primarily to the situation in which the relationship between physicians, as self-employed persons, and their patients is one of free choice; payment of a capitation is used predominantly in the case of physicians who both provide primary care and act as gatekeepers of the health system by having the responsibility of referring their patients to other providers when necessary; physicians employed in establishments supplying them with other inputs, staff, and equipment are paid a salary proportional to the number of hours worked.

If the patient has no health care insurance, few rules govern the payment of physicians, and generally the amount the patient pays is determined by market forces. However, such a situation rarely occurs in OECD countries. At present, some degree of general coverage of health care expenditure exists in all OECD countries in the form of a national health service, statutory insurance agencies, or private insurance arrangements chosen by individuals. In the case of insured health care, the features and operation of each method of remuneration are usually governed by rules negotiated by representatives of the medical profession and the health insurance agencies. Generally speaking, the smaller the proportion of cost borne by the patients themselves is, the greater are the power and influence of third-party payers.

The payment of the physician involves one or more financial transactions. The nature of the payer(s), the proportion that each pays, and the timing of the payment are conditions that, like the basis of the remuneration or the scale of charges, can influence the behavior of the different actors. Describing the methods of physician payment by considering only the last parameter would be an oversimplification and could lead to forgetting the strong incentives and possibilities for control associated with the other factors.

In Figure 1, the four main situations concerned in the case of self-employed physicians are outlined. The physician may receive total payment from the patient (who either is or is not later reimbursed by the agency), total payment from the health insurance agency or agencies, or partial payment from both. Incentives may differ according to who pays and when.

When the patients have to make the initial outlay, they are aware of the cost of health care, sometimes to the extent that it may deter them from calling upon a physician's services. In this case, the health care financing agencies lose some power of control. On the other hand, the system of full coverage might be seen as providing an incentive to higher health care consumption, because the demand from the patient for treatment is no longer regulated by prices. However, although the treatment may be free, in most cases, the patient has to be registered on a doctor's list and cannot consult a specialist without the prior consent of the general practitioner. What is more, full and direct physician payment by the health insurance agencies means that they have greater control over the physician's activity and remuneration. The use of a sliding fee scale in Quebec and the fixing of payments in line with an overall budget in Japan are good illustrations of this ability to control expenditure.

Theory versus reality

In comparing the hypotheses implicit in the theory with the reality observable in the sample of countries considered, we look first, at the consumption of physicians' services; second, at physician workload and prescribing behavior; and finally, at the earnings

Figure 1

Four main forms of remuneration for self-employed physicians

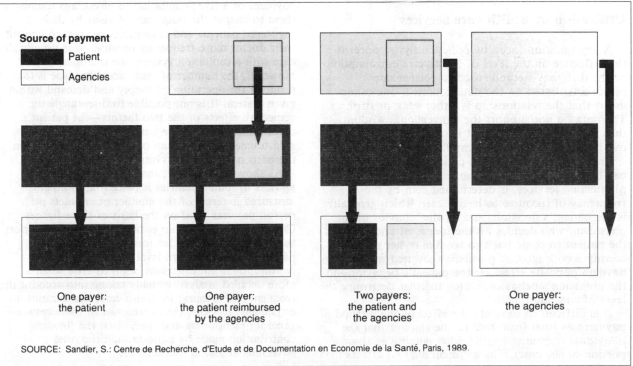

SOURCE: Sandier, S.: Centre de Recherche, d'Etude et de Documentation en Economie de la Santé, Paris, 1989.

43

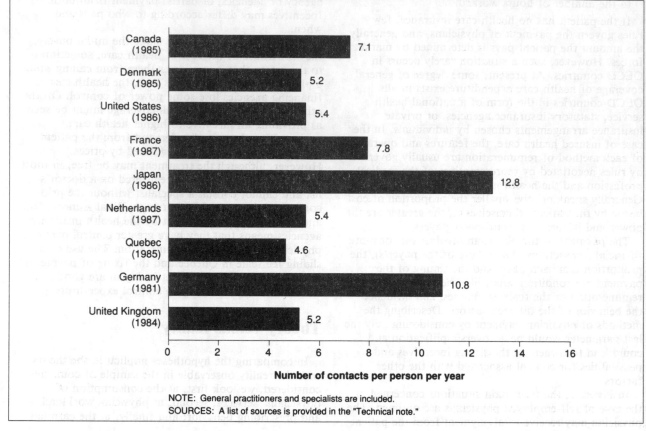

Figure 2
Utilization of physician services: Selected countries, selected years 1981-86

Canada (1985) — 7.1
Denmark (1985) — 5.2
United States (1986) — 5.4
France (1987) — 7.8
Japan (1986) — 12.8
Netherlands (1987) — 5.4
Quebec (1985) — 4.6
Germany (1981) — 10.8
United Kingdom (1984) — 5.2

Number of contacts per person per year

NOTE: General practitioners and specialists are included.
SOURCES: A list of sources is provided in the "Technical note."

of physicians. The sources of the data used are enumerated in the "Technical note."

Utilization of health care services

A key question faced by policy analysts concerns the influence on the level of health care consumption of the different methods used to compensate physicians. Based on the data collected, one cannot assert that the relationship is either weak or strong. The data do not support the conventional wisdom that fee-for-service payment is more conducive to overconsumption than the capitation system is.

The number of physician-patient contacts, which can be regarded as an indicator of the consumption of physicians' services, is determined both by the frequency of recourse to health care, which generally is the patient's decision, and by the behavior of the physician, who decides on the treatment and may ask the patient to come back to see him or her or to consult a colleague. A particular payment method can have an opposite effect on the patient's behavior and the physician's behavior, which together determine the level of consumption.

It is difficult to separate the effect of the method of payment as such from that of the amount that the individual consumer bears (either nothing at all or a portion of the cost). The payment method affects the

physician's behavior; the amount the individual pays affects that of the consumer. For example, in theory, payment of a fixed capitation to physicians tempts them to restrict the frequency of visits by their registered patients and encourages patients to consult their doctor more frequently because, as is usually the case with a capitation system, the treatment is free. However, the number of visits actually made is the result of the operation of supply and demand within a given system. It is not possible to disentangle the respective effects of the two factors—the patient's contribution, on the one hand, and the unit of measurement of physician output, on the other—on the basis of number of visits.

As shown in Figure 2, the use of physicians' services in some countries is twice that in others, measured in terms of the number of contacts per person per year. Just on the basis of these figures, Germany seems to be an example that would support the argument that the fee-for-service system of payment leads to a high level of health care consumption, but questions begin to arise when a more detailed analysis is made taking into account the frequency of recourse to health care, the duration of physicians' services, the breakdown of these between general practitioners and specialists, the financial contribution made by patients, and the rules governing access to specialist care.

Access to health care, measured in terms of the percentage of the population having recourse to physicians' services, varies little among countries with the exception of Japan, where the proportion of consumers (55 percent) appears to be substantially lower than elsewhere. Access seems to be little influenced by the method of payment of physicians or by the financial contribution required of patients. For example, in the United States, where in many cases patients have to bear at least part of the cost of ambulatory care, 76 percent of the population saw a physician at least once during 1986, whereas in Quebec, where health care is free, the figure was 78 percent in 1985. In a detailed analysis of health care use in the Netherlands, Van Vliet and Van de Ven (1985) revealed that the more frequent recourse to physicians by those with statutory health insurance was related to a higher incidence of illness among these patients than among those with private insurance. On the whole, patients with statutory health insurance were older and in poorer health than patients in the other group were.

The number of general practitioner (GP) services per person is generally expected to be lower in countries where the capitation system predominates, with the incentive that this theoretically gives physicians to limit the number of services per registered patient supposed to overweigh the effect on patient demand of having free health care. However, the analysis of different systems existing alongside one another in Denmark and the Netherlands seems to support the opposite conclusion—that the level of consumption is influenced more by the fact that it is free of charge to the patient than by the method whereby physicians are paid. In these two countries, the number of general practitioner services per insured person using a physician paid a capitation and receiving their treatment free is higher than that for persons covered by the other system, who are generally in better health, consult physicians who are paid on a fee-for-service basis, have to pay the physician themselves, and bear part of the cost. The difference in per capita consumption between publicly and privately insured persons in the Netherlands is 40 percent for physicians as a whole, 28 percent for general practitioners, and 53 percent for specialists. In Denmark, the number of general practitioner services for those insured in Group 1 (with no copayment) is twice that for those insured in Group 2 (less extensive coverage). Faced with an inconsistency of this kind and being unable to control the data for the health status of the population concerned, one has to be cautious with conclusions about impacts.

Data on the consumption of specialist services seem to indicate that access to a specialist is more frequent when referral by a GP is not required. The number of annual contacts with a specialist per person is comparatively higher in Germany (5.0), the United States (3.7), France (3.0), and Canada (2.5) than in the Netherlands (1.8), the United Kingdom (1.2), and Denmark (0.6). However, these figures cannot be used as the basis of an analysis of GPs'

referral behavior in relation to the manner in which they are paid because, when access to specialists is free, some consultations are arranged on the initiative of the patients themselves.

The average length of a GP visit in the countries surveyed varied by a ratio of almost 3 to 1: 5 minutes in the Netherlands in 1985, 9 minutes in Germany during 1981-82, and 14 minutes in the United States in 1985 (Figure 3). It is likely that the content of physician encounters of different lengths also differs, with a more or less detailed interview and a varying number of accompanying tests and examinations. Although the number of countries surveyed is too small to provide conclusive evidence, it would seem that procedures tend to be lengthier when the patient pays the fee directly (United States and France) and when GPs compete with specialists (Germany, United States, and France). Encounters tend to be shorter when the physician is paid a capitation by a health insurance agency without any contribution from the patient.

The average time spent with a physician, measured by the number of contacts and their duration, is another indicator of the consumption of health care.[1] For a general practitioner, it can be reckoned at about 1 hour per person per year in France (67 minutes) and in Germany (57 minutes), whereas in the Netherlands and the United Kingdom, it would seem to be no more than 18 and 33 minutes, respectively. The total amount of time spent with physicians of all types would appear to be about 1½ hours in Germany and the United States and roughly 2 hours in France. The ranking of the countries on this basis is thus different from their ranking on the basis of the number of contacts per person and would seem to indicate that the consumption of physicians' time is substantially higher when they are paid on a fee rather than a capitation basis.

Physician workload

The characteristics of the different methods of remuneration play a direct part in determining the income that physicians will derive from their practice for a given amount of work. Conversely, physicians who set themselves an earnings target need to take into account the method of payment for services in determining the output needed to achieve this. Consequently, the method of remuneration is one factor that can influence the way physicians behave when they are providing the health care themselves or referring their patients to other producers of goods and services.

According to the data on physician workload and the number of visits physicians perform in a year, the level of activity differs quite substantially in the countries surveyed. It is not possible to relate these

_____

[1]The estimates used here were derived by multiplying the number of services by their average duration. Because the figures are not always for the same years, the estimates can provide only an approximate idea of the situation.

Figure 3
Number of patient visits per general practitioner per year, average duration of visits, and number of hours worked per week: Selected countries, selected years 1979-87

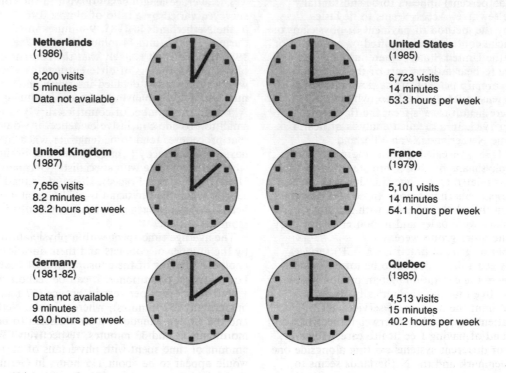

Netherlands
(1986)

8,200 visits
5 minutes
Data not available

United States
(1985)

6,723 visits
14 minutes
53.3 hours per week

United Kingdom
(1987)

7,656 visits
8.2 minutes
38.2 hours per week

France
(1979)

5,101 visits
14 minutes
54.1 hours per week

Germany
(1981-82)

Data not available
9 minutes
49.0 hours per week

Quebec
(1985)

4,513 visits
15 minutes
40.2 hours per week

SOURCES: A list of sources is provided in the "Technical note."

differences to differences in methods of remuneration, because some of the findings are at variance with the theory, the sample is small, and methods of computation may vary.

On the whole, there does not seem to be a strict relationship between the number of visits and the number of hours worked. Visits are shortest in countries where physicians have the most visits. In countries where the average visit lasts less than 10 minutes, i.e., Germany, the Netherlands, and the United Kingdom, the average numbers of visits per general practitioner per year are 10,000, 8,100, and 7,600, respectively. These figures are substantially higher than those recorded for countries where the average visit lasts about 15 minutes: 6,700 visits per GP per year in the United States, 5,100 in France, and 4,500 in Quebec (Figure 3).

Capitation forms the basic remuneration for GPs in the United Kingdom and the Netherlands: Capitation accounts for up to 50 percent of the remuneration of GPs in the United Kingdom and applies to two-thirds of the clientele of GPs in the Netherlands. The fact that GPs in these countries have more visits than their counterparts in the other countries raises doubts as to the theory that the fee-for-service system of payment encourages physicians to increase their output and the system of capitation encourages them to see their

patients less frequently. However, this conflict becomes less apparent if one considers their activity in terms of the number of hours worked: GPs in the United Kingdom devote the least amount of time to the provision of care, 38.2 hours a week, compared with more than 50 hours for GPs in France and the United States.

The workload of physicians should not be related to the method of payment without at the same time taking into account the demand factors, the number of physicians, and the financial procedures associated with the methods of remuneration. Moreover, it should be emphasized again that physicians are not alone in determining their level of activity and that, in a system of capitation, the fact that the patient pays nothing generally tends to lead to a higher demand.

The number and distribution of the medical profession are factors that tend to distort the effects of a method of remuneration. The increase in the number of physicians may be associated with the drop in the number of visits per physician that is apparent in each of the countries for which these figures are available, irrespective of the system of remuneration for physicians. For example, the number of visits per GP decreased during the period 1980-86 from 7,448 to 6,723 in the United States, from 5,327 to 5,101 in France, and from 9,847 to 7,656 in the

46

United Kingdom. Both in the United Kingdom, with its capitation system, and in France, with its fee-for-service system, physicians practicing in regions where there is a high concentration of doctors spend more time on each consultation than do their counterparts in regions where there are fewer doctors.

In Quebec, the scale of charges for services over and above a given level of activity was sharply reduced in the fee-for-service system for GPs. The reduced scale of charges seems to have offset the possible inflationary effect of the fee-for-service system of payment. The time spent by Quebec GPs on the delivery of health care services is low (little more than 40 hours) compared with the time spent by their counterparts in other countries who are paid in the same way. What is more, the number of hours worked has been declining for more than 15 years. It was estimated that, in 1972, general practitioners in Quebec spent an average of 49.7 hours treating patients; the figure dropped to 46.8 hours in 1976, 44.6 hours in 1980, 41.9 hours in 1984, and 40.2 hours in 1986 (Contandriopoulos, Fournier, and Boileau, 1988).

The theory that the fee-for-service system is conducive to higher prescribing rates for pharmaceutical products and additional exploratory examinations than capitation or salary is neither proved nor disproved by the figures that have been compiled. The proportion of GP-patient contacts giving rise to the prescribing of pharmaceutical products ranges from 55 percent in Canada and 66.1 percent in the United States to more than 80 percent in France and the Netherlands; for GPs in the United Kingdom, who are paid a capitation, the figure is 74 percent. Part of the explanation for the differences in this case may be the traditions of medical practice and payment of the cost of pharmaceutical products by health insurance agencies. In the United States, for example, patients pay 75 percent of their pharmaceutical costs out of their own pocket (Letsch, Levit, and Waldo, 1988). In France, GPs' higher prescribing rates for pharmaceutical products (more frequent prescriptions and more products per prescription) may, to some extent, counterbalance the lower-than-average admission rate in hospitals in France.

The figures for referrals to other physicians also tie in with the accepted idea that practitioners who are paid a fee prefer to keep their patients and physicians who are paid a capitation are more prone to refer them to other physicians. In France and the United States, where patients can consult specialists directly, the proportion of patients referred by their GP to another physician is relatively low, 2.8 and 5.2 percent, respectively. In contrast, the figures are 8.6 percent in the United Kingdom, where a specialist can be seen only on the recommendation of a GP, and 7.9 percent in the Netherlands, where the same applies to 70 percent of the population. The figures for both Quebec and Germany (8.7 and 9.4 percent, respectively) tend to confirm that the regulations influence behavior. In both Quebec and Germany,

access to specialist care is theoretically free, but GPs, who are paid on a fee-for-service basis, refer their patients fairly frequently to other physicians. In Quebec, the scale of charges is calculated in such a way that GPs are not encouraged to perform more services and specialists are not encouraged to recruit patients directly because they are paid a higher rate if the patient is referred to them by a general practitioner. In Germany, under the statutory system of health insurance, a patient who wants to consult a physician other than the one to whom he has surrendered his voucher has to ask for a transfer form.

A question arises as to whether methods of payment also affect other aspects of the provision of health care. Such aspects include the skimming (selection) of patients, emphasis on preventive medicine, provision of a comprehensive and lower geared form of treatment rather than intensive use of sophisticated techniques of examination and specialist expertise, spread of technological innovations, and the split between ambulatory and hospital care. It would be even more risky to answer this sort of question on the basis of the macroeconomic data used for these cross-country comparisons than is the case with questions about overall physician activity. Nonetheless, it appears that the scale of charges (nomenclature, in the case of fee-for-service payment) for the different health care services can substantially affect the orientation of medical practice. A number of examples bear out this hypothesis.

The United Kingdom provides an example of the effectiveness of gearing the capitation to the patient's age so that the elderly, whose health care needs are greater, will not be discriminated against. The fact that persons 65 years of age or over represent the same proportion of a physician's workload in the United Kingdom as in France and the United States (about 20 percent) provides evidence of this.

Another example pertains to tariff changes. The proportion of home visits has declined in all countries. However, the number of home visits has risen in Quebec following a substantial uprating of their tariff, demonstrating that medical practice can be influenced through a change in the scale of tariffs (Contandriopoulos and Fournier, 1983).

Medical practice in every country has been placing increasing emphasis on technical diagnosis and treatment procedures, despite the disparities among the relative scales of charges for different countries. However, in some areas, particularly France and Quebec, what was considered an unduly rapid increase in the use of certain technical procedures has been temporarily checked by making changes in the nomenclature (Contandriopoulos and Fournier, 1983). In fact, the spread or abandonment of particular procedures is primarily a reflection of the development of medical technologies for the treatment, relief, or reassurance of patients. However, at the same time, the behavior of physicians in each specialty can be influenced by the relative scale of charges.

Changes in tariff scales affect the relative position of general practitioners and the different specialists on the earnings ladder. In Ontario, for example, the government leaves it to the medical associations to apportion most of the amount set aside for an increase in tariffs among the different types of medical service.

Physician earnings

Physicians' gross income is determined by their output and the corresponding payments they receive based on the system of remuneration in use. The pretax income that a physician derives from the practice is calculated by subtracting from gross earnings the professional expenses incurred for the performance of work.

In most countries, average physician earnings are, in essence, a reflection of the value that society places on physician services. Apart from the United States, in countries where the cost of health care is financed by the government or by powerful health insurance agencies, a physician's scale of earnings is explicitly or implicitly fixed in advance on the basis of the total amount to be allocated among the physicians and a forecast of the level of activity for the coming year. This is true irrespective of whether physicians are paid on a fee-for-service, capitation, or salary basis. The fee-for-service system of payment is, in theory, more conducive to expenditure overshoots because there may be a sharper-than-expected increase in the number of services performed. However, even in such a case, safeguards like those applied in Germany or Quebec can limit such variations, and they can always be offset the following year.

In order to try to make a cross-country comparison of physician earnings and income in relation to methods of remuneration, a number of different parameters have been used. Physicians' gross and net income have been calculated in U.S. dollars adjusted on the basis of purchasing power parities (PPPs) calculated by the OECD. The purchasing power parities used in this case were based on the gross domestic product (GDP). This means that the cross-country comparison of the level of physician remuneration is based on a unit that is more meaningful in economic terms than official exchange rates are.

Physician remunerations have been compared with general economic indicators. For example, in each country, the average earnings of a physician have been compared with per capita GDP, and net pretax income has been compared with the average wage. These variables denote the physician's economic status within the community and allow comparisons among countries.

The long-term trend in earnings has been analyzed using series adjusted on the basis of GDP price deflators. These adjustments were made in order to assess the trend in terms of the purchasing power of physician remuneration in each country and also so that a cross-country comparison could be made on the basis of figures that have been adjusted for inflation.

Separate gross and net income series were compiled for GPs and for total physicians. The latter series is an accurate indicator for the medical profession as a whole. However, in each country, it is made up of differing proportions of the various types of specialists, whose scale of earnings differ widely. Surveys carried out in Germany, the United States, and France have shown that pediatricians and psychiatrists were at the bottom end of the income scale for the medical profession, whereas radiologists and surgeons were at the top. The variance in national distributions tends to distort the analysis.

The data that have been collated[2] are presented in Figures 4-6. Income is given in PPP-adjusted U.S. dollars. In terms of gross income, Japan has the best paid physicians, followed by the United States and Germany. British, Danish, and French physicians have the lowest earnings. By and large, these differences seem to be related more to countries' economic characteristics than to the methods of remuneration in use. To some extent, this calls to mind the more general link that was shown to exist between a country's economic level and the level of its total expenditure on health care (Organization for Economic Cooperation and Development, 1977, and Schieber, 1987).

In the case of general practitioners (Figure 4), the most homogeneous category of physicians considered here, average gross income in 1985 was highest in the United States: $174,400, more than twice the figure for Canada and almost three times that for the United Kingdom. However, these disparities become less marked once the figures are adjusted on the basis of national economic indicators. The ratio of net income per physician to the national average wage, an indicator of physicians' relative economic status within their country, falls within a narrower range, 2 to 3.2, the maximum difference between countries being 60 percent between Germany and France. The national average wage, therefore, seems to be a fairly good predictor. For the countries included in the sample, if general practitioners' average income were estimated on the basis of average wage × 2.6, the difference between these estimates and what is believed to be the true figure would be a maximum of 23 percent in the case of Germany and France and less than 10 percent for the other countries. Even if all of this deviation could be ascribed to certain characteristics of the methods of remuneration, the area of their influence on levels of remuneration would appear to be comparatively restricted.

---

[2]The earnings and income figures for GPs and physicians as a whole have been either derived from national published data or calculated by the author. All variables are available for Canada, the United States, France, and Germany. Some countries have been included only for certain of the variables: general practitioner earnings and income in the case of the United Kingdom, general practitioner earnings in the case of the Netherlands and Quebec, net income for physicians as a whole in the case of Denmark and Japan.

Figure 4

Gross income per physician and ratio of net income per physician to national average wage for general practitioners and all physicians: Selected countries, selected years 1983-85

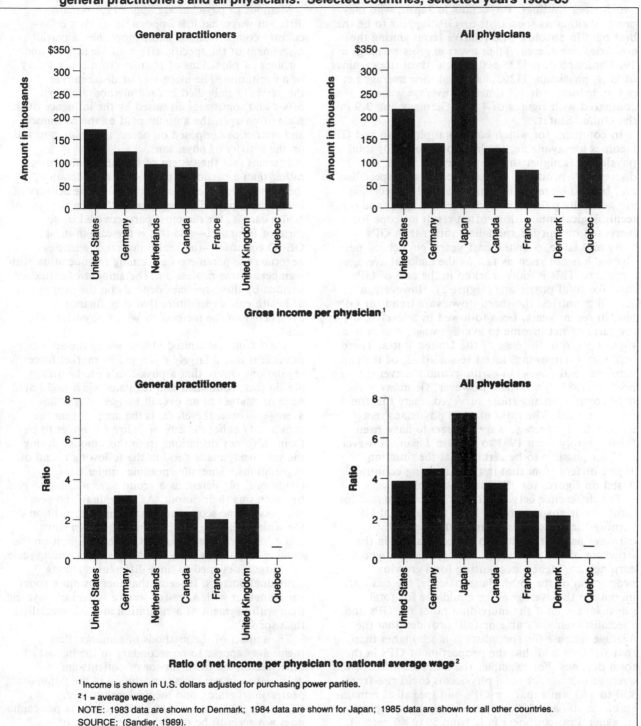

General practitioners

Gross income per physician [1]

All physicians

General practitioners

Ratio of net income per physician to national average wage [2]

All physicians

[1] Income is shown in U.S. dollars adjusted for purchasing power parities.

[2] 1 = average wage.

NOTE: 1983 data are shown for Denmark; 1984 data are shown for Japan; 1985 data are shown for all other countries.

SOURCE: (Sandier, 1989).

The analysis of average earnings for total physicians does not provide any new insight into the role of method of physician remuneration, but it does yield two further findings. Physicians in Japan, who may practice either as specialists or GPs, appear to be the best paid in absolute and relative terms among the countries considered. Their average gross earnings in 1984 amounted to $325,500, or 1½ times the earnings of U.S. physicians ($202,400), and their average net pretax income was 7.3 times the average wage, compared with figures of 4.4 in Germany and 3.9 in the United States.

In countries for which both total physician and GP incomes are available, the level of income for total physicians is higher than that for GPs. This discrepancy primarily reflects the fact that specialists are, by and large, better paid than GPs. Specialists are generally paid on a fee-for-service basis, and technological innovations often result in scope for increased output for specialists rather than GPs.

By and large, over the past years, physicians' net income has not risen as fast as the national average wage has. This is more marked in the case of GPs than for total physicians (Figure 5). However, in several countries, the sharp downward trend for GPs has, in recent years, been followed by a leveling off of the ratio of net income to average wage, and even a slight upturn in the case of the United States. There was also a narrowing, albeit less marked, of the gap between total physician earnings and the average wage prior to 1983. Since then, however, Germany is the only country among those surveyed where this trend has continued. The ratio of total physicians' net income to the average wage appears to have risen fairly sharply from 1981 to 1984 in Japan. However, it is not possible to be certain that the situation in Japan differs from that in the remaining countries based on figures for 1981 and 1984 only.

The difference between the ratios for GPs and for total physicians may result from the fact that GP earnings have risen less sharply than specialist earnings have. It could also reflect changes in the structure of the profession, with specialists, whose earnings are higher, accounting for a growing proportion of the total. Paradoxically, the ratio of income to the average wage could rise for total physicians even if the individual ratios for GPs and specialists remain stable or fall, provided that the average income for specialists is much higher than that for GPs and that the proportion of GPs in the total declines. For example, the index number for the average income for total physicians could rise from 150 to 160 while that for GPs and specialists remains stable at 100 and 200, respectively, if the proportion of general practitioners falls from 50 to 40 percent.

Conclusions

Despite reservations concerning the comparability of the data analyzed, it is possible to draw a number of conclusions from this survey of selected OECD countries. Although these conclusions may have no statistical validity, they are by no means without significance and supplement what can be inferred from the theory.

Methods of payment are applied in so many different ways that it is impossible, from a cross-country comparison, to make more than a partial assessment of the specific effect on the activity and earnings of physicians of payment of a fee, a salary, or a capitation. The incentives or disincentives theoretically embodied in each method are often offset and sometimes disguised by the influence of the scale of charges, the amount paid by the consumer, and restrictions imposed on access to health care and on the activity of physicians.

It seems that the system of funding health care, rather than a particular method of remuneration, is the most potent factor in conditioning the delivery of health care, physician earnings, etc. When the cost of health care is, for the most part, covered by some form of insurance—and this is the case in most OECD countries—the health insurance agencies negotiate the parameters governing remuneration with members of the profession. The amount of influence wielded by these agencies depends on the proportion of health care expenditure that they finance, irrespective of the method by which physicians are paid.

Apart from the United States, where the activity of physicians is still largely governed by market forces, regulations ensure that a physician's total earnings are, in fact, controlled and regulated via a negotiated scale of charges or an overall budget. Physicians' average income, therefore, is the amount that the community either directly or indirectly agrees to pay them, with any deviations from this amount during the year being made good in the following round of negotiations. Generally speaking, under these conditions, physicians as a group have nothing to gain by increasing their output. As individuals, however, they have some scope for improving their position on the scale of earnings for the profession. In some countries, there are provisions, such as a limit on the number of patients on a doctor's list or a sliding scale of charges, designed to limit differences among individual doctors. It seems that there is more room for maneuver with a fee-for-service system of payment than with payment of a capitation and for specialists than for GPs.

The impact of the methods of remuneration themselves appear to be secondary to the impact of other factors on the behavior of patients and physicians—in particular, morbidity in the population, professional ethics, and medical technology.

The number of physician-patient contacts per capita does not seem to be related to the method of remuneration. GPs respond to the quantity of the demand from their patients but seem to have some scope for adjusting the amount of time they devote to them. For example, the duration of medical visits and the average total amount of time spent with a physician are shorter when the physician is paid a capitation by the health insurance agency rather than

Figure 5
Ratio of average net pretax income per physician to national average wage for general practitioners and all physicians: Selected countries, selected years 1970-86

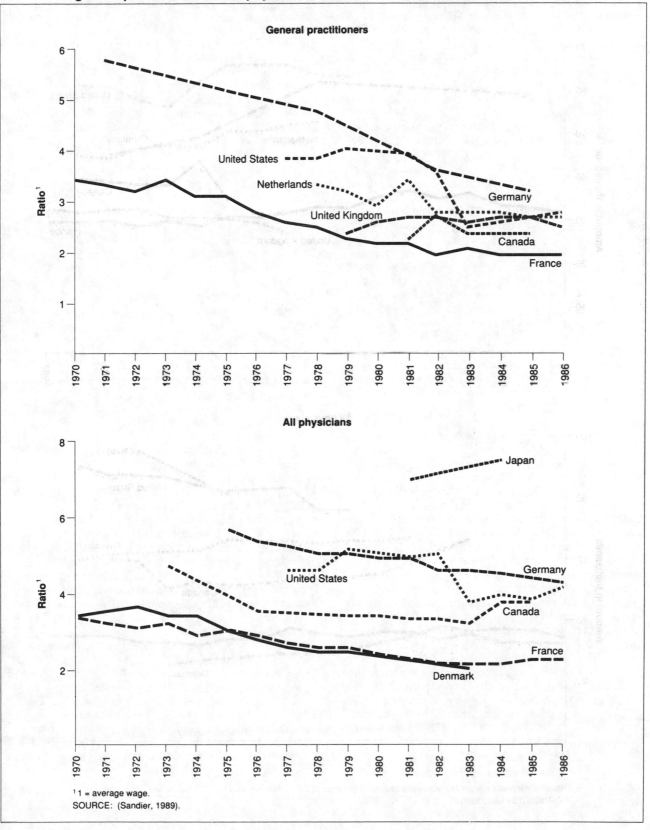

¹ 1 = average wage.
SOURCE: (Sandier, 1989).

Figure 6
Income per physician in relative terms for general practitioners and all physicians: Selected countries, selected years 1970-87

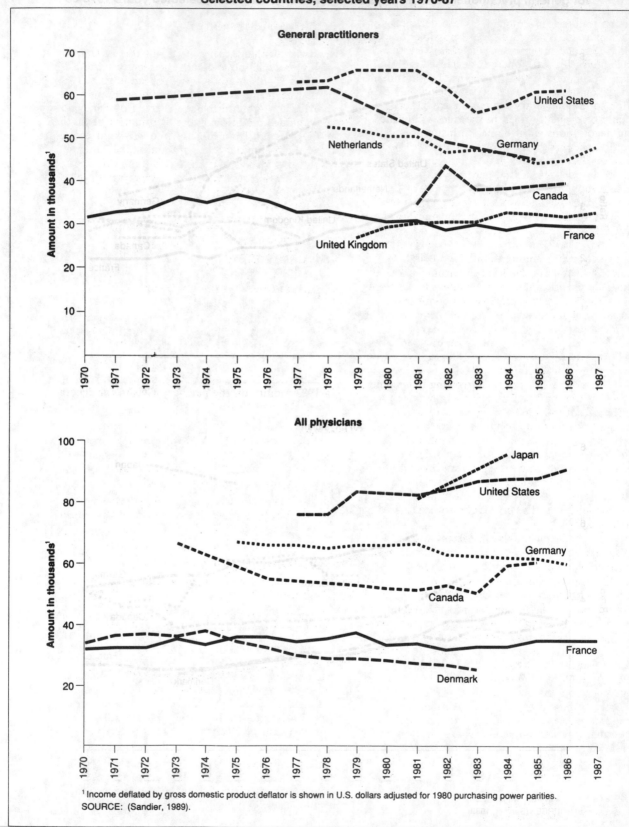

[1] Income deflated by gross domestic product deflator is shown in U.S. dollars adjusted for 1980 purchasing power parities.
SOURCE: (Sandier, 1989).

a fee paid directly by the patient. Similarly, the number of hours worked per week by a physician appears to be shorter under systems of capitation.

The number of medical visits performed by GPs in all of the countries examined has been declining for a number of years. There are several possible reasons for this. Demand may not be sufficiently elastic; average physician workload has decreased with the increase in the number of physicians. The decline in the average number of visits per physician may be a reaction to the budgetary limits that are either implicitly or explicitly fixed in the rules established during negotiations with the health insurance agencies. Therefore, these rules may create an inverse correlation between prices and volume of output, which is the opposite of that generally associated with a classic supply curve.

The national average wage has been shown to be a fairly good predictor of physicians' income. In the case of GPs, it explains more than three-quarters of the variation among countries, thus leaving little room for the method of remuneration as a possible explanatory factor for the level of earnings. A comparable phenomenon in this context is the close and increasing correlation between a country's economic level and its expenditure on health care.

Until the last 4 years, the economic status of GPs, whose income is currently from twice to three times the national average wage (Figure 5) had been deteriorating in most countries (Figure 6). This trend is part of a general pattern of narrowing of income differentials that has been occurring in many countries since the end of the 1960s. Because of this trend, it seems doubtful that physicians have considerable scope to adjust their activity in line with their earnings target. In fact, a number of constraints limit physicians' activity, in particular, those resulting from the increase in their numbers. For physicians as a group, the relative deterioration in economic status is offset by the shift of the profession toward increased specialization.

In recent years, this downward trend has been checked (except in Germany). The ratio of GP income to the average wage has stabilized, and GPs' purchasing power, which had been shrinking, has increased, particularly in the United States. Is this new trend likely to last? The period surveyed here is too short to provide an answer. However, there are three possible explanations of what is happening: a certain loss of enthusiasm for the philosophy of egalitarianism, the perhaps temporary benefits of disinflation, and the comparatively low level to which GP incomes had already descended.

In short, taking into account the difficulties involved in making cross-country comparisons and considering only the countries included in this study, the following conclusion can be made. At present, the influence of the method of remuneration on the behavior of the actors within the health care system seems to be outweighed by other more decisive factors—the coverage of expenditure by health insurance agencies and their powers of intervention, morbidity in the population, medical technology, and the country's economic level.

Acknowledgments

I wish to thank the members of the OECD working party on social policy, both the secretariat and country representatives, for their support, encouragement, and valuable insights. I am particularly grateful to Jean-Pierre Poullier, who not only guided me in obtaining information from the OECD Health Data File but also was kind enough to read the preliminary versions and make valuable comments and suggestions. If, despite this assistance, there are still some errors of interpretation, the responsibility is entirely mine.

Technical note: Sources and computations of parameters

Contacts per capita per year

Canada: Number of physician visits per capita for the period 1984-85, excluding X-rays and analyses: Santé et Bien-Etre Social Canada (1987).

Denmark: Total number of contacts: NOMESKO (1988); OECD data file. Extrapolation of findings of a 1983 inquiry on the number of visits for general practitioners: Chadwick (1987).

France: Author's estimate based on service reimbursement by the Health Insurance Scheme and Centre de Recherche, d'Etude et de Documentation en Economie de la Santé (1989).

Germany: Personal contacts with physicians: Schwartz et al. (1984). Breakdown between general practitioners and specialists derived from Delozier et al. (1989).

Japan: Information received from the Japanese delegation to the OECD.

Netherlands: Health Interview Survey, Aug.-Sept. 1988: Central Bureau voor de Statistiek.

Quebec: Figures compiled by the Regie de l'Assurance Maladie du Quebec.

United Kingdom: Office of Population Censuses and Surveys (1986). According to estimates based on the survey General Medical Practitioners' Workload, 1985-86, the number of GP consultations per person has remained stable since 1981. The figure for specialists is based on hospital consultations (Department of Health and Social Security, 1987).

United States: Data from the 1986 National Health Interview Survey of NCHS. For the GP-specialist breakdown, the ratio of 31 percent to 69 percent was used, based on data from the 1981 National Ambulatory Medical Care Survey of NCIIS.

Percentage of users

Canada: Health and Welfare Canada (1981).

France: Charraud and Mormiche (1986); Caisse Nationale d'Assurance Maladie des Travailleurs Salaries (1982).

Germany: Ingolstadt, quoted in Geissler (1981).

Japan: Information received from the Japanese delegation to the OECD.

Netherlands: Health Interview Survey, Aug.-Sept. 1988: Central Bureau voor de Statistiek.

Quebec: Figures compiled by the Regie de l'Assurance Maladie du Quebec.

United Kingdom: Office of Population Censuses and Surveys (1986); Cartwright and Anderson (1981).

United States: Data from the 1986 National Health Interview Survey of NCHS.

Duration of physician visits

France: Letourmy (1979).

Germany: Duration of 11.3 minutes in the case of interns: Schwartz et al. (1984).

Netherlands: Central Bureau voor de Statistiek (Jan. 1986).

United Kingdom: Department of Health and Social Security (1987).

United States: Data from the 1985 National Ambulatory Medical Care Survey of NCHS.

Physicians' workload

Canada and Quebec: Taylor, Stevenson, and Williams (1984); Contandriopoulos, Fournier, and Boileau (1988).

France: Self-employed physicians: Bui Dang Ha Doan (1980).

Germany: Gesundheitswesen (1988).

United Kingdom: All activities relating to care: Department of Health and Social Security (1987).

United States: American Medical Association (1987). Care includes direct care of patients plus interpretation of results of tests.

Outcome of physician contacts

Canada: Prescription of pharmaceuticals, 1977 data: IMS Canada, 1988. Number of services: Taylor, Stevenson, and Williams (1984).

France: Le Fur and Sermet (1985); Institut National de la Santé et de la Recherche Medicale (1976).

Japan: Information received from the Japanese delegation to the OECD.

Netherlands: Estimates based on findings from the Health Interview Survey: Central Bureau voor de Statistiek (various years).

Quebec: Estimated rate of referral to a specialist: Taylor, Stevenson, and Williams (1984).

United Kingdom: Estimates based on findings from the 1984 General Household Interview Survey: Abel-Smith (1981). Number of services: Department of Health and Social Security (1987).

United States and Germany: Ambulatory care comparisons: Delozier et al. (1989). Number of services in the United States: American Medical Association (1987). Number of services in Germany: Schwartz et al. (1984).

Gross earnings of physicians

Canada: Santé et Bien-Etre Social Canada (1984 and 1985).

France: Centre de Recherche, d'Etude et de Documentation en Economie de la Santé (1989).

Germany: Schneider, Sommer, and Kececi (1987); Brenner (1988).

Netherlands: Author's computation using Ministerie van Volksgezondheid en Milieuhygiene (1985); Central Bureau voor de Statistiek (1988).

Quebec: Contandriopoulos and Fournier (1983).

United Kingdom: Review Body on Doctors' and Dentists' Remuneration (1987) for data since 1980. Earlier data were estimated by Centre de Recherche, d'Etude et de Documentation en Economie de la Santé.

United States: American Medical Association (1987). For GPs: average of GPs and family practice.

Net income before taxes

Canada: 62 percent of gross income (1984 ratio for physicians with at least one visit during each trimester).

France: 60 percent of gross income.

Germany: Brenner (1988); Geissler (1981).

Japan: Information received from the Japanese delegation to the OECD.

Netherlands: 60 percent of gross income.

United Kingdom: Review Body on Doctors' and Dentists' Remuneration (1987).

United States: American Medical Association (1987).

Population, gross domestic product, and deflator

Organization for Economic Cooperation and Development (1988a and 1988b); Poullier, Gillion, and Schieber (1985).

References

Abel-Smith, B.: *Alternative Methods of Physician Compensation and Their Effects on Physician Activity, an International Comparison: Country Report for the United Kingdom.* Paris. Centre de Recherche pour l'Etude et l'Observation des Conditions de Vie, 1981.

American Medical Association: *Socioeconomic Characteristics of Medical Practice, 1987.* Chicago, 1987.

Brenner, G.: Realinkommen weiter Rückläufig. *Arzt und Wirtschaft* 6:11-16, 1988.

Bui Dang Ha Doan: L'activité professionnelle des médecins en 1977. *Cahiers de Sociologie et de Démographie Médicales* 1:1-58, special issue, 1980.

Caisse Nationale d'Assurance Maladie des Travailleurs Salariés: *Qui Consomme Quoi?* Paris. CNAMTS, 1982.

Cartwright, A., and Anderson, R.: *General Practice Revisited: A Second Study of Patients and Their Doctors.* London. Tavistock, 1981.

Central Bureau voor de Statistiek: *Maandbericht Gezondheidstatistiek.* Various issues. S'Gravenhage. Various years.

Centre de Recherche, d'Etude et de Documentation en Economie de la Santé: *ECO-SANTE, un Logiciel pour Analyser l'Evolution du Système de Santé en France.* Software. Paris. Medsi/McGraw-Hill, 1989.

Chadwick, L. K.: Incentives Influencing General Practitioners in Selected European Health Systems: A 1985 Comparative Study. Unpublished report. London. 1987.

Charraud, A., and Mormiche, P.: Disparités de consommations médicales, Enquête Santé 1980-1981. *Collections de l'INSEE (Institut National de la Statistique et des Etudes Economiques).* Series M(118):1-135, 1986.

Contandriopoulos, A. P., and Fournier, M. A.: *Les Services Médicaux au Québec.* Montréal, Canada. Groupe de Recherche Interdisciplinaire en Santé, University of Montréal, 1983.

Contandriopoulos, A. P., Fournier, M. A., and Boileau, H.: *Les Effectifs Médicaux au Québec: Situation de 1972 à 1986 et Projections pour 1990.* Québec, Canada. Corporation Professionnelle des Médecins du Québec, 1988.

Contandriopoulos, A. P., Lemay, A., and Tessier, G.: Les coûts et le financement du système socio-sanitaire. *Les Publications du Québec.* No. 29. Québec, Canada. 1987.

Delozier, J., et al.: Ambulatory care comparisons: France, Federal Republic of Germany, and the United States of America. *Vital and Health Statistics.* Series 5, No. 5. National Center for Health Statistics, Public Health Service. Washington. U.S. Government Printing Office, June 1989.

Department of Health and Social Security: *General Medical Practitioners' Workload.* London. 1987.

Geissler, U.: *Alternative Methods of Physician Compensation and Their Effect on Physician Activity: Country Report for the Federal Republic of Germany.* Paris. Centre de Recherche pour l'Etude et l'Observation des Conditions de Vie, 1981.

Gesundheitswesen: *Medizinische und Ökonomische Orientierung.* Baden-Baden, Federal Republic of Germany. 1988.

Glaser, W. A.: *Paying the Doctor.* Baltimore, Md. The Johns Hopkins Press, 1970.

Health and Welfare Canada: *The Health of Canadians.* Ottawa, Canada. 1981.

Hogarth, J.: *Payment of the General Practitioner.* Oxford, England. Pergamon Press, 1963.

IMS Canada: Personal communication. 1988.

Institut National de la Santé et de la Recherche Médicale: *Les Malades en Médecine Libérale: Qui Sont-Ils? De Quoi Souffrent-Ils?* Paris. 1976.

Kassenärztliche Bundesvereinigung: *Grunddaten zur Kassenärztlichen Versogung in der Bundesrepublick Deutschland.* Bonn, Federal Republic of Germany. Undated.

Le Fur, P., and Sermet, C.: *Clientèle, Morbidité, Prescriptions en Médecine Libérale.* Paris. Centre de Recherche, d'Etude et de Documentation en Economie de la Santé, 1985.

Letourmy, A.: *Etude du Comportement du Médecin Généraliste de Ville.* Paris. Centre de Recherches et d'Etudes sur le Bien-Etre, 1979.

Letsch, S. W., Levit, K. R., and Waldo, D. R.: National health expenditures, 1987. *Health Care Financing Review.* Vol. 10, No. 2. HCFA Pub. No. 03276. Office of Research and Demonstrations, Health Care Financing Administration. Washington. U.S. Government Printing Office, Winter 1988.

Ministerie van Volksgezondheid en Milieuhygiene: *Financieel Overzicht van de Gezondheidzorg.* The Netherlands. Various years.

NOMESKO: *Health Statistics in the Nordic Countries.* Copenhagen, Denmark. 1988.

Office of Population Censuses and Surveys: *General Household Survey, 1984.* London. Her Majesty's Stationery Office, 1986.

Organization for Economic Cooperation and Development: *Les Dépenses Publiques de Santé.* Paris. 1977.

Organization for Economic Cooperation and Development: *Banque de Données sur le Secteur de la Santé.* Data tape. Paris. 1988a.

Organization for Economic Cooperation and Development: *Comptes Nationaux Principaux Agrégats, 1960-1988.* Paris. 1988b.

Poullier, J. P., Gillion, C., and Schieber, G.: *La Santé en Chiffres, 1960-1983, Dépenses, Coûts, Résultats.* Paris. Organization for Economic Cooperation and Development, 1985.

Regie de l'Assurance Maladie du Québec: *Statistiques Annuelles.* Québec, Canada. Various years.

Reinhardt, U., Sandier, S., and Schneider, M.: *Die Wirkungen von Vergütungs-Systemen auf die Einkommen des Ärzte, die Preise und auf die Struktur Ärztlicher Leistungen im Internationalen Vergleich.* Augsburg, Federal Republic of Germany; Paris. BASYS and Centre de Recherche, d'Etude et de Documentation en Economie de la Santé, 1986.

Review Body on Doctors' and Dentists' Remuneration: *Seventeenth Report.* London. Her Majesty's Stationery Office, 1987.

Sandier, S.: *The Payment of Physicians in Selected OECD Countries.* Paris. Organization for Economic Cooperation and Development, Mar. 1989.

Santé et Bien-Etre Social Canada: *Etude sur le Revenu des Médecins par Spécialité*. Ottawa, Canada. 1984.

Santé et Bien-Etre Social Canada: *Les Gains des Médecins au Canada, et Mise à Jour*. Ottawa, Canada. 1985.

Santé et Bien-Etre Social Canada: *Utilisation des Services de Médecins, 1980-81 à 1984-85*. Ottawa, Canada. 1987.

Schieber, G.: *Santé: Financement et Prestations, Analyse Comparée des Pays de l'OCDE*. Paris. Organization for Economic Cooperation and Development, 1987.

Schneider, M., Sommer, J., and Kececi, A.: *Gesundheitssysteme in Internationalen Vergleich. Gesundheitsforschung 160*. Augsburg, Federal Republic of Germany. BASYS, 1987.

Schwartz, F. W., Kerek-Bodden, H. E., Schach, E., et al.: The Ambulatory Medical Care Survey in FRG, 1981-1982, the EVAS-Study. Paper presented at the International Epidemiological Association Meeting. Vancouver, Canada, 1982. Edited in 1984.

Taylor, M. G., Stevenson, H. M., and Williams, A. P.: *Medical Perspectives on Canadian Medicare*. Institute of Behavioural Research, York University, 1984.

Van Vliet, R., and van de Ven, W.: Differences in Medical Consumption Between Publicly and Privately Insured in the Netherlands. Paper presented at the International Meeting on Health Econometrics, Rotterdam, The Netherlands. 1985.

What can Europeans learn from Americans?

by Alain C. Enthoven

In a wide-ranging look at many aspects of health care financing and delivery, the concepts of glasnost and perestroika are used as a framework for presenting ideas from the American system that may have value for European health care planners. These include more uniform approaches to data collection and cost reporting, patient outcome studies, evaluation of service and access standards, publication of information, quality assurance review, decentralization and independent institutions, prepaid group practice, demonstrations and experiments, and managed competition. Suggestions are offered for making health care systems on both sides of the Atlantic more manageable, efficient, and responsive.

Introduction

What can Europeans learn from Americans about the financing and organization of medical care? The obvious answer is "not much." We Americans are spending nearly 12 percent, going on 15 percent, of gross national product (GNP) on health care, while most European countries are spending an apparently stabilized 6 to 9 percent (Division of National Cost Estimates, 1987; Francis, 1989; Schieber and Poullier, 1988). The western European democracies have achieved essentially universal coverage, but some 35 million Americans—17.5 percent of the population under 65 years of age—have no financial protection against medical expenses, public or private (Short, Monheit, and Beauregard, 1989). (Those who cannot pay may get free care from community or public hospitals, after they have paid what they can. This places an inequitable burden on the hospitals that care for the uninsured and motivates them to find ways of avoiding attracting patients who cannot pay, such as by closing emergency rooms.) Millions more have inadequate coverage that leaves them exposed to large risks or to exclusions for care of preexisting conditions. At the same time, our infant mortality rate is higher than that of most of the western European democracies, but life expectancy is about in the middle of the group. A recent public opinion poll found that only 10 percent of Americans agree with the statement "on the whole, the health care system works pretty well," compared with 56 percent of Canadians and 27 percent of the British (Blendon and Taylor, 1989). So it would be, quite frankly,

ridiculous for an American to suggest that we have achieved a satisfactory system that our European friends would be wise to emulate.

Americans like to believe that we have the world's best medical care—at least for those who are insured and can pay for it. I have some doubts. For example, it has been well established that there is a pronounced negative relationship between annual volume in a hospital and mortality for complex surgical procedures such as open-heart surgery (Luft, Bunker, and Enthoven, 1979). The curve relating death rates to annual volume for coronary artery bypass graft (CABG) surgery is still descending at 150 operations a year, indeed at several hundred (Prospective Payment Assessment Commission, 1988). That is why the California Department of Health Services and the American College of Surgeons recommend minimum annual volumes of 150 for open-heart surgery. Nevertheless, in 1986, of 103 California hospitals in which open-heart surgery was performed, 37 did fewer than 150 such procedures (Steinbrook, 1988b.) This helps to explain the high death rates from CABG surgery in some California hospitals, ranging as high as 17.6 percent in 1986 (Steinbrook, 1988a). In Des Moines, Iowa, a metropolitan area with a population of 380,000, two hospitals did kidney transplants, with 1988 volumes of 8 and 15, respectively. At the university hospital about 100 miles away, the volume was 69 cases (Iowa Department of Public Health, 1989).

A recent genre in our medical literature is called "appropriateness." A panel of expert and generalist physicians reviews the literature and determines the indications for surgery: Under what conditions is it appropriate (i.e., clearly beneficial to the patient), equivocal, or inappropriate? Then a team reviews a large sample of medical records and classifies cases. Such studies have recently reported 32 percent of carotid endarterectomies inappropriate, another 32 percent equivocal (Winslow et al., 1988); 14 percent of CABG surgery inappropriate, another 30 percent equivocal (Winslow et al., 1988); 27 percent of hospital days inappropriate (Restuccia et al., 1984); 20 percent of pacemaker implants inappropriate, another 36 percent equivocal (Greenspan et al., 1988.), etc.

Somewhere in America might be found the world's best medical care. But the merits of that claim will not be apparent to the families of hundreds of Californians who have died of inappropriate or equivocal open-heart operations in low-volume hospitals, especially if the widows are being hounded for payment because their deceased husbands did not have insurance.

I could go on. We have much to be humble about.

The difficulties of writing this article are compounded by the fact that European health care

Reprint requests: Alain C. Enthoven, Graduate School of Business, Stanford University, Stanford, California 94305.

systems and practices are not all the same. Their diversity exceeds that among and within the different States in the United States. If there are lessons, their relevance will vary considerably from one country to another. Moreover, our intellectual roots and cultures are intertwined. Americans and Europeans read many of the same books and professional journals. Most, if not all, of the ideas I discuss in this article have some European roots. So identifying some ideas leading to good things in America these days is not meant to deny their European ancestry.

One approach I considered was to recommend that Europeans learn from our mistakes, lest they repeat some of them. For example, various British writers, and lately Her Majesty's Government, have proposed offering tax breaks for the purchase of private health insurance (*Working for Patients*, 1989). The merits of this idea are likely to depend a great deal on exactly how it is done. But in the United States, the open-ended tax break for employer-paid health insurance has had some very negative consequences (Enthoven, 1985a). It greatly weakens the incentive of upper income people to make cost-conscious choices of health care financing plans. Considering payroll and State income taxes as well as Federal income taxes, the tax break reduces by 35 to 40 percent the marginal cost, in net after-tax dollars, of the employee's decision to choose more costly coverage. It costs the Federal budget more than $40 billion a year—an amount that grows about 10 to 15 percent per year, and an amount that substantially exceeds Federal contributions to Medicaid, the Federal-State program that pays for health care for welfare recipients. About 80 percent of the revenue loss goes to households with above-average incomes. This subsidy offers a costly inducement to buy health insurance to many who would buy coverage anyway; at the same time, it offers little to people in low income brackets and nothing to people who have no employer-paid health insurance. There are lessons to be learned from our mistakes. The problem here is that it is hard to find Europeans who need these lessons.

Each country's health care system reflects its own history, culture, political system, and society. And incremental change is one of the most persistent themes in all of our democracies. Labour rhetoric notwithstanding, there is no prospect for the Europeans to adopt the American system or vice versa. And there is no point in discussing whose system is superior. The really interesting questions are how to identify and design politically feasible incremental changes in each country that have a reasonably good chance of making things better. Each country can get useful ideas from others about how to do this.

I like to believe that there are some things in the rich variety of American experiences that may be quite useful to some Europeans, although I recognize that other Europeans are already well informed about such developments. Even the most interesting and promising of these ideas are not uniformly or even widely applied in the United States. In this article, I am pointing to "best practice," not average practice in America. I group these ideas under two headings: Glasnost and Perestroika.

Glasnost

Glasnost, of course, is generally understood to mean "openness," and thus published information. Beginning with this general definition, we can then expand it further to include meaningful evaluated management information, especially in health services research. Some European health care systems—at least those I have visited—struck me by their lack of relevant management information and evaluation studies based on such information. It appears to be a fair generalization that many European health care systems have not developed and put into use the tools of management information and control that any modern industrial enterprise would consider necessary to plan and manage efficiently. Nor do they take much advantage of their opportunities for research. Volvo, Mercedes, and BMW would not be selling nearly as many cars in California as they do if they attempted to conduct their operations with so little information. Nor has our health care system taken advantage of such opportunities on a wide scale.

Until recently, few policymakers have considered efficiency to be a relevant or appropriate goal for the health care system. In the western European and North American democracies, social policy was initially preoccupied with equity, with extending equal financial protection and access to health care services to most or all of the population. In more recent years, as health care expenditures have grown rapidly as a share of GNP, limiting the growth of spending has become the great preoccupation. But until recently, the efficiency with which resources were used has rarely been addressed in any fundamental way. The creation of institutions that would systematically motivate efficient behavior by providers has received even less attention. Efficiency in the use of resources has not been a part of the culture of our medical professions.

Moreover, the problems in defining and obtaining meaningful information about efficiency in medical and hospital care are exceptionally complex and subtle. Many simple measures, such as a hospital's cost per bed-day or in-hospital mortality unadjusted for medical risk, can be quite misleading. Average cost per bed-day can be reduced by needlessly prolonging hospital stays. The patients of the best surgeon in the country may have a high mortality rate because the sickest patients are referred to him or her. So, development of a really satisfactory system of management information will be a formidable intellectual task. Moreover, before the advent of modern information technology, the collection and processing of the types of data I discuss would have been prohibitively costly.

So, my purpose is not to criticize anyone for the lack of management information. There are good reasons why the "information revolution" in medical care did not happen sooner. But Europeans now have great opportunities to take major steps forward by implementing nationally some of the best ideas being developed in America. European health care systems are more organized than ours, and people do not move around as much, so it should be much easier to keep track of what happens to most patients. Europeans could now take advantage of powerful, flexible, and economical information technology to achieve truly valuable systems of medical and financial information for planning, management, analysis, and evaluation. First, I suggest some opportunities for institutionalized production of information; then I identify research opportunities.

Uniform hospital discharge data reports

Apparently uniform reporting to a central authority of all hospital inpatient cases is not mandatory in most European countries. For example, in Sweden I learned that there are discharge reports but that not all hospitals report, nothing compels them to report, and the reports are not very detailed. It is therefore difficult to compare efficiency by hospital or region without reliable summary reports on many aspects of hospital operations (e.g., per capita admission rates · by age and sex, procedure rates per capita, death rates by procedure).

One good place to begin such information production would be with a system of mandatory reporting to a national data bank of all hospital discharges, including the following information:

- Personal identification.
- Date of birth.
- Sex.
- Residence.
- Hospital identification.
- Dates of admission and discharge.
- Identification of attending physician and operating physician, if there was a procedure.
- Diagnoses.
- Procedures and dates.
- Disposition of patient (i.e., alive or dead, discharged to home or to an institution).

This list comes from the Uniform Hospital Discharge Data Set (UHDDS), which must be reported for all care paid for by Medicare and Medicaid (two large Government programs that pay for care for the aged, disabled, and welfare recipients) and for all hospital cases in some States, such as California and Maryland (U.S. Department of Health and Human Services, 1985). In addition to these data, it may well be that additional information, such as some key diagnostic measurements, should also be included. The UHDDS has served as a foundation for developing diagnosis-related groups (DRGs), comprehensive longitudinal records, risk-adjusted measures of outcomes, outcomes management, utilization review, and peer review, which are discussed later in this article. For these developments to take place, it has been necessary that these data,

with individual patient identification removed, be available for use by health services researchers.

Mandatory reporting alone is not enough to produce good data. The data have to be put to significant uses for the people who prepare it, so that they will be motivated to make it accurate. Both doctors and medical records technicians must be involved in coding. American experience suggests that there is a substantial potential for error (or at least disagreement) among people who prepare discharge reports. The Institute of Medicine of the National Academy of Sciences did a study in which specially trained medical records technicians prepared new abstracts from hospital records for discharges in 1974 and then compared them with reports already submitted by leading private abstracting services. The study found that the old and new abstracts agreed on principal diagnoses in 65 percent of cases and on procedures in 72 percent of cases (Institute of Medicine, 1977). Therefore, a data commission or board is needed to provide leadership in a continuing effort to improve the coding of information, including clarifying definitions, ruling on disagreements, and requiring audits to check on accuracy. There will be some hospitals that will be reluctant to report on a timely basis. So there must be some real penalty that actually can and will be applied, such as the nonpayment of State subsidies, if timely reports are not submitted. In the American Medicare program, the hospital is not paid for a case until it has submitted a satisfactory discharge report signed by the attending physician.

National uniform hospital cost accounting

I have asked a number of people in Britain, France, the Netherlands, and Sweden to tell me how the average costs per case for particular types of cases compared among hospitals. I was told that such information was not available. (American hospitals can all say what they charge for various types of cases, but few can say what their costs are, and many of their managers do not know the difference.) If European hospital managers had such information, they could analyze and compare medical and management practices in different hospitals to identify the best, i.e., the most cost-effective, practices. Regional and county managements could use the same information as a guide for resource allocation, as, for example, in deciding which services to expand. In the United States, there can be quite wide variations in the charges and apparent costs among hospitals for similar cases, e.g., more than a threefold variation in median charges for CABG surgery among Los Angeles hospitals in 1986 (Steinbrook, 1988a). At least one American management consulting firm has developed a successful business by working with groups of hospitals to identify "best demonstrated practice" in each department (Johnson, 1983). They found variations averaging 40 percent in the cost to treat the same kind of case, and thus substantial opportunities for savings.

The European health care systems could open up significant opportunities for efficiency enhancement by developing and implementing systems of hospital cost accounting capable of producing cost reports for "intermediate products" (such as laboratory tests and X-rays) and "final products" (individual patient cases). With such a system, it would be possible to compare cost per test and cost per case (e.g., CABG surgery in different hospitals) to pinpoint just how and where less costly hospitals save money. As an example of such a system, Sweden's Uppsala Academic Hospital has contracted with Transition Systems, Inc., for installation of a cost-accounting system developed at the New England Medical Center in Boston.

In the European nonmarket systems, I believe there is a case for a uniform national system, at least down to the level of cost per case by type of case, despite the preferences of many hospital administrators to be free to develop their own systems. In a market system, people use prices as indicators of the costs of goods and services they are thinking of buying. It does not matter whether all producers use the same system of cost accounting, because their customers will compare quoted prices. But in the nonmarket systems, such as in the United Kingdom and Scandinavia, there are few or no prices. Cost comparisons must be based on cost information. In this case, there are two reasons to prefer uniform national systems. First, without a truly uniform system, every proposed cost comparison is likely to bog down in detailed arguments about why one hospital's data are not comparable with another's. People who do not want to be compared can prevent comparisons by raising issues of accounting definition. Second, such systems are costly to design and implement. It would be more economical for each country to use a single system. American experience suggests great resistance to such uniformity. Attempts by the U.S. Government to require uniform cost reporting in the early 1980s failed in part because hospitals consider detailed cost information to be trade secrets in our competitive, pluralistic system. As in the case of discharge data reports, auditing and supervision by an accounting principles board would be needed to put life into this idea.

Diagnosis-related groups

In the 1970s, a team at Yale University developed a system for describing a hospital's production called diagnosis-related groups (DRGs) (Fetter et al., 1980). In 1983, the Medicare program adopted the prospective payment system (PPS), based on DRGs. All inpatient cases are classified in one or another of about 470 DRGs that are relatively homogeneous with respect to resource use, and hospitals are paid a fixed price per case, depending primarily on the assigned DRG. Medicare DRGs are now updated each year, based on the latest available information. PPS has not solved all of Medicare's cost problems. The physician fee and outpatient care part of Medicare remains

open-ended and out of control. But PPS has had great success in slowing the growth of real inpatient cost per beneficiary. From 1980 to 1983, real Medicare inpatient costs per beneficiary rose 6.8 percent per year; from 1983 to 1984, they rose 2.7 percent.

Kaiser Permanente, our largest nongovernmental medical care organization, uses DRGs as a management tool. Hospital administrators in their Southern California Region are evaluated on the basis of their ability to control their cost per case, with DRGs used to measure case mix. Hospital administrators with costs per case above the average have been directed to bring their costs down to the level of costs in the low-cost hospitals. I have been told that this innovation has led administrators in the high-cost hospitals to become very interested in how the low-cost hospitals achieve their favorable results, and that cost differences have been narrowed considerably.

DRGs are being studied actively in Europe. The most promising use for DRGs in Europe that I can see is as an indicator of a hospital's total inpatient workload or output, to serve as a denominator in a calculation of cost per case. Although it is not perfect, it is the best available indicator of hospital inpatient case load. There are continuing unresolved issues about differences in severity of illness within DRGs, and research is under way to produce a more refined system. Medicare has experienced some "DRG creep," that is, a change in reported case mix for what appears to be in fact the same case mix. But these problems have proven to be relatively minor. Again, regular audits are needed.

Like Kaiser Permanente, European health care systems might evaluate and compensate hospital managers in part on the basis of their ability to control and reduce growth in cost per case, using DRGs. Europeans would need to develop their own sets of DRGs, based on their own medical practices. To get an adequate sample size, the smaller countries would need to form groupings.

Research is now under way in the United States to develop systems for long-term care and ambulatory care that would be somewhat similar in purpose.

Studies of medical practice variations

John E. Wennberg, M.D., professor of medicine at Dartmouth Medical School, has pioneered in the study of geographic variations in medical practice patterns. In an early study of variations in incidence of surgery in different hospital service areas in Vermont, he found a greater-than-eightfold variation in the per capita incidence of tonsillectomy and adenoidectomy from the lowest to the highest areas (Gittelsohn and Wennberg, 1977). Nonphysicians used to think that there were well-established scientifically based standards for medical practice. Wennberg's studies made us aware that this was not the case. As Wennberg has effectively illustrated with data, there is great uncertainty and differing opinion associated with much of medical practice. And there is a widespread lack of scientific data, especially on the quantitative aspects of medical decisionmaking.

In addition, Wennberg found that feeding data back to doctors led the high users of some procedures to cut back (Wennberg et al., 1977).

Wennberg has teamed up with Europeans to study variations in common surgical procedures in New England, England, and Norway. Similar degrees of variability in surgery rates were found in England and Norway as were found in New England (McPherson et al., 1982). McPherson and colleagues at Oxford have done similar studies (McPherson et al., 1981). With a national uniform hospital discharge report, it should be possible for each country to prepare regular reports of age-sex standardized per capita rates of hospitalization by DRG and procedure, by district, department, or county of patient origin. Such reports, when fed back to doctors, would help "outliers" to see where they are. These data might complement cost-per-case reports. A "low-use" district might justify higher costs per case in certain diagnoses, because fewer patients are hospitalized there than in other districts and only when they are sicker. These data could be used to target for further study areas of high medical uncertainty affecting large numbers of patients.

Comprehensive longitudinal patient records

One of the large handicaps under which American physicians work is a lack of longitudinal data on outcomes of care. Unfortunately, most surgical patients can be followed systematically only to the hospital door. Registries are kept for some patients in some institutions, but these are quite limited in scope. Continuous comprehensive records exist for long-term members of some health maintenance organizations, but usually these are not electronically stored and easily retrievable. Patients in some controlled clinical trials are followed for years. Dr. Wennberg has recently linked Medicare inpatient and outpatient records and Social Security records (which record survival) for Medicare beneficiaries in New England. This has enabled him to follow histories of surgical patients over an 8-year period to see what happens to them. For example, a recent study of patients who had undergone transurethral resection of the prostate found a considerably greater incidence of mortality, complications, and reoperation than previous professional consensus held (Wennberg et al., 1988). Similar records exist in the Provinces in Canada.

The development of standardized longitudinal records has been inhibited in the United States by the decentralized and pluralistic nature of the American health care system. Nobody is in charge to direct such a development. Americans regularly change insurance carriers and providers as they move, change jobs, or merely exercise their choices. Medicare may offer us our most promising data source, because practically all Americans are enrolled in Medicare at age 65 and remain in it for the rest of their lives. Because

European health care systems are more homogeneous and people do not move around as much, it should be far more feasible for Europeans to keep track of each patient's medical history in a standardized way. Wennberg's work shows that problems such as preserving confidentiality can be managed and that analysis of such longitudinal data—possibly supplemented by followup questionnaires and other studies—can provide very important information about the outcomes of different treatments.

Risk-adjusted measures of outcomes

An important and promising new development in the United States has been called risk-adjusted measures of outcomes (RAMO) by Dr. Mark Blumberg of the Kaiser Permanente Medical Care Program (Blumberg, 1986). The steps in this process as he describes it are as follows:

- Select a study population.
- Select a clinical care subject (e.g., a procedure or event).
- Select appropriate measures of outcome.
- Identify independent variables that measure risk of adverse outcome (e.g., birthweight, age, presence of multiple diagnoses).
- Develop a technique to estimate expected risk of adverse outcome (e.g., multiple regression, recursive partitioning).
- Estimate the probability of adverse outcome for each case.
- Compare the actual number of adverse outcomes with the expected number for each provider.
- Where there are significant differences, investigate them.

The first example of a risk-adjusted measure of outcomes was R. L. Williams' study of perinatal mortality in California (Williams et al., 1980). The Williams study is now an annual report that compares actual with expected perinatal mortality for every hospital in California. Blumberg has recently analyzed mortality from elective surgery in Maryland (Blumberg, 1988). And the Health Care Financing Administration, which administers the Medicare program, is reporting risk-adjusted mortality by hospital for Medicare patients.

This research is still in its infancy. As Blumberg emphasizes, there are many difficult problems to be overcome, including data accuracy, development of good risk-adjustment models, identification of appropriate outcome measures, and overcoming statistical bias in estimation. Publication of RAMO studies in the United States has been criticized by some physicians on the grounds that "it could be misleading." But analysis of such data, interpreted by people using informed judgment, is really all we have to go on in evaluating outcomes of care. There is no other scientific way of evaluating the quality of care. In the United States, providers have resisted publication of any data that could link results with specific providers. But growth in health care expenditures has forced government and employers to take cost-cutting measures. In response, providers have argued that cost containment would threaten the quality of care. This, in turn, has led government and employers to start measuring the quality of care directly and to take action to correct poor quality care. When significant variations in risk-adjusted outcomes are identified, they should be investigated. In California, risk-adjusted mortality rates for CABG surgery in 1986 ranged all the way from 1.0 percent to 17.6 (Steinbrook, 1988a). The methods used by the best hospitals should be considered for adoption by the worst hospitals. Prospective patients should have a right to such information.

European health care systems ought to designate at least one center in each country for RAMO and embark on a systematic well-funded research and development program to monitor outcomes of care. American experience shows this could be done.

Outcomes management

Dr. Paul Ellwood, chairman of the influential health policy research institute InterStudy, has recently proposed a bold concept he calls "outcomes management . . . a common patient-understood language of health outcomes; a national data base containing information and analysis on clinical, financial, and health outcomes that estimates . . . the relation between medical interventions and health outcomes . . . and an opportunity for each decision-maker to have access to the analyses that are relevant to the choices they must make" (Ellwood, 1988). InterStudy is now working with participating medical centers to implement outcomes management by defining the common data set. The proposed data base will include patient description, diagnostic information, therapies, periodic reports by the patient on quality of life, specific medical results, and complications peculiar to the patient's illness or therapy (InterStudy, 1988).

Dr. William Roper, until recently head of the Health Care Financing Administration, and associates responded to Ellwood's proposal with an "effectiveness initiative" . . . " a four-step process involving monitoring, analysis of variations, assessment of interventions, and feedback and education. In Step 1, monitoring, an ongoing universal data base composed of all Medicare claims is used to characterize the health status of the population involved, . . . monitor the outcomes of various interventions, . . . and screen for emerging beneficial or adverse trends. . . . In Step 2, the goal is to describe and define variations in medical care, in terms of both practice patterns and outcomes. Such studies may be population-based . . . or may examine the effect of certain interventions. . . . In Step 3, interventions are assessed. . . . Step 4 concerns feedback and education" (Roper et al., 1988).

This is an important idea, not yet an achievement. As with the other ideas I have mentioned, this one has European antecedents. Florence Nightingale first proposed this more than 100 years ago, so this is not particularly an American idea. If successful, this initiative could open up large and valuable sources of data regarding what does and does not work and for whom. This could lead to substantial improvements in medical practice. As mentioned earlier, progress in the United States has been inhibited by the diversity, independence, and pluralism of our health care financing and delivery arrangements. Europeans would have an easier time of it, because of their unified comprehensive health care system, and should pursue outcomes management aggressively.

Service and access standards

British and Swedish people complain about access to doctors and about insensitivity of the health care system to reasonable patient demands. Saltman and von Otter (1987) summarized the Swedish problems in these terms: " . . . non-medical characteristics of service delivery often respond more to the internal interests of the provider organizations rather than valid concerns of the patient . . . the continued rationing by queue of certain elective surgical procedures . . . inability to accommodate fundamental differences in treatment preferences . . . long waiting room times, inconvenient appointment hours, . . . complicated regulations regarding delivery sites, poorly coordinated services, and so forth." Dr. David Owen has written of the British situation, "The public concern about NHS [National Health Service] is expressed by 'waiting': waiting for an appointment; waiting then in hospitals or in surgeries for the doctor; waiting to come into hospital; waiting at home for the promised visit. Those who work in the NHS, particularly doctors, have grown to accept too easily that waiting is inevitable." (Owen, 1988).

Poor service to patients is not an inevitable part of medical care, even in large institutional settings. All of our health care systems could learn important lessons from the best companies in service industries such as hotels, restaurants, and airlines. In the United States, large multispecialty group practices have had to work hard on the design and operation of their systems to improve patient access to compete effectively with solo and small group practices. Kaiser Permanente has experimented with detached primary care clinics of various sizes and with primary care panel systems. They have found that waiting times can be reduced and patient satisfaction improved by implementing procedures designed on the basis of management engineering and operations research studies. For example, appointment scheduling has been improved through use of a computerized "airline reservation" type of system. Access to doctors on the same day that the request is made has been improved by reserving a number of places in each doctor's schedule for same-day appointments; the actual number reserved is equal to the statistically estimated demand for that day. Knowing that Monday morning is a time of exceptionally heavy telephone demand, the organization cross-trains some personnel to answer telephones on Monday mornings, while performing other duties the rest of the time. Improved systems of electronic storage and retrieval of records offer great potential for saving doctors' and patients' time.

NHS regions and Swedish county governments could contract with independent market research organizations to measure patient preferences regarding different combinations of service aspects of the health care system. Based on the results, they could develop and publish service and access standards, create systems of measurement of performance in relation to those standards, and regularly publish the results. Examples of such standards might be along the following lines:

- Patients should not have to wait more than 3 months for elective surgery.
- Ninety-five percent of telephone calls to primary care centers should be answered by the sixth ring.
- Primary care centers should be open and staffed a certain number of evening and weekend hours.
- Waits for appointments (excluding routine physical and eye examinations) should not exceed 3 weeks.
- Ninety-five percent of in-office waits to see the doctor should be less than 30 minutes from the scheduled time.

These data must be interpreted with judgment. Waiting lists can be manipulated by providers to strengthen their case for more resources. But these data can be used to assess relative service efficiency in different centers. Comparative performance can be assessed, and poor performers can be encouraged to adopt the practices of the best performers.

Measuring patient satisfaction

As a part of the Health Insurance Experiment, Allyson Davies and John Ware at the RAND Corporation developed a patient satisfaction questionnaire to evaluate the impact of different health care financing arrangements on patient satisfaction (Davies and Ware, 1988). Some American employers are now polling their employees about their perceptions of the quality of their health care and feeding back the results to the health care organizations that serve them. This is intended to identify needs and motivate improvements in service and care. To provide useful information, the questions should be focused quite sharply on specific aspects of service delivery. For example, one employer asks whether employees have experienced a wound infection after surgery or a medical problem at the end of a stay in the hospital that they didn't have before they entered the hospital. Researchers know that the answers depend on how the questions are framed. So it makes sense for the questionnaires to be designed and administered by organizations that are independent of the health care system and that have a consumer point of view. Patients themselves are a great potential source of information about the quality of care and service they receive. The practice

of obtaining such information and using it is not yet well developed in America. But I believe it is potentially important, and I include it for the sake of completeness of the glasnost story.

Publication of information

European voters and public policymakers would be helped in their decisions if the results of all this data gathering and analysis could be interpreted and published in a way that would be accessible to them. For example, it would be very helpful if newspapers would make the investment to develop a corps of a few journalists with the special background needed to understand and responsibly interpret data on the health care system for the general public. This type of reporting might be done by physicians with some postgraduate education in quantitative management tools.

For example, the *Los Angeles Times* has employed Robert Steinbrook, M.D., as a medical writer. Here are some examples of headlines and lead sentences from Dr. Steinbrook's recent articles: "Care for Newborns Varies, Studies of Hospitals Show . . . California's hospitals vary widely in their ability to provide quality medical care to newborn babies, according to a sophisticated hospital-by-hospital analysis of perinatal death-rate data by researchers at the University of California, Santa Barbara." (Steinbrook, 1987.) This article reports the results of R. L. Williams' RAMO study for the years 1980-84. "Heart Surgery Death Rates Found High in 1 in 6 Hospitals . . . Nearly one-sixth of California hospitals with heart surgery programs had significantly high death rates for heart bypass patients in 1986, according to a *Times* analysis of data covering all such operations in the state" (Steinbrook, 1988a). This article reported the results of a study actually commissioned by the *Times* and performed with the assistance of three leading academic health services researchers at the University of California. A third, "U.S. Issues Data About Hospitals' Death Rates," described a risk-adjusted mortality study of Medicare beneficiaries published by the Health Care Financing Administration (Steinbrook and Rosenblatt, 1987). This article published mortality rates for California hospitals significantly above and below average, for all Medicare patients, and for patients with several specific diagnoses. The names of the hospitals were published, and the sky did not fall in. Nor have the patients fled the poorly performing hospitals, which is a disappointment to those of us who believe informed consumer choice is potentially a powerful force for good. If Europeans are looking for incentives to improve efficiency and effectiveness in their health care systems, it seems reasonable to suppose that the professional pride of doctors and managers would motivate many of them to take energetic and imaginative action to avoid appearing on the list of the worst departments or hospitals.

Utilization review

In the 1970s, our Congress created professional standards review organizations (PSROs) to review the use of services in the Medicare and Medicaid programs. These were local nonprofit cooperatives of doctors in each of about 200 health service areas. Studies in the late 1970s showed that these organizations were ineffective in reducing Medicare utilization (Ginsburg and Koretz, 1979). This was not surprising. There was no incentive for PSROs to be effective. A dollar saved in Medicare in California, at the expense of California doctors and hospitals, was a dollar returned to Washington.

In the 1980s, PSROs were replaced by peer review organizations (PROs). These are independent organizations in each State that contract with the Health Care Financing Administration to review the quality and appropriateness of care. These organizations compete to win and keep PRO contracts, so they have a real incentive to produce results. They use statistical "screens" to identify problem areas meriting detailed examination, and they use experienced physicians in the appropriate specialty to evaluate the care given. We do not have broadly based studies evaluating the effectiveness of the PROs.

Our many private sector insurance carriers engage in a great deal of utilization control and review activities, mostly for inpatient hospital care. They engage in preadmission review and authorization for nonemergency admissions, concurrent review, and discharge planning. There is little controlled evaluation of all this activity. One controlled study reports that a Blue Cross utilization review program reduced hospital admissions by 12.3 percent, inpatient days by 8.0 percent, and hospital expenses by 11.9 percent (Feldstein, Wickizer, and Wheeler, 1988). We have no documented evidence of effects on quality. In any case, inpatient hospital admissions and days have been declining markedly in this decade. For example, total admissions for people under 65 years of age fell about 9.0 percent from 1984 to 1986.

The utilization review approach to quality and economy of care in the United States attempts to correct the deficiencies in a system the basic incentives of which do not motivate quality and economy to begin with. This approach has several fundamental defects. First, it looks for outliers, "bad apples" that can be identified, punished, and removed. There is no doubt that we have bad apples that ought to be removed. But this approach contributes to an atmosphere of fear, defensiveness, and resentment among physicians, and this atmosphere may be counterproductive in the quest for better quality. By definition, outliers are a small minority. And this month's outlier may be next month's average performer. Removal of outliers will not do much to improve average performance. A second defect in the utilization review approach is that it is too costly, if not impossible, to detect and control the behavior of doctors who are motivated to defeat the utilization

control system. Such controls may have a useful effect on inpatient care, but ambulatory care is another matter. The indications for care are too numerous, too uncertain, and too changeable for a police force of reasonable size to be able to keep up. Some system of auditing and real public accountability is needed. But negative restraints in the face of inappropriate incentives seem unlikely to be nearly as effective as positive incentives to do the right thing to begin with. What we all need are systems of organization of care that include evaluation and feedback as a positive incentive to motivate continuous improvement in average performance. For the most part, American systems of utilization review and control are symptoms of the fact that we have not yet achieved that desirable state. We all need to think carefully how this can best be done.

Perestroika

Decentralization and independent institutions

American health care may suffer from an excess of pluralism, diversity, and innovation, without an effective market system to encourage the high-quality economical providers while driving out the low-quality and costly providers. But European health care systems, either of the public or highly regulated private variety, often appear frozen, resistant to innovation and change in financing or organization of delivery.

This is not surprising. There are several reasons public systems in Europe or the United States are especially resistant to change. First, there is what Charles Schultze has called the rule of "Do no direct harm. . . . we cannot be seen to cause harm to anyone as the direct consequence of collective actions" (Schultze, 1977). Thus we find it extraordinarily difficult to close an unneeded public hospital or military base. Second, politicians are understandably risk-averse. Most of the innovations people think of prove not to be good ideas, despite the positive connotation of the word. But this can often be discovered only in actual practice. So if politicians try something, the odds are it will fail and they will be blamed. If it succeeds, the rewards are usually quite limited. In the private sector, people can take risks with their own money. In the public sector, the risk-reward ratio often does not favor innovation. And third, most public sector services are monopolies.

On the whole, we have benefited from our Federal system of government. Health care finance and regulation is a mixed Federal-State responsibility. Californians can try many things that appeal to them without being blocked by New Yorkers, who are culturally quite different from Californians. Unitary states in Europe give proposed innovations an "all or none" character.

In the spirit of 1992 (when the trade barriers come down), the different countries of Europe can fill the role of the separate American States. Europeans should build on their practice of studying and learning from each other's experiences, while avoiding legislation that would force uniformity. And within their own countries, Europeans would do well to think more seriously about decentralization, to accommodate more diverse preferences, and to create a climate more tolerant of experimentation.

In the United States, we benefit greatly from the existence of independent nonprofit institutions in the fields of health, education, and social welfare. Indeed, most of our famous universities and hospitals are in that category. These institutions depend on a variety of sources of support, including payments from those they serve, tax-deductible contributions, and grants and contracts from foundations and governments. The element of consumer and provider choice is important. All this creates a framework that fosters diversity and innovation. For example, in health care, we have benefited greatly from the existence of independent nonprofit prepaid group practices (as discussed in the next section). Doctors in the traditional sector tried hard to stop them, including using the power of the State. We never would have had this important innovation, if health care had been entirely provided or controlled by the public sector. The public sector is inherently the protector of the status quo. The established interests have all the power. Our independent nonprofit institutions are usually more socially responsible and long-term oriented than the for-profit sector, but less rigid than the public sector.

Of course, independent (nongovernmental) institutions in health care and finance also exist in Europe. The sickness funds of Belgium, the Netherlands, and the Federal Republic of Germany are independent nonprofit institutions, as are many of their hospitals. Britain has independent provident associations as well as independent hospitals, both nonprofit and investor-owned. The challenge for European societies is to find ways to expand the roles of independent institutions to take advantage of their flexibility and potential for innovation, without sacrificing the social goal of universal access. For example, the British Government is now proposing to transform NHS hospitals into self-governing NHS Trusts, potentially a very productive step in the direction of greater decentralization and greater tolerance of innovation (*Working for Patients*, 1989).

Prepaid group practice

There has been a great deal of European interest in American multispecialty prepaid group practice, (e.g., Kaiser Permanente, Harvard Community Health Plan, and Group Health Cooperative of Puget Sound). I use the term "prepaid group practice" rather than "health maintenance organization" (HMO), because the latter is quite nonspecific and is also used to describe what amounts to insurance arrangements with little actual organization and management of care. There has been a great deal of research and documentation of the performance of these organizations (Luft, 1981; Manning et al., 1984).

Prepaid group practices combine multispecialty group practice and periodic, per capita payment set in advance in a competitive marketplace. The patients always have an annual choice of health plan, so the prepaid group practice has some incentive to solve patients' medical problems while holding down the cost—in short, to give value for money. This feature probably makes prepaid group practice unique, and therefore understandably an object of considerable interest. Their incentive to seek efficiency in the United States is often attenuated by a lack of serious competitors and by employer practices and features of our tax laws that subsidize employees' choice of more versus less costly health care arrangements. Nevertheless, these organizations have developed a number of characteristics worthy of study and emulation by others.

Prepaid group practices have attracted the loyalty, commitment, and responsible participation in management of their doctors. They have managed to bridge the cultures of medicine and management. Doctors and managers work together in an atmosphere of mutual respect. Management principles are applied to matters of quality and economy of care. The opportunity for continuous quality improvement is enhanced by the fact that the doctors are full-time salaried members of the organization, not independent operators with no organizational commitment. In prepaid group practices, making the correct diagnosis promptly and treating the patient without causing complications are rewarded. (In the fee-for-service system, failure to make a prompt diagnosis results in more visits and more money for the doctor.) These organizations have been leaders in systematic quality measurement and control. They match resources used to the needs of the population served, including numbers and types of doctors. Thus, in each specialty, doctors have full schedules seeing and treating patients whose problems fit their specialty. This is good for proficiency and economy. Doctors can make a good living at a low cost per case because they have lots of cases, and they are not under economic pressure to do procedures that are not really indicated. All this is in marked contrast to our fee-for-service solo practice system, which now has an excess of doctors and no effective way of aligning numbers of doctors to patients' needs. The prepaid group practices concentrate specialized services in regional centers to assure economies of scale and experience. They have pioneered the use of treatment settings less costly than inpatient hospital care: outpatient day surgery, many other treatments on an outpatient basis, and home nursing. They have orderly processes for technology assessment and organized responses to changes in technology. (Doctors in fee-for-service solo practices have powerful incentives to deny the validity of new information that is negative about their "bread and butter" procedures. A large multispecialty group can assist the doctors to retrain in other procedures.) Also, these organizations have innovated efficient use of paramedical personnel, such as nurse practitioners.

A unique feature of prepaid group practice is systematic regular professional interaction of generalist and specialist physicians. With relative ease, the generalist can call on the specialist for consultation in which they can examine the patient and discuss the treatment together. This contributes to the professional education and stimulation of the generalist and keeps the generalist's perspective of the whole patient in the picture when the specialist becomes involved. The generalist need not fear "losing the patient" when he or she makes a referral, and the specialist need not fear a loss of business from assisting the generalist to care for the patient. Professional checks and balances help to moderate single specialty points of view.

Some of these features can be found in some European health care systems, but not in others. For example, with respect to regional concentration of specialized services, Kaiser Permanente probably resembles the British and Swedish systems more than the typical American setting.

Some European countries may find it advantageous to attempt to create similar organizations. For example, Launois et al. (1985) have proposed an adaptation of the idea as an experiment in France. The recent proposal of the British Government to create some budget-holding general practitioner (GP) group practices draws some inspiration from the same idea. Alternatively, many Europeans would do well to examine prepaid group practices for detailed ideas on how to improve efficiency.

None of our countries will achieve a truly satisfactory health care system until we find a way to create internal incentives and dynamism for quality, economy, and good customer service. The model of prepaid group practice in a competitive environment comes as close to that as we have seen.

Demonstrations, pilot projects, and experiments

In the United States, we have gained a great deal of useful information from demonstration projects and social experiments in health care and other fields. The Office of Research and Demonstrations of the Health Care Financing Administration directs and supports more than 300 research, evaluation, and demonstration projects related to the management, organization, and finance of Medicare and Medicaid, our public health care financing programs for the aged and the poor (Health Care Financing Administration, 1989). And other agencies such as the National Center for Health Services Research and Health Care Technology Assessment sponsor and conduct many more. Faculty members from leading research universities and institutes participate in the research designs, and generally a high standard of research design is achieved. Some examples follow:

Medicare and health maintenance organizations— Until 1985, care for Medicare beneficiaries was paid for on the basis of fee-for-service and cost reimbursement (or DRGs), even if the beneficiary got his or her care from an HMO. In the 1970s, there were legislative proposals to pay HMOs on a per capita basis, but no action was taken until the late 1970s, when a new law was proposed, providing for Medicare per capita prepayment of HMOs. The Health Care Financing Administration (HCFA) contracted with four HMOs to test the proposed payment method. The test was a success (Greenlick, Lamb, and Carpenter, 1983). Many fears expressed by the critics were shown to be unfounded. A new law was enacted in 1982 to implement the results of the experiment, and the law went into effect in 1985. Subsequently, 1 million Medicare beneficiaries joined HMOs on a "risk-basis" capitation contract. Now HCFA is sponsoring a dozen followup studies of refinements to the Medicare HMO payment methodology.

The health insurance experiment—Does requiring patients to pay 25 percent of their medical bills, up to an annual limit on out-of-pocket costs (as compared with free care), reduce the use of services? Is it more likely to reduce inappropriate, rather than appropriate services? Does it harm patients' health? The RAND Corporation, under a long-term contract with the Department of Health and Human Services, conducted a long-term, multisite, randomized controlled trial of alternative health insurance arrangements. They found that requiring a 25-percent coinsurance payment reduced spending by about 19 percent, compared with no coinsurance requirement and, with a few small exceptions, had no discernable effect on health (Newhouse et al., 1981; Sloss et al., 1987; Brook et al., 1983). This put to rest debates about whether coinsurance was penny-wise and pound-foolish. They compared fee-for-service with a prepaid group practice HMO and found the HMO cut total resource use by 28 percent and hospital use by 40 percent, with no significant negative effect on health (Manning et al., 1984). This was important in settling debates as to whether or not HMO economies could be explained as the consequence of favorable selection of patients.

Preferred provider insurance—Preferred provider insurance (PPI) was effectively outlawed in most of the United States until a coalition of business, labor, and the insurance industry defeated organized medicine in the California legislature in the summer of 1982. Subsequently, most of the larger States have also changed their laws to authorize PPI. The Health Care Financing Administration recently announced a demonstration project to test PPI for Medicare beneficiaries in five different cities (U.S. Department of Health and Human Services, 1989). If someone attempted to pass a law requiring all physicians serving Medicare patients to accept the Medicare-approved fee as payment in full, organized medicine would doubtless be able to block it. But they have not been able to block this demonstration. And it seems likely that if this experiment succeeds, it will be replicated on a much larger scale, at which point it may acquire a momentum of its own.

Of course, such demonstration and pilot projects are far from unknown in Europe. A recent paper by Kirkman-Liff and van de Ven (1989) describes more than 20 very interesting local demonstration projects in the Netherlands in the areas of monitoring and feedback of medical care utilization and costs, incentives for cost-effective care, community care (substituting home nursing for hospital), and coordination of care. The British National Health Service has attempted clinical budgeting experiments and is now doing pilot projects of indicative prescribing budgets for general medical practitioners. Launois, Majnoni d'Intignano, Stephan, and Rodwin (1985) proposed experimental réseaux de soins coordonnés, (networks of coordinated care) an idea inspired by American HMOs adapted to French circumstances. However, established interests in France were too entrenched to permit a potentially threatening idea to get a start, even as an experiment. (Of course, entrenched vested interests are not unknown in America.)

My general recommendation to Europeans would be to make more widespread and large-scale use of pilot and demonstration projects and to make less use of coercive decree, to foster a process of continuous incremental improvement rather than discrete "great leaps forward" ordered from the center. For example, in 1983, the Griffiths inquiry made a number of very sensible recommendations regarding NHS management in Britain, including competitive tendering by commercial contractors for catering, cleaning, and laundry services. The government attempted to implement this by decree, requiring all districts to submit programs and meet tight schedules. In 1985 I wrote that, " . . . it would have made far more sense to begin with a dozen pilot Districts whose managements were enthusiastic about the idea, develop and test the methods, with plenty of expert advice from private sector hospital groups, . . . from airlines and hotels that have much relevant experience, then push tendering to the maximum, display the benefits for all to see, then write the manuals and sample contracts, and develop the short training courses" (Enthoven, 1985b). In 1989, the British Government again proposes some promising and innovative ideas, such as NHS Hospital Trusts. But they announced tight timetables for implementation of ideas that have not been pretested and shown to be workable in practice (*Working for Patients*, 1989). I believe that in the long run, a phased pilot-project approach would be more effective.

Managed competition

The two best known simple conceptual models for organizing the health care economy are at opposite ends of a spectrum: the free market and the tax-supported public sector monopoly. Proponents of each like to point to the evident deficiencies of the other in support of their own preference. In fact, a free market cannot work in health insurance and health care. There are too many ways in which these markets depart from the conditions necessary for a market to produce an efficient outcome: pervasive uncertainty, great asymmetry of information, moral hazard, adverse selection, many not-truly-voluntary transactions, etc. A free market in health insurance cannot produce either equity or efficiency (Enthoven, 1988). In the United States, for the most part, we do not have a free market in health insurance at the individual level. We have mainly collective purchases by groups, in which the elements of tax subsidy and other government regulations are important. We do have roughly 40 million or so Americans who do not get their health insurance through employment-related groups or public programs. Most of them are uninsured and must rely on public hospitals and clinics.

On the other hand, public sector monopolies have their problems, which any impartial observer will admit. They generally contain no serious incentives to improve efficiency. Indeed, they are likely to contain perverse incentives that punish efficiency (Enthoven, 1985b). They are unresponsive to consumer preferences regarding times and places and modalities of treatment. They are guided much more by provider preferences and convenience than consumer preferences. They ration by queues. They lack accountability.

So it is understandable that people are searching for intermediate possibilities, institutional arrangements that capture some of the advantages of markets without their disadvantages, arrangements that can motivate efficiency while safeguarding equity.

A desirable arrangement would separate the demand side from the supply side so that an independent demand side could present the desires of consumers and taxpayers to the providers, set standards, measure performance, and make choices. A desirable arrangement would allow the demand side to become well informed about the costs and the benefits produced by different providers. Thus it would allow the demand side to compel glasnost as described earlier.

A desirable arrangement would also allow choices at two levels: at the level of large group purchasers and at the level of individual choice. The large group purchaser would be able to bring to bear the information and expertise to evaluate all suppliers and exclude those with unacceptable performance; such a purchaser could also structure the market for individual choices so that consumers could make well-informed choices and so that consumers would be guided by correct signals to choose those suppliers that produce high-quality economical care. The element of consumer choice would make the system responsive to responsible consumer preferences regarding quality of care and service.

A desirable arrangement would thus allow the demand side some choice of supplier. It would systematically select and promote the organization and delivery of high-quality, economical, responsive care. How this goal is to be approached in any given country must reflect the cultural preferences, history, and institutional realities of that country. Useful policy proposals must represent politically feasible incremental change. A model that makes sense in one country may have little apparent relevance to another. However, insights gained in one country's experience may be usefully adapted to another.

For the United States, I have been working out and proposing a concept I call managed competition (Enthoven, 1988). Managed competition joins two ideas. First, as previously noted, we now have in the United States a rich variety of schemes that join health care financing and delivery, schemes of varying success in organizing high-quality economical care. Each, in its way, is trying to innovate to find ways to control cost without cutting quality of care or service. Second, managed competition is based on the recognition that the market for health insurance in the United States involves three types of parties: consumers, health insurers (including prepaid group practice and other arrangements), and sponsors. The sponsors are the large group purchasers: employers and the public programs such as Medicare and Medicaid. In managed competition, the sponsor's job is to structure the marketplace, to design and actively manage a process of informed, cost-conscious consumer choice, to motivate the participating health care financing and delivery schemes to produce a favorable combination of efficiency and equity. Efficiency here means value for money as seen by informed consumers. Equity means that the sick do not have to pay much more than the well for coverage and care. Perfect efficiency and equity are of course far from possible. Thus, the sponsor should manage a process of consumer choice that rewards with more subscribers those health care financing and delivery schemes that produce better quality, less costly care, and that does not reward them for selecting good risks, segmenting the market, or doing anything that does not contribute to high-quality economical care.

We have some prototypical examples of managed competition in actual operation. There is the Federal Employees Health Benefits Program, in which more than 400 health plans of various types compete to serve about 9 million Federal employees, dependents, and retirees. This program has been in operation since 1960. In recent years, it has suffered from various correctable design deficiencies that make it vulnerable to risk selection, segmentation, and other problems (Enthoven, 1989a). In California, we have a similar system for public sector employees. And many large private sector employers offer multiple choice of health plan to employees. Richard Kronick and I have recently shown how these concepts might be generalized into a model of universal health insurance for the United States (Enthoven and Kronick, 1989).

Much of managed competition as described here is specific to the American scene, where we have multiple competing health care financing and delivery schemes and strong cultural preference for such pluralism. But some Europeans have been watching this development with interest, to see if similar ideas can be adapted to their situations.

In March 1987, the Committee on the Structure and Financing of Health Care, an advisory committee set up by the Netherlands Government, chaired by Dr. W. Dekker, published a report that proposed major changes to the Dutch health care system (Ministry of Welfare, Health and Cultural Affairs, 1988). In this proposal, market forces would be used to motivate the search for efficiency, especially through better coordination of health and social services, and flexible substitution of more effective, less costly services. In the words of the Ministry of Welfare, Health and Cultural Affairs, English summary, "Market forces provide an answer to the organizational inflexibility and cumbersome operation of the health system in the Netherlands, characterized as it is by high costs, lack of choice and lack of incentives for change." In the Dekker scheme, all citizens would become free to choose among health insurers. Insurers would be paid in two ways. First, a central fund would collect an income-related premium from all those able to pay, and it would pay insurers a risk-related premium contribution based on the characteristics of its subscribers. (This is an important sponsor function in managed competition.) Second, each insurer would charge a flat-rate premium to all insureds. Insurers would compete on this flat-rate component and would be free to negotiate selectively with providers for pay and scope of services. Insurers would no longer be obliged to contract with all providers. They could select those they considered to be efficient. And guaranteed funding for providers would be eliminated. After much public debate, the Netherlands Government indicated broad agreement with the Dekker proposals, and, in March 1988, issued a plan for their cautious and gradual implementation. This Dutch version of managed competition will give Europeans a "demonstration project" to watch much closer to home.

In January 1989, the British Government published a white paper outlining its strategy and proposals for restructuring the National Health Service (*Working for Patients*, 1989). Broadly speaking, one might characterize it as a strategy for separating the demand and supply sides of the market and for strengthening the ability of the demand side to make informed choices. In the government's strategy, District Health Authorities (DHAs), which are now monopoly suppliers of services to the people in their districts, are to be recast as purchasers of services on behalf of the populations they serve, which services are to be supplied competitively. That is, DHAs will be free to seek value for money outside their districts and even outside the NHS, in the private sector. Regions will actually receive their main budget allocations on the basis of population, adjusted for age, morbidity, and other demand-related factors, with the present adjustments for cross-boundary flows replaced by direct payments for services between regions. Regional targets have long been based on such a formula, but actual payments followed targets only gradually, because of fear of disrupting the supply side. In the new plan, district budgets will be based on estimated need, not influenced by the services they produce.

The government's strategy includes allowing hospitals to opt out of district control and to become independent self-governing NHS Trusts. These hospitals will be free to set their own pay, contract with their own personnel, and compete to serve several districts. A key idea is that "money follows patients." Today, a hospital that does an excellent job of producing high-quality care efficiently, thereby reducing or eliminating its queue, is likely to attract more patients without correspondingly more money— a perverse disincentive. Under the new scheme, such a hospital will be able to contract with sending districts for a prompt payment per case. The government's plan also includes strengthening medical audit, and experimentation with the idea of large GP practices holding budgets for a broad range of services beyond primary care. All this is sometimes referred to as an "internal market" for health care, compatible with universal tax-supported provision of comprehensive care (Enthoven, 1985b; Owen, 1988).

The Swedish health care system seems even less amenable to concepts of managed competition than the British. And the geographic pattern of very large county hospitals seems almost a guarantee of territorial monopolies for inpatient care. However, introduction of some elements of managed competition is not beyond the realm of conceivable political reality. I have recommended a program of glasnost like the one described in this article, combined with a policy of rewarding with pay and promotion those physicians and managers who demonstrate superior performance (Enthoven, 1989b). Beyond this, it might be productive to consider competition within the public sector at the primary care level, along the lines proposed by Saltman and von Otter. Moreover, the Swedish Government instituted an arrangement whereby patients waiting for certain procedures could obtain care from other counties if the waiting time in their own county exceeded certain limits, with the patient's county paying the providing county, and the government throwing in a bonus. I understand that this appreciably reduced waiting times. What is needed is the political will for the Swedish people to create an institution independent of the health care providers, with the power to compel production of information and the resources and charter to take initiatives to get more informed choice into the system.

What these ideas and experiences illustrate is that intellectual discourse on health policy does not need to be limited to debates over the merits of polar opposites. Nor is it useful to argue abstractly over the merits of regulation versus competition. Every health care system is likely to have elements of both. The really interesting questions today are about the merits of marketlike incremental changes intended to make our systems more efficient and responsive to consumers. In this realm, American research and debate have produced what ought to be a good deal of interesting reading for Europeans.

Acknowledgments

This research was supported by a grant from the Henry J. Kaiser Family Foundation. The author also gratefully acknowledges comments and suggestions from Bradford Kirkman-Liff, Victor Rodwin, and Peter Van Etten.

References

Blendon, R., and Taylor, H.: Views on health care: Public opinion in three nations. *Health Affairs* 8(1):149-157, Spring 1989.

Blumberg, M.: Risk adjusting health care outcomes: A methodologic review. *Medical Care Review* 43(2):351-396, Fall 1986.

Blumberg, M.: Measuring surgical quality in Maryland: A model. *Health Affairs* 7(1):62-78, Spring 1988.

Brook, R., Ware, J., Jr., Rogers, W., et al.: Does free care improve adults' health? *New England Journal of Medicine* 309(23):1426-1433, 1983.

Davies, A., and Ware, J.: *GHAA's Consumer Satisfaction Survey*. Washington D.C. Group Health Association of America, Oct. 1988.

Division of National Cost Estimates, Office of the Actuary, Health Care Financing Administration: National health expenditures, 1986-2000. *Health Care Financing Review*. Vol. 8, No. 4. HCFA Pub. No. 03239. Office of Research and Demonstrations, Health Care Financing Administration. Washington. U.S. Government Printing Office, Summer 1987.

Ellwood, P.: Shattuck Lecture—Outcomes management: A technology of patient experience. *New England Journal of Medicine* 318:1549-1556, June 9, 1988.

Enthoven, A.: Health tax policy mismatch. *Health Affairs* 4(4):5-14, Winter 1985a.

Enthoven, A.: *Reflections on the Management of the National Health Service*. Nuffield Provincial Hospitals Trust Occasional Papers 5. London, 1985b.

Enthoven, A.: The 1987 Professor Dr. F. de Vries Lectures. *Theory and Practice of Managed Competition in Health Care Finance*, New York. North Holland Publishing Company, 1988.

Enthoven, A.: Effective management of competition in the federal employees health benefits program. *Health Affairs* 8(3):33-50, Fall 1989a.

Enthoven, A.: *Management Information and Analysis for the Swedish Health Care System*. Lund, Sweden. The Swedish Institute For Health Economics, 1989b.

Enthoven, A., and Kronick, R.: A consumer-choice health plan for the 1990s: Universal health insurance in a system designed to promote quality and economy. (In two parts.) *New England Journal of Medicine* 320 (1 and 2): 29-37 and 94-101, Jan. 1989.

Feldstein, P., Wickizer, T., and Wheeler, J.: The effects of utilization review programs on health care use and expenditures. *New England Journal of Medicine* 318:1310-1314, May 19, 1988.

Fetter R., Shin Y., Freman, J., et al.: Case-mix definition by diagnosis-related groups. *Medical Care* 18 (Supplement), Feb. 1980.

Francis, S.: Health services. *U.S. Industrial Outlook, 1989*. Washington. U.S. Department of Commerce, Jan. 1989.

Ginsburg, P., and Koretz, D.: The effect of PSROs on health care costs: Current findings and future evaluations. Washington. Congressional Budget Office, June 1979.

Gittelsohn, A., and Wennberg, J.: On the incidence of tonsillectomy and other common surgical procedures. In Bunker, J. P., Barnes, B. A., and Mosteller, F. *Costs, Risks, and Benefits of Surgery*. New York. Oxford University Press, 1977.

Greenlick, M., Lamb, S., Carpenter, T. M., et al.: Kaiser Permanente's Medicare Plus project: A successful Medicare prospective payment demonstration. *Health Care Financing Review*. Vol. 4, No. 4. HCFA Pub. No. 03152. Office of Research and Demonstrations, Health Care Financing Administration. Washington. U.S. Government Printing Office, Summer 1983.

Greenspan, A., Kay, H., Berger, B., et al.: Incidence of unwanted implantation of permanent cardiac pacemakers in a large medical population. *New England Journal of Medicine* 318(3):158-163, 1988.

Health Care Financing Administration: *Status Report: Research and Demonstrations in Health Care Financing, Fiscal Year 1988*. HCFA Pub. No. 03277. Office of Research and Demonstrations, Health Care Financing Administration. Washington. U.S. Government Printing Office, Mar. 1989.

Hostage, G.: Quality control in a service business. *Harvard Business Review*, July-August, 1975. Reprinted in *Service Management*, Harvard Business Review Reprint Department, Soldiers Field, Boston, Mass. 02163.

Institute of Medicine: *Reliability of hospital discharge abstracts*. Washington, D.C. National Academy of Sciences, Feb. 1977.

InterStudy: An introduction to Quality Quest's outcomes management system development plans. Quality Quest, Inc., P.O. Box 600, 5715 Christmas Lake Road, Excelsior, Minn., 55331. 1988.

Iowa Department of Public Health: Chronic Renal Disease Program, telephone survey conducted Feb. 1, 1989. Personal communication.

Johnson, D.: Baxter shows hospitals how to use cost data to prepare for price competition. *Modern Health Care* 34-42, Aug. 1983.

Kirkman-Liff, B., and van de Ven, W.: Improving efficiency in the Dutch health care system: Current innovations and future options. *Health Policy* 13(1), Oct. 1989.

Launois, R., Majnoni d'Intignano, B., Stephan, J., and Rodwin, V.: Les réseaux de soins coordonnés (R.S.C.): Propositions pour une réforme profonde du system de santé. *Revue Française Des Affaires Sociales* 39(1):37-62, Jan-Mars, 1985.

Launois, R., Majnoni d'Intignano, B., Rodwin, V., et al.: Les réseaux de soins coordonnés, une autre idée de libre choix. In Launois, R., ed. *Des Remèdes Pour La Santé*. Pour une nouvelle politique économique de la médecine. Masson, Paris, 1989.

Luft, H. S.: *Health Maintenance Organizations*. New York. Wiley, 1981.

Luft, H., Bunker, J., and Enthoven, A.: Should operations be regionalized? *New England Journal of Medicine* (301):1364-1369, Dec. 20, 1979.

Manning, W., Leibowitz, A., Goldberg, G., et al.: A controlled trial of the effect of a prepaid group practice on use of services. *New England Journal of Medicine* 301:1505-1510, June 7, 1984.

McPherson, K., Wennberg, J., Hovind, O., et al.: Small-area variations on the use of common surgical procedures: An international comparison of New England and Norway. *New England Journal of Medicine* 307:1310-1314, Nov. 18, 1982.

McPherson, K., Strong, P. M., Epstein, A., and Jones, L.: Regional variations in the use of common surgical procedures: Within and between England and Wales, Canada and the U.S.A. *Social Science in Medicine* 15A:273-288, 1981.

Ministry of Welfare, Health and Cultural Affairs: *Changing Health Care in the Netherlands*. Rijswijk, Sept. 1988.

Newhouse, J., Manning, W., Morris, C., et al.: Some interim results from a controlled trial of cost sharing in health insurance. *New England Journal of Medicine* 305:1501-1507, Dec. 17, 1981.

Owen, D.: *Our NHS*. London. Pan Books, 1988.

Prospective Payment Assessment Commission (ProPAC): *Medicare Prospective Payment and the American Health Care System*. Report to the Congress. Washington, D.C., June 1988.

Restuccia, J., Gertman, P., Dayno, S., et al.: The appropriateness of hospital use. *Health Affairs* 3(2):130-138, Summer 1984.

Roper, W., Winkenwerder, W., Hackbarth, G., and Karkauer, H.: Effectiveness in health care: An initiative to evaluate and improve medical practice. *New England Journal of Medicine* 319:1197-1202, Nov. 3, 1988.

Saltman, R., and von Otter, C.: Revitalizing public health care systems: A proposal for public competition in Sweden. *Health Policy* 7:21-40, 1987.

Schieber, G., and Poullier, J. P.: International health spending and utilization trends. *Health Affairs* 7(4):105-112, Fall 1988.

Scitovsky, A., and Snyder, N.: Use of hospital services under two prepaid plans. *Medical Care* 18(1):30-41, Jan. 1980.

Schultze, C.: *The Public Use of Private Interest*. Washington, D.C. The Brookings Institution, 1977.

Short, P., Monheit, A., and Beauregard, K.: Uninsured Americans: A 1987 Profile. National Center for Health Services Research and Health Care Technology Assessment, Public Health Service. Rockville, Md. Jan. 1989.

Sloss, E., Keeler, E., Brook, R., et al: Effect of a health maintenance organization on physiologic health. *Annals of Internal Medicine* 106(1):130-138, Jan. 1987.

Steinbrook, R., and Rosenblatt, R.: U.S. Issues Data About Hospitals' Death Rates. *Los Angeles Times*. Dec. 18, 1987.

Steinbrook, R.: Care for Newborns Varies, Studies of Hospitals Show. *Los Angeles Times*. Nov. 9, 1987.

Steinbrook, R.: Heart Surgery Death Rates Found High in 1 in 6 Hospitals. *Los Angeles Times*, Part 1. July 24, 1988a.

Steinbrook, R.: Third of Hospitals Perform Too Few Heart Operations. *Los Angeles Times*, Part I. Dec. 27, 1988b.

U.S. Department of Health and Human Services: *The Federal Register*. Vol. 50, No. 147:31,038-31,039, July 31, 1985. American Hospital Association, Division of Quality Control Management, Coding Clinic for ICD 9 CM, Vol. 2, No. 4, July-Aug. 1985.

U.S. Department of Health and Human Services: News Release, Jan. 13, 1989.

Wennberg, J. D.: Dealing with medical practice variations: A proposal for action. *Health Affairs* 3(2):6-32, Summer 1984.

Wennberg, J., Blowers, L., Parker, R., and Gittelsohn, A.: Changes in tonsillectomy rates associated with feedback and review. *Pediatrics* 59:821-826, 1977.

Wennberg, J., Roos, N., Sola, L., et al.: Use of claims data systems to evaluate health care outcomes. *Journal of the American Medical Association* 257(7):933-936, Feb. 20, 1987.

Wennberg, J., Mulley, A., Hanley, D., et al.: An assessment of prostatectomy for benign urinary tract obstruction. *Journal of the American Medical Association* 259(20):3027-3030, May 27, 1988.

Williams, R., Cunningham, G., Norris, F., and Tashiro, M.: Monitoring perinatal mortality rates: California 1970 to 1976. *American Journal of Obstetrics and Gynecology* 136:559-568, Mar. 1, 1980.

Winslow, C., Solomon, D., and Chassin, M., et al.: The appropriateness of carotid endarterectomy. *New England Journal of Medicine* (318)12:721-727, 1988.

Winslow, C., Kosecoff, J., and Chassin, M., et al.: The appropriateness of performing coronary artery bypass surgery. *Journal of the American Medical Association* 260(4):505-509, July 22/29, 1988.

Working for Patients. London. Her Majesty's Stationery Office, Jan. 1989.

Respondents:

Jeremy W. Hurst

Introduction

It is particularly appropriate for a British health economist to be asked to comment on Enthoven's article "What can Europeans learn from Americans?" The British Government has just undertaken "the most far reaching reform of the National Health Service in its forty year history" (*Working for Patients*, 1989). The government's announcement was preceded by an unprecedented public debate about the future of the National Health Service (NHS) (Brazier, Hutton, and Jeavons, 1988; Goldsmith and Willetts, 1988; The Institute of Health Services Management, 1988; King's Fund Institute, 1988; Robinson, 1988). This debate made frequent references, both positive and negative, to the U.S. experience. More specifically, several commentators put forward ideas based on Enthoven's "Reflections on the Management of the National Health Service" (Enthoven, 1985), and some have suggested that, in key respects, the government's final proposals bear a striking resemblance to his suggestions.

I wish I could write as confidently about the situation in other European countries, but, as Enthoven has indicated, their health care delivery arrangements are very diverse. Several countries have recently undertaken or are considering reforms, but my knowledge does not extend to the lessons they have learned, if any, from the United States. Accordingly, my remaining remarks tend to be dominated by a British perspective.

Growth of health expenditure

Enthoven begins his article by conceding some shortcomings in the American health care system.

The opinions expressed in this article are those of the author and do not necessarily represent the views of the Department of Health in England.

Reprint requests: J. W. Hurst, Department of Health, Friars House, 157-168 Blackfriars Road, London SE1 8EU, United Kingdom.

Here he illustrates neatly the rule that Americans are usually more authoritatively critical of institutions in the United States than are foreigners. However, it is true that Europeans tend to feel superior about their universal health insurance coverage, and they look with mixed feelings at the growth rate of American health expenditures.

I was a little surprised that Enthoven did not bring us more news on cost containment. There is much interest in European countries, with their predominantly public sources of finance, in the growth rate of total health expenditures. This is especially so in those countries with relatively open-ended social insurance systems, such as the Federal Republic of Germany, France, and Belgium. They, presumably, would be curious to know what, if anything, has been learned in the United States from the long debate about competition and regulation. To what extent have the new developments, such as payment based on diagnosis-related groups (DRGs), health maintenance organizations (HMOs), and utilization reviews, influenced total health expenditures? Is there still optimism that competition will secure cost containment?

In countries such as Britain and Sweden, where governments, central or local, have taken upon themselves the awesome responsibility of setting the overall level of most health expenditures, there are invariably painful debates about the right level of health spending and considerable uncertainty about the criteria for reaching decisions. In this connection, I found Enthoven's summary of findings from the literature on appropriateness particularly thought provoking. What is missing from public decisions on the level of health expenditures is some measure—however partial—of the marginal health outcome per increment of spending. The new work in the United States on appropriateness and outcome offers a glimpse of how we might establish a relationship between outcome and expenditure, at least for certain programs.

Glasnost

Enthoven devotes the bulk of the first half of his article to an informative and stimulating report on certain recent developments in management information in U.S. medical care under the general heading of "glasnost." In my own research (Hurst, 1985), I have been struck by the general similarity (if not the equal accessibility) of management information in the United States and the United Kingdom, putting aside payment methods. Thus, picking up four of Enthoven's recommendations, the United Kingdom has had uniform hospital discharge reports and a uniform national system of hospital cost accounting since soon after the formation of the NHS. The latter now provides specialty costs but not yet DRGs for inpatients.

England has had a long-standing trial of comprehensive longitudinal patient records in the Oxford Region. There have been regular national polls of patient satisfaction with the NHS (Davies, 1989), and there has been an ongoing, high-quality debate about the achievements and failings of the NHS and private medicine in some British newspapers. I could go on: The United States and the United Kingdom have similar health and vital statistics, similar household surveys, and similar data on health expenditures and manpower. True, I have only examined data collected nationally in the United States, but I assume that the superstructure gives important clues to the foundations.

On the other hand, there is, so far, a desperate lack of health outcome and quality data in both countries. This leaves consumers (and governments) short of information with which to make rational choices. What is now being confirmed, from studies of medical practice variations, is that doctors themselves are often uncertain about the indications for and effectiveness of treatments. It is sometimes said that there is a major asymmetry of information on the two sides of health care markets (consumers and providers). On some occasions, it looks more like a symmetry of uncertainty.

Meanwhile, European countries often look to the United States for advances in management information. Several have already started their own work on DRGs and on variations in medical practice. In Britain, experts have also done a good bit of work on some other imports from the United States, especially avoidable mortality (Charlton et al., 1986) and the idea and practice of quality-adjusted life years (Williams, 1985). The latter has helped to focus (and sometimes to inflame) some debates about the allocation of resources; the former is now used as a performance indicator for the NHS (*The Government's Expenditure Plans*, 1989).

The recent review of the NHS has underlined the importance of the measurement of health outcome, clinical audit, and achievement of consumer satisfaction. Hence, I would expect the Department of Health (in England) to look carefully at risk-adjusted measures of outcomes, outcomes management, utilization review and peer review organizations, and the development of service and access standards. I would add to this list the important American work on appropriateness and risk-adjusted capitation payments.

A major concern about such advances, however, is what they will cost. Enthoven does not attach price tags to his proposals. It has been estimated that America already devotes about 22 percent of its health expenditures to administration (Himmelstein and Woolhandler, 1986). It is sobering to learn that the available management information is nevertheless not enough. The same authors estimate that the share of British health expenditure devoted to administration is about 6 percent. There is an expectation in some quarters that this figure will rise, because the reforms call for, and will demand, better management information. Nevertheless, the whole exercise will, as usual, be governed by a tight budget. It would have been nice to know which bits of glasnost, if any, have been shown to represent particularly good value for the money in the United States.

This leads me to a final point about management information. There seems to be a certain tension between the two parts of Enthoven's article—in particular, between his plea for uniformity and centralization (of information systems) in the first part and his plea for diversity and decentralization (of organizational structures) in the second part. Is it that the production of information is to some extent a public good and that, therefore, we cannot rely on the market to produce the optimum quantity? Will perestroika fail to produce glasnost? Later in his article, Enthoven argues that a desirable arrangement would allow large group buyers of health care to become well informed about performance and to compel glasnost. But would large group buyers necessarily have either the incentive or the power to do this adequately? Is this one area in which there is an inescapable role for government?

Perestroika

In the second half of his article, Enthoven recommends that Europeans think seriously about decentralization, the accommodation of more diverse preferences, and the creation of a climate more tolerant of experimentation. He suggests that we steer between the extremes of the free market and the tax-supported public sector monopoly. He recommends managed competition, which would involve a separation of the demand side of health markets from the supply side and would offer two levels of choice: choices by individuals among large group purchasers and choices by large group purchasers among providers. Such arrangements could " . . . motivate efficiency while safeguarding equity."

The recent reforms in Britain seem to follow some of these prescriptions. From 1948 to date, the NHS has provided medical care to all, when needed, mainly free of charge to the patients. It has been funded out of general taxation. There has been only a small, but growing, private sector. Primary care has been supplied by independent general practitioners (GPs), remunerated partly by capitation fees and under contract with the NHS. Individuals have been able to choose their GP and about 75 percent of episodes of medical care have started and finished with the GP. Hospital care has been supplied by public hospitals managed by District Health Authorities (DHAs), funded by block grants from central government. Apart from emergencies, access to specialist doctors and to hospitals has been through the GP gatekeeper.

The reforms retain tax funding, and services will continue to be available to all patients mainly free of charge. But, as Enthoven has reported, the reforms introduce a new separation of the demand side from the supply side for hospital services within the NHS.

On the demand side, there will be two levels of choice: level 1, where the existing arrangements for individuals to choose their GP will be strengthened; and level 2, where DHAs will now become mainly buyers of hospital services, able to contract with both local and more distant hospitals, public and private, for services to their resident populations. In addition, large GP practices can volunteer to have transferred to them part of the DHA's hospital budget, thereby allowing them for the first time to back up with cash their referrals of patients to hospitals.

On the supply side, public and private hospitals will be encouraged to compete for the business of both DHAs and those GP practices holding hospital-referral budgets. In addition, well-managed public hospitals will be able to volunteer for self-governing status within the public sector.

Such arrangements should offer an opportunity to increase efficiency without reducing equity. Moreover, taken together with those features of the NHS that have been retained, they seem to qualify for the title of "managed competition."

Despite the parallels with American thinking here, it is not clear that Europeans have as many lessons to learn from the United States about perestroika as they do about glasnost. One difficulty is that it is hard to draw conclusions when institutions are quite different on either side of the Atlantic. Another difficulty, of which Enthoven warns us, is that America is still wrestling with the appropriate mix of management and competition in her own health markets. It would have been nice to know more about whether the ". . . prototypical examples of managed competition in actual operation" in the United States (from Enthoven's article) have provided answers to the sort of questions that tend to be posed about managed competition, such as:

- How can information and administration costs be prevented from eating into the savings that result from effective competition among providers?
- How can cost-conscious competition avoid focusing on cost at the expense of quality, when cost is more easily measured than quality?
- To what extent can adverse selection be dealt with by using either risk-related capitation payments or regulations, when there is consumer choice among providers?
- How can the right balance be struck between consumer choice and agency choice in health care?

On the last of these topics, it is interesting to read in Enthoven's article that in California patients have not fled poorly performing hospitals (in terms of mortality), despite negative publicity. Can we take it that Californians are more concerned about the convenience of hospital care than about its clinical quality, or have these patients been poorly advised by their agents? What is the appropriate scope for consumer choice and agency choice, respectively, in hospital care?

Convergence

One of the most striking facts about the financing and organization of medical care is the extent to which it varies among developed countries. With the arrival of ideas that amount to managed competition in several countries simultaneously, may we now expect some convergence?

I think it is premature to talk about convergence. One of the features of managed competition is that it seems to be capable of coexisting with some very different financing regimes—with private insurance in the United States, with social insurance in the Netherlands, and with tax-funded global budgets in the United Kingdom. Countries with private and social insurance will no doubt look to managed competition to deliver overall cost containment, among other things. Britain will ask less of it. There is no sign that Britain will abandon its reliance on tax-funded global budgets: They seem to be the surest way of limiting the burden of health care on the taxpayer while such care continues to be available to all mainly free of charge to the patients. Also, managed competition is capable of coexisting with some major differences in organizational arrangements, ranging from specialty doctors with hospital admitting privileges and mainly private hospitals in the United States, to strong primary care, the GP gatekeeper, and mainly public hospitals in the United Kingdom.

So, I believe that diversity will continue. Nevertheless, it is clear from this exchange that Europeans and Americans still have a lot to learn from each other as we continue to pursue our somewhat separate ways.

Acknowledgments

I am grateful to Andrew Burchell, Mike Parsonage, Jean-Pierre Poullier, and Clive Smee for comments on the first draft of this article.

References

Brazier, J., Hutton, J., and Jeavons, R.: Reforming the U.K. Health Care System. Centre for Health Economics, Health Economics Consortium, 1988 Discussion Paper 47. York, United Kingdom. University of York, 1988.

Charlton, J., Lakhani, A., and Aristidou, M.: How have "avoidable death" indices for England and Wales changed? 1974-78 compared with 1979-83. *Community Medicine* 8(4):304-314, 1986.

Davies, P.: The NHS goes to the opinion polls. *The Health Service Journal* 99(5156):750-751, 1989.

Enthoven, A. C.: Reflections on the Management of the National Health Service. Nuffield Provincial Hospitals Trust Occasional Papers 5. London, 1985.

Goldsmith, M., and Willetts, D.: *Managed Health Care*. London. Centre for Policy Studies, 1988.

The Government's Expenditure Plans, 1989-90 to 1991-92. Chapter 14-Department of Health. Cm 614, London. Her Majesty's Stationery Office, 1989.

Himmelstein, D. U., and Woolhandler, S.: Cost without benefit: Administrative waste in U.S. health care. *New England Journal of Medicine* 314(7):441-445. 1986.

Hurst, J. W.: *Financing Health Services in the United States, Canada and Britain*. London. King's Fund, 1985.

Institute of Health Services Management: *Working Party on Alternative Delivery and Funding of Health Services, Final Report*. London, 1988.

King's Fund Institute: *Health Finance, Assessing the Options*. London, 1988.

Robinson, R.: *Efficiency and the NHS: A Case for Internal Markets*. London. The IEA Health Unit, 1988.

Williams, A.: Economics of coronary artery bypass grafting. *British Medical Journal* 291(6491):326-329, 1985.

Working for Patients. London. Her Majesty's Stationery Office, 1989.

Björn Lindgren

Introduction

As Enthoven emphasizes in the introduction to his article, there is not one single European health care system, but many. The ways in which health care is financed, organized, managed, and delivered vary probably even more within and among the countries of Europe than in the United States, with its great variety of health care institutions. The relevance of the advice and suggestions given in Enthoven's article thus depends very much from which country's perspective they are seen.

These circumstances call for some caution on my part. I do not know enough about every country in Europe to be able to speak for all of them. I must be more modest and limit my comments to the experience of a country I know fairly well—Sweden.

Thus, the first question to be asked and answered in response to Enthoven's suggestions is whether the Swedes need his advice or not. I am personally totally convinced that we do; otherwise, I would not have invited him to Sweden to critically review the Swedish health care system (Enthoven, 1989). For the readers of this journal, however, the need for advice may not be so obvious. Let me, therefore, begin this response with a brief description of the Swedish health care system: structure, relation to the overall economy, variations in efficiency, and lack of consumer choice. The second issue concerns the practicality of reforms in Swedish health care. I do share Enthoven's pragmatic view: "The really interesting questions are how to identify and design politically feasible incremental changes that have a reasonably good chance of making things better." Thus, I discuss Enthoven's proposals from these perspectives.

Reprint requests: Professor Björn Lindgren, Director, IHE, The Swedish Institute for Health Economics, P.O. Box 1207, S-221 05 LUND, Sweden.

The Swedish health care system

Structure

A characteristic feature of the Swedish health care system is the dominant role played by the county councils. The 26 county councils (including some independent larger cities) are by law responsible for health care delivery within their geographical boundaries. They are also empowered to impose a proportional income tax on their residents. Moreover, health care is practically the county council's sole responsibility; health care accounts for 85-90 percent of the operating costs of a county. Inpatient care is almost completely financed through county-council taxes and delivered by hospitals owned by the county councils.

During the last 25 years, the role of the county councils has actually been strengthened. Mental hospitals used to be a central government responsibility but were transferred to the county councils in 1963. Another important change occurred in 1970, when the ability of hospital physicians to have private outpatients treated at county council facilities was abolished. Since 1980, public vaccination programs are no longer the responsibility of central government but of each county council. Also, the two university hospitals still owned by the State at the time (the Karolinska Hospital of Stockholm and the Academic Hospital of Uppsala) changed from State to county council ownership in 1982 and 1983, respectively. Furthermore, the Swedish Health Care Act of 1982, revised in 1985, places the prime responsibility for all health care planning on the county councils. This responsibility implies, for instance, that the county councils have the authority to negotiate the establishment of a new private practice and the maximum number of patients that the private practitioner will be allowed to see per year. Without an agreement with the appropriate county council, visits to private physicians are not reimbursed from social insurance. Thus, the county councils also regulate and, to a high degree, control the market for private health care.

Each county has at least 1 central general hospital, with more than 1,000 beds and between 15 and 20 specialties, as well as several minor district hospitals. There are also nine regional hospitals in Sweden. These are affiliated with medical schools and serve as centers for research and teaching. A regional hospital provides specialized services such as neurology, neurosurgery, dermatology, thoracic surgery, plastic surgery, radiotherapy, urology, and pediatric surgery. It serves residents of several counties, so there are cooperative agreements among the counties on provision and financing of these highly specialized services.

Two additional things should be noted. First, in addition to its duties to serve the whole region with specialized services, the regional hospital also functions as a district hospital or a central general hospital for those people who live in the town or city where the hospital is situated. Second, all hospitals in Sweden have large outpatient departments; in fact, about 40 percent of the 27 million yearly visits to physicians in Sweden take place at hospitals. Besides, to a large extent, patients are allowed to make appointments with the hospital outpatient departments even without having a referral from a general practitioner. This is also true of regional or university hospitals. Hospital based inpatient and outpatient care accounts for more than 70 percent of total health care costs in Sweden.

Most health care in Sweden is provided by the public sector, i.e., by the county councils; 97 percent of hospital admissions, for instance, are public. About 20 percent of all physicians (one-third of these in occupational health) and 50 percent of all dentists are privately employed; their incomes normally depend on how many patients they see. Publicly employed physicians and dentists are all salaried. The pharmacies were privately owned until 1971, when they became nationalized and organized as one national corporation. More than 60 percent of all pharmaceuticals are imported. The Swedish pharmaceutical industry is private with one exception, Kabi, which was nationalized in the late 1960s. Medical schools are financed and administered by central government.

Direct consumer charges for health care are only nominal; for visits to the public health care facility, for prescribed medicines, and for visits to private doctors associated with the social insurance plan, the charges are less than the price of a man's haircut. In total, consumers' out-of-pocket expenses account for 9.5 percent of total health care expenditures. The proportional county council personal income tax rate has increased from an average of 8 percent in 1970 to 13.5 percent in 1985. County council taxes finance 65 percent and central government 6.5 percent (through subsidies to county councils) of the total health care bill. The remaining part is paid for by social insurance: 8.5 percent of the total bill is for privately provided medical and dental care and prescribed medicines, and 10.5 percent is for publicly provided health care.

The health insurance part of social insurance is mainly a sickness cash-benefit system; sickness cash-benefit payments account for about 65 percent of the total social health insurance expenditures. However, social insurance pays a nominal charge per bed-day to hospitals but contributes more substantially for prescribed medicines and private or public outpatient health care. Swedish social insurance is a centralized system; central government is the supreme decisionmaker. Social health insurance is financed mainly by a proportional payroll tax; some transfer payments from central government (15 percent of the total expenditure for social health insurance) are also involved. The social insurance plan covers all Swedish citizens as well as foreigners residing in Sweden. Residents are automatically insured, and, in general, the insurance is compulsory.

Relation to the overall economy

Health care represents the largest subsector within the public sector and, apart from the social sector, it is also the fastest growing. In 1985, expenditures for health care were nearly 75 billion Swedish Krona (SKr), or SKr 9,000 per inhabitant. Additional expenditures associated with sickness and disability are also significant; sickness cash benefits totalled SKr 18 billion, and early retirement pensions SKr 15 billion in 1985, i.e., SKr 3,940 per inhabitant (National Swedish Social Insurance Board, 1987). As a percentage of gross national product (GNP) in current prices, health care consumption appears to have stabilized at a level just below 9 percent.

Whereas health care consumption reached a constant share of GNP in nominal terms in the 1980s, the development looks somewhat different in real terms. Real health care consumption increased at an annual rate of 2.2 percent from 1980 to 1985, compared with 1.8 percent for real GNP, hence, increasing its share of real GNP. Thus, in real terms, health services not only used more resources but also a greater share of all resources. The tendency, however, was not as pronounced as it was during the last half of the 1970s, when annual real health care consumption increased three times faster than did real GNP.

The impression of a large and expanding sector is strengthened by a look at labor statistics. Employment in the health care sector increased rapidly during the 1980s; annual increases averaged 2.4 percent, for both persons employed and hours worked. Granted, this is less than it was during the 1970s, when the annual increase averaged 5.6 and 3.6 percent, respectively. Nevertheless, employment in health care increased much more rapidly than did employment generally in Sweden, raising its share of total employment from 9.9 percent of all hours worked in 1980 to 11.1 percent in 1985.

The explanation for the divergent trends in health care consumption in nominal and real terms, respectively, is obviously to be found in the development of prices. Before 1980, salaries for health care staff increased as rapidly as they did for other groups in Sweden. Between 1980 and 1985, salaries rose only 6 percent per year, on average, compared with 9 percent for the rest of the economy. It is clear, however, that the labor markets for health care personnel were not in equilibrium, so future increases in payments would be expected (Lindgren, 1989b).

Variations in efficiency

Despite the absence of a relevant and consistent management information and control system, which Enthoven emphasizes in his article, some data and statistics are produced regularly or on an ad hoc basis. A number of comparative studies have been made, and these indicate significant differences among hospitals and hospital departments concerning the costs for comparable output, productivity, production technique, and quality. Of course, inefficiency is not the sole explanation of observed variations, but in most studies, the differences are significant enough to reveal an efficiency problem.

Thus, Eckerlund, inspired by the works of Wennberg (1984), studied variations in practice at departments of gynecology (Eckerlund and Gårdmark, 1986) and dermatology (Eckerlund and Swanbeck, 1987). In gynecology departments, the average length of stay in the maternity ward varied between 4.4 and 8.2 days, averaging 6.5 days. The rate of cesarean section varied from 7.5 percent to 19.2 percent of all deliveries. A comparison of dermatology departments in Sweden found that the number of dermatology beds varied between 2.5 and 11.3 per 100,000 inhabitants in a catchment area. Lindgren and Roos (1985) found significant differences in the development of productivity among Swedish hospitals form 1960 to 1980, ranging from − 9 percent to + 3 percent change in productivity per year. There was no evidence that hospitals with low costs and a rapid increase in productivity neglected the quality of services.

Lack of consumer choice

There are considerable deficiencies in consumer choice in Swedish health care. The opportunities for a Swedish citizen to influence his or her own situation and the general development of society have been studied by one of the research projects associated with the 1985 government committee on power and democracy in Sweden (Petersson, Westholm, and Blomberg, 1989). The analysis was based on more than 2,000 interviews in which persons 16-80 years of age were asked about the degree of influence they had over their own situations in six essential dimensions: housing, consumer, patient, parents with small children, parents with school-aged children, and employee. Of the six areas investigated, health care showed the greatest tendency toward "silent

powerlessness"; widespread dissatisfaction existed but was relatively seldom expressed by independent action. For example, patients and families felt they had little opportunity to choose their physician or to change to another hospital department or primary health care center. This attitude contrasted sharply with the area that ranked highest in terms of consumer influence, i.e., the role of the consumer.

Furthermore, Otter, Saltman, and Joelsson (1989) asked each of the 26 county council health service managers in Sweden about their patients' opportunities to choose a primary health care center or physician within the county council's domain. The responses showed a wide gap between patients' hypothetical and actual opportunities for free choice. Free choice seemed to be regarded as something difficult, something that creates administrative problems, and that therefore should be permitted only as a last resort after a patient has lost all confidence in the physician assigned to him or her.

Enthoven's proposals

Enthoven's advice is separated into two parts: one concerned with management information, evaluation, and control; the other with changes in the financing and organization of health care that might be considered in the European countries. Enthoven presents a detailed argument for developing advanced management information systems and explains in detail the role market incentives might play in improving the efficient provision of health care, often with direct reference to Sweden. Therefore, I shall not repeat all the arguments here. In principle, the arguments are no different in Sweden than anywhere else. Furthermore, it would add little, because I fully agree with Enthoven that the Swedes should have much to learn from the American experience, not least from "best practice" as he presents it. So, instead, I try to concentrate most of my discussion of Enthoven's proposals on what is actually happening in the Swedish health care system and on the political feasibility of introducing "glasnost" and "perestroika."

Management information, evaluation, and control

Information by which performance can be measured should, naturally, be as important to the public health care sector as it is to private industry, a necessary internal management instrument on which to base incentives for efficiency. Normally, consumers do not concern themselves with how private firms measure their performance or how they provide quality assurance for their products. This is up to the individual firm. The market test of survival serves the purpose of external control. Only the efficient producers will, in the long run, find consumers willing to buy their products at prices that cover their costs of production. Inefficient companies will run at a loss and, if things do not change, they will have to close and leave the market.

For activities within the public sector, there is a second purpose for information on performance in terms of productivity, efficiency, and quality. Because the monopolistic public health care sector does not have to face competition in the market and, hence, cannot go bankrupt, there is a need for detailed information for decisionmakers and taxpayers to ensure the greatest health care value for the money spent. In place of the market test, comparisons of costs, productivity, and quality become important. The information is then no longer just a private affair, but a social concern. As such, a large amount of openness is required.

Enthoven presents an 11-point program for management information, evaluation, and control. The core of the information system consists of uniform hospital discharge data reports and a national uniform hospital cost accounting system, which could be linked to each other via the use of DRGs, diagnosis-related groups. For long-term care and ambulatory care, similar-in-purpose systems are not yet available, but are presently being developed in the United States. Based on the information produced, a number of examples of possible ways to compare productivity and quality and to set standards for service and access are given by Enthoven.

I doubt that there is much controversy in Sweden, at least in principle, about the possible usefulness of this kind of information and evaluation studies. Studies of medical practice variations are performed from time to time; there are a few regional and national registries of longitudinal patient records for some surgical and orthopedic surgical procedures; there are quality assurance study groups in some hospitals; DRGs are being adapted to Swedish conditions; and comparisons of costs per case and so on are being done now and then.

These studies reveal a spontaneous curiosity and a natural interest among some physicians and administrators to evaluate their own work. Yet there are no regular evaluations, no consensus as to how to do the evaluations, and still very little public openness about the results. And the studies are made difficult by the fact that Swedish health care lacks the uniform cost-accounting system necessary to compare costs for patients, treatments, hospitals, and hospital departments. Nor is there a good working system for reporting on patients according to diagnosis, treatment, health status, etc., which could be interfaced with a cost-accounting system. True, providers are obligated to report patient information to the Swedish National Board of Health and Welfare, but there is little incentive for accurate reporting, hence, these reports contain errors of importance for planning (Berglund, Cederlöf, and Höglund, 1985; Nilsson, 1988). It is also true that the Federation of County Councils has issued guidelines for the cost-accounting systems to be used by the county councils. These recommendations, however,

give wide latitude for different interpretations, which make direct comparisons difficult.

To produce good data, data collection and processing must appear meaningful to those who do the job. As Enthoven emphasizes, mandatory reporting to national data bases will never be successful, if the local hospital or hospital department does not have incentives to use the information in the first place, or if it does not get any useful feedback from the national central agency. Within the context of the present Swedish health care system, however, I would guess that one must think more about positive incentives to do it right than about penalties for not doing it. The strong independence of tax-raising county councils makes them less sensitive to the nonpayment of central government subsidies, which Enthoven suggests in order to ensure accurate and timely reports.

There must be created a self-interest for hospitals and hospital departments to report information properly and promptly. A majority of physicians, other health care personnel, and administrators—or, because of their key role in Sweden, the relevant trade unions—should therefore be persuaded to accept that promotion possibilities and pay should be related to performance in terms of productivity, efficiency, and quality. To evaluate performance properly is not possible without a fairly large sample of hospitals with which to make comparisons. This would require uniform national reporting systems. Some system of independent auditing would also be needed.

The central government in Sweden seems to be aware of the need for better management information and for evaluative studies. In May 1988, a government committee was established to propose a uniform (national and county council) health care information system that meets the basic informational needs for different levels of planning, management, monitoring, and assessment. However, despite the fact that information will be collected and used only if it appears meaningful for the decisions to be made at the local level, the committee (which is still working) is not supposed to deal with the issues of proper incentives.

It is quite obvious from Enthoven's article that it is certainly not impossible to create systems for information, evaluation, and control that better utilize existing knowledge, experience, and initiatives. The internal systems of information, evaluation, and control, however, reflect conditions in the external environment—the way in which health care is financed and organized. Thus, internal reforms would be facilitated, or rather, made necessary, by changing the external conditions. If sensible changes in financing and organization could be introduced, and if the survival and success of providers were to depend on how well they met the requirements formulated by consumers, then there would also be a good chance that the internal management and control structure would adapt and develop accordingly.

Financing and organization options

I strongly sympathize with Enthoven's view that "the really interesting questions today are about the merits of marketlike incremental changes intended to make our systems more efficient and responsive to consumers." So, what changes in finance and organization could be made? Could consumer choice and provider competition be introduced in Sweden to improve efficiency, while at the same time satisfying equity considerations to a degree not less than today? In principle, the answer is yes, and I do believe that there are important lessons to be learned from the American experience and from the ideas presented by Enthoven. Moreover, Swedish economists have shown how the concepts of prepaid group practices, health maintenance organizations, and managed competition might be used in the Swedish context (Blomqvist, 1980; Jönsson and Rehnberg, 1986; Lindgren, 1989a; Ståhl, 1979 and 1983; and Svalander, 1982).

Consumer choice and influence could certainly be increased within the framework of the present organization. Without shaking the system down to its foundations, patients might very well be allowed to freely choose a primary care center, physician, and hospital to a much greater extent than what, according to present studies, is currently the case. Patients could also be given more opportunity to feel that they can influence decisions and to speak up concerning conditions that they believe are not satisfactory. This would be particularly effective if they could be supported, as Enthoven suggests, by strong independent organizations—sponsors—with a consumer point of view (Enthoven, 1988).

The opportunity to choose is important per se to consumers and, hence, is a source of well-being. However, in order to result in more than marginal improvements in efficiency, consumer choices must have an influence on the revenues or budgets of the health care providers. This would then create competition among individual health care providers, who might look for ways of acquiring patients by delivering high-quality care at lower cost.

Competition can never work if the roles of the consumer and provider are not separated. This is definitely true in health care. In Sweden, however, the county councils are by law the main providers of health care, while at the same time, they have constitutional rights to tax their citizens. Thereby, the county councils finance their own production, while at the same time, elected county politicians are expected to represent the interests of their consumers or voters. Potential and actual conflicts between consumer and provider interests are innumerable, and there is a tendency for the provider interests to dominate. The county council is the sponsor, insurance organization, and provider—all in one.

Technically, it would be quite possible to create a system in which the three roles of the county councils would be separated. The most natural role for the county councils would be that of sponsor. As before, the county councils could have the right to tax their citizens, and insurance for all citizens could be mandatory. But rather than having only one provider, the county councils should offer their citizens a selection of different arrangements. No health care institution would remain under county council ownership. Hospitals and other health care institutions could instead be owned by insurance companies, consortia of private companies, not-for-profit trusts, or companies owned by the central government. These arrangements could be so designed that they stimulate cost-conscious consumer choices. Then consumers would be motivated to try to obtain the best buy for their money.

There may be several reasons why proposals on changes in the organization and financing of health care have not gone very far from mere academic discussion in Sweden. First, the existing system enjoys, despite all, a certain advantage in public opinion. There is always a resistance to change in the health care system. Not only politicians but also voters are highly risk-averse. Second, except for dental care, health care in Sweden is a public monopoly; over the years, more and more power has been concentrated in the county councils. Third, many people in Sweden are opposed to competition for strictly ideological reasons, especially competition in health care. Fourth, legislation today gives the county councils and their elected officials direct responsibility for providing health care; the county councils are supposed to not only finance health care but also run the hospitals. Existing legislation is thus an obstacle, and new laws would be needed. However, in overhauling the legislation, it would be important to also make an investigation into what, for instance, the optimal sponsor would look like. There are several alternatives that seem natural to investigate. One would be to let the local communities be the sponsors. Another alternative would be to let health care finance be incorporated within the same central government system as social insurance.

There are certainly many lessons to be learned by Europeans from Americans about the financing and organization of health care. But I wonder whether the best lesson to be learned, especially for the Swedes, might be the willingness of Americans to experiment and to set up demonstration projects. The number of projects mentioned by Enthoven is impressive. I personally do not believe that it is possible to choose one optimal approach based solely on a priori reasoning and available empirical evidence. Thus, if we Swedes are not totally convinced that we have found the best organizational solution for supplying ourselves with the health services we want—and much indicates that we are no longer as convinced as we were—then we must allow ourselves to experiment in order to explore alternatives to the present organization. Because the present system is a rigid public system, market incentives seem natural candidates to be tried. The evidence from carefully evaluated experiments could be used to make more global decisions about how to provide health care most effectively.

Closing remarks

I am sure that Europeans have much to learn from Americans, not least from what seems to be best practice in the health care business. There is no doubt about that. However, every society has its own social, cultural, economic, and political goals and traditions. The relevance of the American experience is then very dependent on from what country's perspective it is seen; how health care is presently financed and organized in that country; and the kind of political environment in which health care must work.

Swedish economists have shown a great interest in adapting and transforming the best American experience and ideas into suggestions as to how Swedish health care might change its financing and organization to improve consumer choice, introduce provider competition, and increase efficiency. The discussion of alternatives has not reached far beyond academia, and the economists' arguments have mostly been met with political counterarguments based on worst American experience. The need for better information should, however, be self-evident in a country in which all official documents, including the Health Care Act, emphasize the need for planning in health care. Naturally, the Swedes could afford to spend some share of their huge health care bill to create one of the best health care information systems in the world. It is really not a question of resources, but a matter of political will.

For other countries in Europe, a minimum of necessary information may seem to be enough, taking into account the limited resources available for health care. To yet other countries, i.e., countries such as Belgium, the Netherlands, and the Federal Republic of Germany, with long traditions of strong independent institutions, marketlike incremental changes should look more tempting. Come 1992, all member states of the European Economic Community (EEC) will probably be much more oriented toward consumer choice and provider competition in the financing and organization of health care.

1992 will be important for the Swedes, too, even if Sweden were to continue to stay outside the EEC. The member states may be able to provide the Swedes with good examples of how more competition could be introduced in health care, without completely destroying the foundations on which the welfare state has been built. A number of good examples close to home might more than balance the bad experiences of the United States in the political debate. Consumers-voters-taxpayers might then acquire the experience and information necessary to demand the changes that will be required.

References

Berglund, K., Cederlöf, R., and Höglund, D.: *Epidemiologisk bevakning. Om användningen av register för sluten somatisk vård som datakälla.* Stockholm. Statens miljömedicinska laboratorium, 1985.

Blomqvist, Å. G.: Konsumentönskemål och effektivitet i sjukvården, *Ekonomisk debatt* 8(1), 1980.

Eckerlund, I., and Gårdmark, S.: *Ekonomiska konsekvenser av skillnader i praxis: jämförande studie av kvinnokliniker.* Spri report 204. Stockholm, 1986.

Eckerlund, I., and Swanbeck, G.: *Ekonomiska konsekvenser av skillnader i praxis: jämförande studie av hudkliniker.* Spri report 218. Stockholm, 1987.

Enthoven, A. C.: *Theory and Practice of Managed Competition in Health Care Finance.* North Holland, Amsterdam, 1988.

Enthoven, A. C.: *Management Information and Analysis for the Swedish Health Care.* Lund, Sweden. The Swedish Institute for Health Economics, 1989.

Jönsson, B., and Rehnberg, C.: *Effektivare sjukvård genom bättre ekonomistyrning.* Rapport till Expertgruppen för studier i offentlig ekonomi, Ds Fi 3, 1986.

Lindgren, B.: *Consumer Choice and Provider Competition in Swedish Health Care - Is It Possible?* Lund, Sweden. The Swedish Institute for Health Economics, 1989a.

Lindgren, B.: Sjukvårdskostnaderna, hälsoekonomin och framtiden. *Överläkaren* 1(1):8-10, 1989b.

Lindgren, B., and Roos, P.: *Produktions- kostnads- och produktivitets-utveckling inom offentligt bedriven hälso- och sjukvård 1960-1980.* Report to the Group of Experts for Studies in Public Economics, Ds Fi 3, 1985.

National Swedish Social Insurance Board: *Socialförsäkringsstatistik. Fakta 1987.* Stockholm RFV, 1987.

Nilsson, C. A.: DRG i svensk tillämpning: Stora fel och brister i diagnostiken. *Journal of the Swedish Medical Society*: 34:2621-2624, 1988.

Otter, C. von, Saltman, R., and Joelsson, L.: Valmöjligheter, konkurrens, entreprenader mm inom landstingens sjukvård. Enkätresultat. (mimeo) Stockholm, Arbetslivscentrum, 1989.

Petersson, O., Westholm, A., and Blomberg, G.: *Medborgarnas makt.* Stockholm. Carlsson Bokförlag, 1989.

Ståhl, I.: Sjukvården - problem och lösningar. *Ekonomisk Debatt* 7(7):476-482, 1979.

Ståhl, I.: Sjukdom och socialförsäkringar, i *Inför omprövningen. Alternativ till dagens socialförsäkringar.* Stockholm. Liber Förlag, 1983.

Svalander, P. A.: *Primärvårdspolitikern och makten.* Delegationen för social forskning. Rapport 1982:3. Stockholm, 1982.

Wennberg, J. E.: Dealing with medical practice variations: A proposal for action. *Health Affairs* 3(2):6-32, 1984.

Robert G. Evans and Morris L. Barer

The American predicament

Enthoven takes on a formidable challenge. Rehearsing the stylized facts of the American health care system—an immodest system with much to be modest about—his summary is blunt. " . . . [I]t would be, quite frankly, ridiculous . . . to suggest that we have achieved a satisfactory system that our European friends would be wise to emulate." Agreed. A more plausible proposition might be that most European countries have achieved a reasonably satisfactory system of health care funding and delivery, any one of which the United States would be wise to emulate. If only they could.

The long-standing American problems of cost escalation and grossly inequitable coverage are well known and widely deplored. But Enthoven emphasizes an additional point often obscured in the partisan rhetoric. Many Americans comfort themselves with the belief that, even if their system is by far the most costly and least equitable of any in the industrialized democracies, at least it provides "the world's best care" for those who can afford it. But if "best" is defined in terms of outcomes achieved, rather than as a simple linear function of cost, then the evidence suggests that even this is wishful thinking. "More" is not the same as "better." What America provides is not the world's best, but the world's most, and most highly priced. (Providers of health care, in the United States and out of it, assiduously promote the illusion that the quality of health care is a simple linear function of expenditure, with a significant (positive) slope coefficient. This relationship certainly holds for provider incomes, which are in total identically equal to health expenditures; the activity and outcome data are rather more refractory.)

This is an important lesson for all of us. For the past decade, most western European countries have limited the expansion of their health care systems to a roughly constant share of (growing) national incomes (Schieber and Poullier, 1988). Providers, habituated to the rapidly rising shares of earlier years, have grown increasingly restive over these "cutbacks," and their ambitions press ever more strongly upon the restraints imposed by payers. Everywhere they seek "just a bit more" (than everyone else), to do ever more good, and allege growing threats to the health of patients if their claims are denied. But only in America have providers succeeded in commanding an ever-growing share of national economic resources. Hence, the importance of Enthoven's point: Americans are not better served, or healthier, as a result.

But are they nevertheless more satisfied with their

Reprint requests: Robert G. Evans, Ph.D., Department of Economics, #997-1873 East Mall, Vancouver, B.C., Canada V6T 1W5.

system? After a decade of growing divergence between the United States and Europe (Abel-Smith, 1985), a poll of individual Americans has found a substantial majority who say they would like to trade their system for someone else's—specifically that of Canada (Blendon, 1989). This extraordinary finding suggests that a majority of the American public shares the assessment of external observers and of Enthoven.

Necessity—the mother of invention

Yet in spite, or more probably because, of its overall difficulties, the United States appears to be far and away the most fertile field of major institutional innovation in health care delivery and finance. Its experience presents, Enthoven suggests, many examples of the good as well as the bad and the ugly. He offers a selection of promising American innovations from which others might " . . . identify and design politically feasible incremental changes . . . that have a reasonably good chance of making things better."

His category labels for these innovations—glasnost and perestroika—are both eyecatching and functional. Unexpected and foreign, they emphasize the system independence of the issues involved. But the categories themselves are very old and very familiar—information and incentives. The behavior of individuals and organizations is determined by what they (think they) know about their environments and capabilities and how (they believe) their behavior will further their objectives. To modify a system, one must change the information held by and/or the incentives bearing on the actors in that system. At this level of generality, it makes no difference whether one is contemplating the economy of the U.S.S.R., the health care system of the United States, or a private corporation such as Exxon or Philips.

Glasnost: More information for whom?

But who are the critical actors for whom better information is to be provided? Proposals such as uniform discharge abstracts and cost accounting, or patient coding by diagnosis-related groups (DRGs), are improvements in MIS, management information systems. They presuppose a health care system with a well-defined management structure, whose managers are to be enabled and encouraged to achieve the best possible health outcomes for the resources that the rest of society hands over to them—or rather, through them to the providers of care. American employers, health maintenance organizations (HMOs), and insurers, Canadian provincial governments, German Krankenkassen, and British District Health Authorities are all, in different ways, financially at risk for the behavior of their health care systems and need much better information than they now have to ensure that they are getting value for money. Enthoven suggests that the United States is farther ahead in developing appropriate information systems, and, on balance, we believe he is right.

On the other hand, publication of outcome information, and the development of risk-adjusted measures of outcomes (RAMOs), peer review organizations (PROs), and standard-setting processes that will generate the publishable information, presuppose a much more powerful role for the individual citizen, either as actual or potential patient, or as voter, employee, and tax or premium payer. In Enthoven's proposals for the United States, individual choice and system management are subtly interlocked (Enthoven and Kronick, 1989a and 1989b). The choices (and political pressures) of better informed individuals create incentives to keep the system managers up to scratch, while the improved MIS not only provides the latter with the necessary tools but becomes the source of improved information for the former.

The glasnost strategies thus address two distinct audiences, through a combination of MIS and public information, though the two are powerfully linked and interdependent in a way that represents an important lesson for both the United States and Europe. Better management may require better management data, but from whence arises the demand for better management?

Who wants to know?

This interconnection requires emphasis, because comparative system performance suggests that MIS improvements—more, better, and especially more timely data—have heretofore been neither necessary nor sufficient for better results. They were not necessary, as indicated by Enthoven's argument that European systems are significantly better than that of the United States, despite a management information base that no private firm would or could tolerate for 20 minutes. And they have not been sufficient, because, in fact, many of the MIS-type innovations that Enthoven describes (uniform discharge abstracts and accounting systems, comprehensive population-based utilization data) have been in place, or within easy reach, in the Canadian provinces for roughly 20 years. As an MIS, the Canadian health care data bases have a number of inadequacies. But the key point is that, for roughly two decades, the provincial agencies that generate these administrative data have not judged it worthwhile to improve them. The constraints have not been technical ones. Yet critiques of the Canadian health care system have consistently emphasized that, despite its important advantages, it is seriously undermanaged and displays substantial room for improved performance (e.g., Rachlis and Kushner, 1989).

Better tools for management do not themselves lead to better management. In Canada, the payers for care (provincial governments) have not had the political legitimacy or will to engage in the more detailed, microlevel system management that such better data would make possible. The extraordinarily underdeveloped state of European data bases may reflect similar inhibitions felt by governments and social insurance agencies (Evans, 1989). After all, it is hard to believe that, over a time span of decades, Europeans have simply not noticed that their information base was somewhat scanty.

Who is in charge here?

At present, in Europe, Canada, and, to a large extent, still in the United States, the providers of health care, particularly physicians, regard themselves as the only legitimate managers. If "there [are] well-established scientifically based standards for medical practice" that form part of professional training, then obviously only professionals are competent to interpret and apply those standards, to decide what shall be done, to whom, and by whom. Insurers and governments are there to pay the bill, not to direct the performance. What Enthoven (and we) would regard as more cost-effective management, most providers would—do—regard as wholly unwarranted and inappropriate lay interference with professional autonomy.

Not only do professionals believe this, it is even more important that most of the general public agree. The illusion of physician omniscience has been much eroded in recent years, but physicians still enjoy a great deal more public confidence than health researchers, insurance agencies, or bureaucrats.

Shifting the locus of control

As Enthoven points out, students of health care utilization have long ago exploded the myth that patterns of care are based on coherent professional standards of any sort, much less on standards based on scientific evidence. Indeed, the sorts of data that are generated through his glasnost proposals have played an important role in undermining that myth.

Moreover, managerial control is implicitly shared between payers and providers, in countries with universal payment systems, because governments impose direct or indirect controls on the physical and financial resources available to the health care system that clearly affect patterns of medical practice. But payers have largely shied away from direct intervention (Evans, Lomas et al., 1989). Only in the United States have private payers, under extreme pressure and without access to the sorts of global controls applied in other countries, begun to intervene in the clinical decisions of the individual physician.

One can make a strong case, as sketched by Enthoven, for more detailed intervention. There are many opportunities for improving the efficiency and the effectiveness of health care delivery on both sides of the Atlantic. Furthermore, it seems unquestionable that better data on which to base clinical and managerial decisions are essential to this process (e.g., Roper et al., 1988). But to become policy-relevant, this view must not merely be shared by the payers for and regulators of care. In addition, they must believe that there is a political consensus among the general public that will support, or at least not strongly oppose, such intervention.

Political costs and benefits

The opposition of providers, and particularly of their organizations, can be taken as automatic. More effective and efficient management will, must, mean diminution, on average, of professional autonomy and incomes. The key question is whether any responsible political authority will be prepared to confront that opposition, data in hand, and argue a case for better management before the general public. Up until now, the answer in both Canada and Europe has been "no." Nor can the academic, comfortably isolated from both the battle and the consequences of defeat, honestly blame them. After all, the first man over the barricade gets the spear through the chest.

In such a political environment, with popular health care systems functioning at a bearable cost, why should Europeans go to the trouble of acquiring information that might be very dangerous to use? The evidence for significant potential improvement in efficiency and effectiveness may be compelling, but neither patients nor voters know that. Physicians will vehemently deny it. Better data might be a political embarrassment! Better management of health care is not, at root, a scientific problem requiring more research and more data, but a political problem of mobilizing support for intervention against the opposition of powerful and genuinely threatened interests. (These interests include private insurers, drug and equipment manufacturers, and hospitals and clinics, as well as physicians.)

The suggestion that Europeans would find it easier to establish mechanisms to improve the quality and effectiveness of medical practice, because they already have unified, comprehensive health care systems, reflects a technical view of the issue. The real question is whether, in a unified system, the opponents of such oversight mechanisms can mobilize more or less effectively to resist or subvert them.

The Canadian provinces, for example, have all had physician practice monitoring programs for a number of years. But they compare each physician's profile against norms defined by the contemporaneous behavior of his or her peers. By definition, therefore, the average practice pattern is the right one, and other patterns over broad ranges on either side are acceptable; as Enthoven notes, outliers are very few. There is no exogenous standard in this process, only consensus. As one (American) physician said, "We protect each other by all agreeing to make the same mistakes."

Perestroika: Restructuring the incentive environment

In all systems, many of those responsible for reimbursing and regulating providers of care have now come to the same conclusions, in general terms if not in specific details, as the research community. Health care utilization (and cost!) does not result from the application of "well-established scientifically based standards," and in aggregate appears fundamentally arbitrary. But effective policy based on this understanding depends on the development among the general public of a broader political constituency that recognizes the tenuousness of the connection (in both directions) between health states and medical interventions. In Marmor's terms, the "political market" is at present seriously imbalanced on this issue (Marmor, Wittman, and Heagy, 1983).

As long as a large section of the public provides a receptive audience for allegations that quality is a linear function of expenditure, or at least of activity, and that only professionals know what is to be done, then payers and would-be managers of health care will have to intervene in "Stealth and Total Obscurity" (the alternative British name for the Department of Health and Social Security), if at all. The public information aspects of glasnost thus form a bridge between MIS and perestroika. Changing public perceptions through more and better information may—perhaps—restructure the environment of political incentives that presently constrains both public and private management. The feasibility of improved system management depends less on improved data per se than on the creation of a more supportive political environment in which to take managerial action. (Better data are, of course, relevant to this process, in that detailed management based on obviously faulty information loses credibility rather rapidly, especially in an adversarial environment.)

The lesson for Europeans, and Canadians, appears to be an old one: "You must educate your masters." But this process of information transmission is little developed or understood. Enthoven is undoubtedly correct that the United States has more examples of attempts to communicate directly with the public on medical matters over the heads of the professionals. But it is not at all clear that this has resulted in, or is moving in the direction of, a more supportive environment for the management of clinical activity. Intrusions on physician autonomy are increasingly occurring, but through private institutions that have no counterparts outside the United States, and the motivation and balance of benefit are contentious.

But there is much more to Enthoven's perestroika than public information campaigns. Attempts to graft various forms of managed competition onto European systems and to decentralize the payment and control processes are attempts both to change the incentive structures in which decisions are made, and also, importantly, to raise up new organizational allies for the existing payers. If governments alone do not have the credibility to challenge providers on matters that can be interpreted as falling within the scope of medical practice, then national variants of the sponsors, which Enthoven has described in more detail elsewhere (Enthoven and Kronick, 1989a and

1989b), may be called into existence or molded out of preexisting institutions to serve as counterweights to the health care delivery system itself. The progressive evolution of the District Health Authorities in the United Kingdom, partly under the influence of Enthoven's ideas, toward being purchasers of services on behalf of their populations rather than monopoly suppliers, is a clear example (*Working for Patients*, 1989).

But is it working?

There is, however, a critical distinction between the American experience as it is and Enthoven's vision of what it might become. He recommends, in the United States and in Europe, the creation of institutions independent of the health care system, "to get more informed choice into the system"—prudent purchasers on the patient's behalf, yet without the political constraints that inhibit governments. But he would be the first to admit that this has not yet happened in the United States. Despite the rapid expansion of various forms of managed care, now covering more than one-half of the employed and privately insured population, and even in those regions where perestroika is most extensive and longest established, the anticipated benefits—equity, efficiency, and cost control—have yet to emerge (Gabel et al., 1988).

Enthoven's reference to the "big success" of the prospective payment system (PPS) based on DRGs is premature; its impact on costs between 1983 and 1985 now looks like a one-time effect that did not influence the overall trend.[1] He might argue, and very justly, that the full structural requirements of informed and cost-conscious choice have not yet been put in place—his system has not really been tried. But the same might be said for Christianity—or communism.

The jury is still out on managed care in the United States. There is certainly a school of thought (e.g., Amara, Morrison, and Schmid, 1988) that argues that most such programs have placed little risk on providers and that the real "deep capitation," provider-at-risk revolution, is yet to come. But others are losing heart—most notably the Chrysler Corporation—and national health insurance is, in 1989, back near the top of the American political agenda, after over a decade in the wilderness. This fact is itself a commentary on both the effectiveness of present forms of managed care and the perceived political feasibility of Enthoven's much more sophisticated form. Europeans should take note.

Decentralization: Accountability to whom?

Furthermore, there seems to be an essential ambiguity in the argument for decentralization. Do decentralized structures change the information and objectives of the general public—empowering the expression of more informed choice? Or do they merely weaken the expression of the views of the general public by eliminating centralized political accountability? Citizens of most European countries, which in this context includes Canada, are at root very satisfied with their health care systems, and have well-developed channels of accountability through which to express dissatisfaction in specific cases. Americans are unique in that they are not, and have not.

It may well be that Europeans should be less satisfied, and, in particular, much less confident in the professional institutions and decisions that determine their patterns of care. If they knew more, they would want less, and perhaps different things. But it is not clear, at least to this point, that decentralized reimbursement and control structures have been developed, anywhere, that empower more informed "market" choices rather than simply disempowering (however badly informed) political ones.

There is certainly room for improvement in all the European systems, and particularly in their balances of provider and patient convenience, as Enthoven points out. But—and this is the crux of the debate over the recent British White Paper (*Working for Patients*, 1989)—if provider incentives are changed, to which patients do they become more sensitive? Those with the greatest needs? Or those whom it is most profitable or professionally satisfying to serve (cream-skimming, or moving up-market . . .)? No one should underestimate the power of incentives. But it is easy to overestimate our ability to control or even predict their direction of effect, particularly if we rely on economic models of human behavior that are grossly oversimplified both in their postulates of objectives, and in their specification of the range of possible behaviors.

None of this is news to Enthoven; nor are we so naive as to imagine that existing systems of political accountability yield (nearly) ideal results. But it does suggest a good deal of caution in introducing restructuring proposals that may have unpredictable and far-reaching effects, into systems that appear to be basically satisfactory. Careful monitoring, piloting, and some clear idea of how one can withdraw if things work out badly would seem at least prudent.

Copayments: How not to decentralize

The varying national approaches to user charges provide a good example of the risks of decentralization. European and Canadian experience demonstrates that centralized financial controls over fees, budgets, and new capital outlays ("sole source funding") are relatively successful and politically acceptable, if not always popular. Decentralization of funding, in the form of substantial charges to individual patients or widespread private insurance, destroys this control. Providers of care in all

[1] It may also be relevant that a substantial decline occurred in acute care hospital use in Canada in the 1980s, without any change in the payment system—but under substantial administrative pressure (Evans, Barer et al., 1989). There may be several ways to skin a cat.

countries, recognizing this relationship very clearly, press for increased private funding and particularly greater charges to patients, explicitly in order to increase the flow of funds into health care.

The results of this form of decentralization—which is not at all what Enthoven is advocating—are displayed in the American experience. The poor, the elderly, and the sick spend a much larger share of their incomes on health care than does the general population. There is no evidence that Americans generally approve this distribution of burden, which most other societies would find, have found, unacceptable, any more than they favor the steady escalation of health care costs. Both emerge, not from anyone's conscious choice, but from a whole series of decisions by employers, insurers, providers, and patients. No one can control, or be held accountable for, the overall outcome.

Amazingly, many Americans continue to believe that at least user charges hold down overall health care costs, a view strengthened by the RAND study to which Enthoven refers. Yet this is clearly inconsistent with the observations that only in the United States, where such charges are most prevalent and most significant, are costs out of control, and that the loudest advocates of such charges in other countries are the providers of care, whose incomes would suffer if charges really did moderate the growth of health care costs.[2] Moreover, international comparisons suggest that the more rapid escalation of costs in the United States is traceable to more rapid price inflation (Poullier, 1989), consistent with the interpretation that user charges serve not to constrain utilization, but to undermine collective price controls.[3]

The RAND findings, that direct charges reduce care-seeking by patients, cannot be generalized to systemwide levels of utilization. That experiment, by design, excluded the effects of provider responses to changes in patient-initiated behavior, and consequent changes in provider workloads and incomes. Yet those responses, the information and advice given to patients, are the critical determinants of overall utilization. Attempts to interpret the RAND results as support for greater allocations of burden through user charges represent an elementary fallacy of composition and teach a strong negative lesson in both research and policy. (This negative lesson is reinforced by more recent reports from the RAND study (Lohr et al., 1986), which are much less sanguine about the impact of user charges on access to "needed" care and the distribution of their burden across the population, than those cited by Enthoven.)

The paradox: Why restructure success?

So we have something of a paradox. The serious weaknesses of the American system are rooted in its decentralized structure; the advantages of European systems are rooted in their centralized funding control. Enthoven's perestroika suggestions imply greater decentralization. Might not a European (or a Canadian) reply: "If it ain't broke, don't fix it."? To what question is Enthoven providing answers?

Only diamonds are forever

Several, we think. Although Europeans are, in the main, satisfied with their systems, these are far from perfect and very expensive. Enthoven's MIS comments are well taken, and in a world of scarce resources should not lightly be dismissed. Further, his emphasis on "user friendliness" is also important. The convenience and comfort of the patient, although perhaps secondary to results achieved, are not trivial considerations. They can easily be neglected in the tug-of-war between payers and payees. Providers in all systems will respond that better service requires more resources; as a long-time student of management, Enthoven points out that the real answer is different incentives.

Perhaps most important, the political resistance to top-down global financial and capacity controls does appear to be growing. Such controls may, over time, become less effective and/or more expensive to maintain—the status quo may not be an option for the long term.[4] A failure to develop the political and informational base for improved management could conceivably result in a slow drift towards "privatization" on the uncontrolled, inequitable, and expensive American model. There is no reason to believe that Europeans (much less Canadians) are immune to "the American disease."

Decentralized incentives within central controls

The trick is, exactly as Enthoven says, to find "politically feasible incremental changes" with "a reasonably good chance of making things better." These probably will take the form of increased decentralization of decisionmaking, but within a continuation of the quite-tight centralized constraints that apply in one form or another in the successful European systems. These critical constraints will continue to include:

---

[2]International opinions differ. In France, it seems widely believed that the "ticket moderateur" paid by patients helps to hold down costs. In the Federal Republic of Germany and Canada, patients are not charged for hospital or medical care. Health expenditure levels and trends are roughly similar in all three countries.
[3]Lest one fear the starvation of the health care sector, it is important to recall that the American experience is one of health care price increases that are much more rapid than general inflation rates (Levit, Freeland, and Waldo, 1989). Centralized controls in other countries manage to keep health care inflation more closely aligned to general inflation (e.g., Barer, Evans, and Labelle, 1988).

[4]On the other hand, one must beware of being stampeded by Chicken Little cries that "the sky is falling"—the health care system in Country X is on the verge of collapse. Such claims are part of the everyday litany of providers negotiating for more resources in politically controlled systems—"orchestrated outrage" (Evans, Lomas et al., 1989).

- Global controls on health spending (not just public sector spending.)
- Separation of individual contributions from either illness experience or health status.
- Protection of the de facto universality of the European financing and delivery systems (some countries have separate arrangements for the wealthy, but not for the poor) against fragmentation.

Decentralization of funding, American-style, has strongly promoted competitive cost shifting, and concomitant escalation, and made overall control virtually impossible. (Do not worry about the size of the bill, you cannot do anything about it anyway. Just get someone else to pay.) At the same time, it has encouraged the distribution of the burden of health care costs according to both actual and expected illness experience—user charges and risk-related premiums—rather than according to ability to pay. Those with the greatest needs carry the greatest financial burdens or do without.

But this does not have to be the case—or at least so Enthoven believes (and we agree). Nor does he advocate a continuation of this pattern of financing in the United States, much less its extension to Europe; as noted above, he is one of the most clear-eyed critics of the present American situation. More sophisticated organizational design can make it possible to reconcile decentralized and better informed management of the specifics of care with centralized defense of the essential principles.[5] Such changes will not be easy; they are both inherently technically difficult and will be strongly opposed or subverted. Among their opponents will be those who advocate decentralization precisely to break out of spending controls, and/or to redistribute the burden of costs back from the more to the less healthy and wealthy. But the process will certainly be interesting, and the stakes are high enough to justify the effort.

---

[5]The British White Paper, *Working for Patients* (1989) appears to represent such an effort, whatever one thinks of its chances for success.

References

Abel-Smith, B.: Who is the odd man out? The experience of western Europe in containing the costs of health care. *Milbank Memorial Fund Quarterly* 63(1):1-17, 1985.

Amara, R., Morrison, J. I., and Schmid, G.: *Looking Ahead at American Health Care*. Washington, D.C., McGraw-Hill Healthcare Information Center, 1988.

Barer, M. L., Evans, R. G., and Labelle, R. J.: Fee controls as cost control: Tales from the frozen north. *Milbank Quarterly* 66(1):1-64, 1988.

Blendon, R. J.: Three systems: A comparative survey. *Health Management Quarterly* 11(1):2-10, 1989.

Enthoven, A., and Kronick, R.: A consumer choice health plan for the 1990s: Universal health insurance in a system designed to promote quality and economy. (First of two parts). *New England Journal of Medicine* 320(1):29-37, 1989a.

Enthoven, A., and Kronick, R.: A consumer choice health plan for the 1990s: Universal health insurance in a system designed to promote quality and economy. (Second of two parts). *New England Journal of Medicine* 320(2):94-101, 1989b.

Evans, R. G.: The dog in the night time: Medical practice variations and health policy. In Andersen, T. F., and Mooney, G., eds. *The Challenge of Medical Practice Variations*. London. Macmillan Press, 1989.

Evans, R. G., Lomas, J., Barer, M. L., et al.: Controlling health expenditures: The Canadian reality. *New England Journal of Medicine* 320(9):571-577, 1989.

Evans, R. G., Barer, M. L., Hertzman, C., et al.: The long good-bye: The great transformation of the British Columbia hospital system. *Health Services Research* 24(4):435-459, Winter 1989.

Gabel, J., Jajich-Toth, C., de Lissovoy, G., et al.: The changing world of group health insurance. *Health Affairs* 7(3):48-65, 1988.

Levit, K. R., Freeland, M. S., and Waldo, D. R.: Health spending and ability to pay: Business, individuals, and government. *Health Care Financing Review*. Vol. 10, No. 3. HCFA Pub. No. 03280. Office of Research and Demonstrations, Health Care Financing Administration. Washington. U.S. Government Printing Office, Spring 1989.

Lohr, K. N., Brook, R. H., Kamberg, C. J., et al.: Use of medical care in the RAND Health Insurance Experiment: Diagnosis and service-specific analyses in a randomized controlled trial. *Medical Care* 24(supplement), 1986.

Marmor, T. R., Wittman, D. A., and Heagy, T. C.: The politics of medical inflation. In Marmor, T. R., ed. *Political Analysis and American Medical Care: Essays*. Cambridge, United Kingdom. Cambridge University Press, 1983.

Poullier, J. P.: The Chicago Tunnel doesn't connect. Paper presented to the Annual Meeting of the Association for Health Services Research. Chicago. June 20, 1989.

Rachlis, M., and Kushner, C.: *Second Opinion: What's Wrong with Canada's Health Care System and How to Fix It*. Toronto. Collins, 1989.

Roper, W. L., Winkenwerder, W., Hackbarth, G. M., and Krakauer, H.: Effectiveness in health care: An initiative to evaluate and improve medical practice. *New England Journal of Medicine* 319(18):1197-1202, 1988.

Schieber, G., and Poullier, J. P.: International health spending and utilization trends. *Health Affairs* 7(4):105-112, 1988.

Working for Patients. London. Her Majesty's Stationery Office, 1989.

What can Americans learn from Europeans?

by Bengt Jönsson

In this article, the opportunities for Americans to learn from Europeans regarding the pros and cons of a comprehensive health care system, the role of regionalization in achieving cost control, efficiency, and equity, and the management of new expensive technologies are discussed. One conclusion is that there is a convergence of health care systems, at least in terms of means to achieve cost containment and efficiency. European health care systems will increasingly provide interesting information on how different health policies—many of them devised in the United States—work under different economic and regulatory conditions.

Introduction

The United States, with its great plurality of organizational, ownership, and financing forms in health care, has been described as a laboratory for experimentation in health service organization and financing. The variety of institutions and financing mechanisms is enormous, and it has, over time, produced many interesting experiments that have been of great interest to European countries looking for models to reform their health care systems. During the last decade, concepts such as HMOs (health maintenance organizations), DRGs (diagnosis-related groups), and MTA (medical technology assessment) have become part of the standard vocabulary in most European countries.

It is therefore a somewhat strange situation, for an economist who has devoted a significant amount of time and effort to looking for opportunities to learn from the U.S. health care scene, to reverse his perspective and look for lessons that Americans can learn from European systems. Because there is so much variety in U.S. health care, it is also difficult to find new ideas and approaches that have not already been tried somewhere at some time in the United States. There is also the risk of being irrelevant. Means cannot be judged without reference to the goals. It is obvious that the moral bases or values on which health care systems are based differ between the United States and European countries. In the United States, personal responsibility, freedom of choice, and pluralism are the major moral commitments. In European countries, goals related to population health and equality of access to health services have been relatively more important. Centralized health planning and a large governmental

role in health care financing have therefore been me generally accepted in Europe.

As has been pointed out by others (e.g., Culyer, Maynard, and Williams, 1981), it is unhelpful to seek to learn from a system that is seeking to accomplish different aims. However, this should not be overstated: After all, a means may serve more than one end or may be adopted more appropriately to serve another end. Therefore, even though the ideological bases may vary between countries, it does not follow that neither has anything to learn from the other. So without appearing presumptuous, I hope to identify some areas or issues in which I think the experience of European countries can be of value in the development of U.S. health policy. I concentrate on issues that I can substantiate with data from the Organization for Economic Cooperation and Development (OECD) data base on international differences in health care (Organization for Economic Cooperation and Development, 1989).

Common aspects of European systems

Europe, as well as the United States, shows a great variety in health care systems and consequently also in health care policies. In addition to learning from its own diversity, the United States can learn from the specifics of different European systems at different points in time. There are also many studies in which U.S. researchers have looked at particular types of policies, such as physician reimbursement and cost containment (Reinhardt, 1981) or have focused on individual countries. For Sweden alone, it is easy to find more than a dozen publications in which U.S. researchers have looked at various aspects of the Swedish health care system and made comparisons with the United States (e.g., Lembcke, 1959; Anderson, 1972; Navarro, 1974; and Rosenthal, 1986 and 1987).

In this article, I concentrate on a number of aspects that are common to most, if not all, European health care systems. There are many from which to choose. The most obvious to start with is the financing and delivery of health care to the elderly. The populations of Europe are significantly older than that of the United States; therefore, Europe can give interesting evidence of what is to come in the United States. As shown in Table 1, the proportion of the population 65 years of age or over is 13.8 percent in Europe, compared with 12.2 percent in the United States. In some countries, such as Sweden, it is more than 17 percent.

An increasing share of health care resources spent on the elderly dramatically alters the conditions for health care financing and delivery. The insurance function becomes more of an intertemporal allocation

Reprint requests: Bengt Jönsson, Department of Health and Society, Linköping University S-58183, Linköping, Sweden.

Table 1

Percent of the population in each of three age groups: Selected countries, 1987

Country	Years of age		
	65 or over	75 or over	80 or over
	Percent		
United States	12.2	5.0	2.6
Europe[1]	13.8	6.0	3.0
Austria	14.7	6.9	3.4
Belgium	14.3	6.4	3.3
Denmark	15.4	6.7	3.4
Finland	12.9	5.3	2.5
France	13.5	6.5	3.5
Germany	15.9	7.3	[2]3.4
Greece	13.5	5.7	[2]2.8
Iceland	10.3	4.4	[2]2.5
Ireland	11.0	4.2	2.0
Italy	12.9	5.4	[3]2.5
Luxembourg	13.3	5.7	[2]2.7
Netherlands	12.4	5.2	2.7
Norway	16.1	6.8	3.5
Portugal	12.5	4.9	2.2
Spain	12.4	5.1	2.5
Sweden	17.7	7.7	3.9
Switzerland	14.4	6.5	3.4
United Kingdom	15.5	6.6	3.4

[1]Unweighted average.
[2]Data from 1986.
[3]Data from 1985.

SOURCE: (Organization for Economic Cooperation and Development, 1989).

problem, similar to the pension system, than a traditional health insurance. In the Federal Republic of Germany (hereafter called Germany), the public pension funds transfer money to the sickness funds to subsidize health care expenses for retired members. In 1975, these transfers accounted for 27 percent of total revenues for sick funds (Henke, 1980.) An increasing amount of total health expenditures is spent on the last years of life, and almost everyone reaches the average life expectancy (Le Grand and Rabin, 1986).[1] For the provision of health care, this means that nursing home care becomes relatively more important, as does the integration of social and medical services. In order to study health care for the elderly in different countries, age-specific cost and utilization data are needed. These data are not yet available, so this topic will have to wait for further refinements of the international comparative health statistics.

Another aspect of great interest is the quality of care. Systems of quality control are different in Europe from those in the United States. The use of litigation to deal with medical malpractice is considerably more common in the United States than in Europe. This affects health care costs directly, through insurance premiums paid by doctors, and indirectly, through its effect on physician behavior—

[1]The results shown by Le Grand and Rabin (1986), a decline during the past 50 years in the Gini coefficient for variation in the age of death, can be described as a "rectangularization" of mortality. For a discussion of rectangularization of morbidity, see Fries (1980). Please note that rectangularization is not caused by changes in demography but by changes in the epidemiology of disease, partly caused by medical interventions.

the practice of defensive medicine. It would be of great interest to know more about the consequences for quality of care of the different ways of practicing medicine. In addition, it would be helpful to look at measures of quality assurance in the United States and Europe. However, international comparative statistics provide only scant information for such exercises.

Instead, I concentrate on three general aspects of European systems for which there are existing international statistics: the comprehensiveness of these systems; the role of regionalization in achieving cost control, efficiency, and equity; and the management of new expensive medical technologies.

A comprehensive health care system

The most striking difference between European systems, taken as a whole, and that in the United States is the comprehensiveness of the European systems. In most European countries, everyone is eligible for coverage of medical expenses through a public plan—usually public both in the sense of finance and in the sense of provision. This is the case for hospital care, ambulatory care, and medical goods, though the element of copayment is usually higher for the latter two categories. Even in countries with a significant amount of private insurance, such as Switzerland and the Netherlands, the share of the population eligible for coverage through public plans is close to 100 percent for hospital care (Table 2). Those not covered are mainly the more affluent members of the population, who may choose not to participate in the public plans.

Table 2

Percent of population eligible for public health insurance, by type of coverage: Selected countries, 1987

Country	Hospital care	Ambulatory care	Medical goods
	Percent		
Austria	99	99	90
Belgium	98	93	68
Denmark	100	100	100
Finland	100	100	90
France	99	98	92
Germany	92	92	97
Greece	100	100	90
Iceland	100	100	—
Ireland	100	37	95
Italy	100	100	99
Luxembourg	100	100	95
Netherlands	77	72	80
Norway	100	100	100
Portugal	100	100	100
Spain	98	97	84
Sweden	100	100	100
Switzerland	98	98	100
United Kingdom	100	100	99
United States	40	25	—

NOTES: Most countries do not publish data on the number of people covered by, or benefits received under, public health insurance plans. These are crude Organization for Economic Cooperation and Development Secretariat estimates based on descriptive evidence.

SOURCE: (Organization for Economic Cooperation and Development, 1989).

In Switzerland, three partners share the expenditures for the health care system. In 1984, public funds accounted for 6.2 billion Swiss francs, sickness funds and social insurances for 5.1 billion francs, and privately insured and uninsured persons for 5.2 billion francs (Gygi and Frei, 1986). In the Netherlands, about 70 percent of the population is insured with the sickness funds, which operate the social insurance system of the Sickness Funds Insurance Act. Individuals with an income of more than a certain amount (approximately 43,000 Dutch guilders in 1982) have to acquire private health insurance, but employees with an annual income under that level are mandatorily insured by sickness fund insurance. Private financing accounted for about 25 percent of total health expenditures in 1980. Insurance for greater risks, i.e., exceptional expenses, is governed by the General Special Sickness Expenses Act. This is a national insurance plan applying in principal to all residents of the Netherlands (Rutten, 1982). At present, the health care system in the Netherlands is in a period of transition. In October of 1988, the Dutch parliament approved the implementation of the first steps in the new direction. Two major issues are the introduction of national health insurance ("basic insurance") and regulated competition among insurers and among providers. For a review of the recent developments, see van de Ven (1989).

In the United States, the coverage rate of public plans is estimated to be only 40 percent of the population for hospital care and 25 percent for ambulatory care. Even if a higher degree of private

insurance, subsidized through tax exemptions for employers or individuals, partly compensates for this, a significant part of the population lacks coverage or is inadequately covered for health care. It has been estimated (Davis, 1989) that as many as 37 million people, 15 percent of the population, lack adequate insurance coverage; many lack coverage of any kind and are dependent on private charity. However, other sources show that 14.5 percent of the poor, 15.6 percent of the near-poor, 11.9 percent of other-low-income people, and 4.5 percent of all others lack insurance coverage (Kasper, 1986). This is a total of 17 million people, or 7 percent of the population, who are uninsured.

The coverage rate is only one aspect of the comprehensiveness of a system. We also have to look at what benefits are provided. In Table 3, the average or typical percent of a bill paid by public insurance is shown for several European countries and the United States. It can also be seen that the copayment rate is lower in European countries than in the United States.

The advantages as well as the problems associated with a system that provides insurance coverage for everyone probably provide the most significant lessons for the United States.

Differences in total health expenditures

A higher coverage rate and a greater share of public financing in Europe may be thought to imply significantly higher total expenditures. However, this is not the case. On the contrary, the health expenditures share of the gross domestic product (GDP) is significantly higher for the United States than it is for any European country (Table 4). (Gross domestic product is the gross market value of the goods and services attributable to labor and property located in a given nation.)

In 1986, total health expenditures, as a percent of GDP, were 10.9 percent in the United States, compared with a European average of 7.2 percent. Sweden, the European country with the highest share, had 9.1 percent. Also in absolute terms, using exchange rates or purchasing power parities (PPPs) for conversion of national currencies, the expenditures in the United States are significantly higher than in any European country.

Does this mean that the level of expenditures in the United States is totally inconsistent with the experiences of the European countries? To answer this question, we must look more closely at the determinants of health care expenditures. The major determinant of such differences is GDP per capita. (See Gerdtham et al., 1988, for a review and some new estimates.) Taking into account that GDP per capita is higher in the United States than in Europe, are the expenditures still higher than would be expected?

In Table 5, the actual and predicted 1986 health expenditures for 18 European countries and the

Table 3
Average percent of bill paid for by public insurance, by type of benefit received: Selected countries, 1987

Country	Hospital care	Ambulatory care	Medical goods
	Percent paid		
Austria	90	80	50
Belgium	68	50	52
Denmark	100	76	45
Finland	90	70	61
France	92	62	58
Germany	97	85	56
Greece	90	85	75
Iceland	—	—	—
Ireland	95	47	48
Italy	99	65	63
Luxembourg	95	98	83
Netherlands	80	67	58
Norway	100	—	—
Portugal	100	100	67
Spain	84	—	77
Sweden	100	90	75
Switzerland	100	86	90
United Kingdom	99	88	93
United States	55	56	—

NOTES: Most countries do not publish data on the number of people covered by, or benefits received under, public health insurance plans. These are crude Organization for Economic Cooperation and Development Secretariat estimates based on descriptive evidence.

SOURCE: (Organization for Economic Cooperation and Development, 1989).

Table 4

Total health expenditures expressed as a percent of gross domestic product (GDP) and as expenditures per capita: Selected countries, 1986

Country	Real GDP index[2]	Percent of GDP	Expenditures per capita[1] Converted using purchasing power parities	Converted using exchange rate
Austria	64	8.3	$ 929	$1,023
Belgium	66	7.2	825	883
Denmark	75	6.0	777	962
Finland	70	7.4	900	1,069
France	71	8.7	1,068	1,142
Germany	73	8.1	1,031	1,183
Greece	36	5.3	331	212
Iceland	82	7.5	1,063	1,192
Ireland	41	7.8	550	553
Italy	66	6.6	764	702
Luxembourg	80	7.0	962	928
Netherlands	68	8.3	983	1,002
Norway	86	6.8	1,021	1,144
Portugal	33	5.5	310	158
Spain	46	6.1	486	358
Sweden	75	9.1	1,193	1,429
Switzerland	88	7.6	1,162	1,573
United Kingdom	57	6.1	706	594
United States	100	10.9	1,886	1,886

[1]In U.S. dollars.
[2]United States = 100.
SOURCE: (Organization for Economic Cooperation and Development, 1989).

Table 5

Actual and predicted health expenditures[1] per capita, differences, and upper and lower bounds of a 95-percent confidence interval: Selected countries, 1986

Country	Actual	Predicted	Difference	Lower bound	Upper bound
Austria	929	810	+ 119	644	1,018
Belgium	825	844	− 19	671	1,061
Denmark	777	997	− 220	791	1,258
Finland	900	909	− 9	722	1,143
France	1,068	918	+ 150	730	1,156
Germany	1,031	963	+ 68	765	1,213
Greece	331	363	− 32	277	477
Iceland	1,063	1,122	− 59	886	1,421
Ireland	550	431	+ 119	334	557
Italy	764	842	− 78	670	1,059
Luxembourg	962	1,081	− 119	856	1,367
Netherlands	983	873	+ 120	694	1,098
Norway	1,021	1,198	− 177	943	1,521
Portugal	310	321	− 11	241	426
Spain	486	516	− 30	405	659
Sweden	1,193	1,003	+ 190	795	1,265
Switzerland	1,162	1,230	− 68	967	1,563
United Kingdom	706	850	− 144	676	1,069
United States	1,886	1,472	+ 414	1,145	1,894

[1]Expenditures converted from national currency units to U.S. dollars using purchasing power parities.
SOURCE: Jönsson, B.: Linköping University, Linköping, Sweden, 1989.

United States are shown. A logarithmic function has been used (Gerdtham et al., 1988). The regression equation is:

$$HEXP = -5.99 + 1.36 \text{ GDP} \quad (R^2 = 0.89)$$
$$t\text{-ratio} \quad (-5.6) \quad (11.9)$$

The constant elasticity is 1.36, which means that a 1-percent increase in GDP will give a 1.36-percent increase in total health expenditures. Both the elasticity and the constant are strongly significant. As

can be seen in Table 5, the actual health expenditures for the United States are 28 percent higher than predicted. This is close to the upper bound of a 95-percent confidence interval. (The comparability of health care expenditures data among countries is, despite significant improvements, still not exact. The lower-than-predicted levels of expenditures for Denmark, Luxembourg, and Norway can be explained partly by underreporting of certain types of expenditures, mainly nursing home care.)

Table 6

Actual and predicted health care expenditures[1] for the United States in 1986, based on data for 18 European countries

Log function: $HEXP = -5.30 + 1.29\ GDP$ $R^2 = 0.89$

Actual	Predicted	Difference	Lower bound	Upper bound
1,886	1,466	+420	1,041	2,064

Linear function: $HEXP = -139 + 0.0853\ GDP$ $R^2 = 0.83$

Actual	Predicted	Difference	Lower bound	Upper bound
1,886	1,341	+545	1,064	1,617

[1] With 95-percent confidence interval.

NOTE: *HEXP* is health expenditures. GDP is gross domestic product.

SOURCE: Jönsson, B.: Linköping University, Linköping, Sweden, 1989.

The expenditure levels of 18 European countries were used as a basis to predict health expenditures for the United States (Table 6). The result is very similar for the logarithmic specification of the regression function, although the elasticity is slightly reduced. For the linear specification, the prediction is lower and the level of actual expenditures is significantly outside the 95-percent confidence interval.

We can conclude that the higher share of public financing in European countries does not result in higher expenditures than in the United States. In fact, there is evidence to the contrary.[2] Details on the cost-containment policies used in Europe are covered in the article by Culyer in this issue; therefore, they are not discussed here. Instead, let us look at other

---

[2] This does not necessarily mean that the United States is "overspending." This is a normative concept, which cannot be judged with reference to international comparisons only. Studies indicate that a significant part of the higher expenditures in the United States are the result of higher relative prices for health care, rather than greater volume of services (Parkin, 1989).

---

aspects of health policy that relate to the comprehensive nature of European systems. However, it is necessary to relate these aspects to expenditure restraint, because this is the major mechanism by which resources are allocated in European systems.

Preventive versus curative services

The most important question for any health care system is how well it is achieving the basic health objectives of the population. The difficulties in comparing the objectives of health care systems are well known. Health is difficult to measure and is determined to a major extent by factors outside the control of the health care system. However, one area in which health care can make a directly measurable difference is in the reduction of infant mortality, although it is difficult to document exactly the relative contribution of various factors.

The World Health Organization (1981) states that the infant mortality rate "is a useful indicator of the health status not only of infants but also of whole populations and of the socioeconomic conditions under which they live. In addition, the infant mortality rate is a sensitive indicator of the availability, utilization, and effectiveness of health care, particularly perinatal care." Waaler and Sterky (1984), examining trends in infant mortality, perinatal mortality, and gross national product in four Scandinavian countries, suggest that perinatal mortality (late fetal and neonatal deaths per 100 live and still births) is preferable to infant mortality (death rates of infants under 1 year of age per 100 live births) as an indicator of the quality of heath care. However, examining the relationship between infant mortality and perinatal mortality in 1986 and changes from 1960 through 1986 in European countries and the United States gives no support for this hypothesis.

Table 7

Infant and perinatal mortality rates: Selected countries, selected years 1960-86

Country	1960 Infant	1960 Perinatal	1970 Infant	1970 Perinatal	1980 Infant	1980 Perinatal	1986 Infant	1986 Perinatal
				Rate per 100 live births				
Austria	3.75	3.5	2.59	2.7	1.43	1.4	1.03	0.9
Belgium	3.12	3.2	2.11	2.3	1.21	1.4	0.97	—
Denmark	2.15	2.6	1.42	1.8	0.84	0.9	0.82	0.8
Finland	2.10	2.8	1.32	1.7	0.76	0.8	0.58	0.6
France	2.74	3.1	1.82	2.3	1.01	1.3	0.80	—
Germany	3.38	3.6	2.34	2.6	1.27	1.2	0.87	—
Greece	4.01	2.6	2.96	2.7	1.79	2.0	1.22	1.5
Iceland	2.17	2.0	1.33	1.9	0.77	0.9	0.54	0.8
Ireland	2.93	3.8	1.95	2.4	1.11	1.5	0.87	—
Italy	4.39	4.2	2.96	3.1	1.43	1.8	1.01	—
Luxembourg	3.15	3.2	2.49	2.5	1.15	1.0	0.80	0.7
Netherlands	1.79	2.7	1.27	1.9	0.86	1.1	0.64	1.0
Norway	1.89	2.4	1.27	1.9	0.81	1.1	0.78	0.8
Portugal	7.75	4.1	5.51	3.7	2.43	2.4	1.59	1.8
Spain	4.37	—	2.81	—	1.23	1.4	0.87	—
Sweden	1.66	2.6	1.10	1.6	0.69	0.9	0.59	0.7
Switzerland	2.11	—	1.44	1.8	0.91	1.0	0.68	0.8
United Kingdom	2.25	3.4	1.85	2.4	1.21	1.3	0.95	—
United States	2.60	2.9	2.00	2.3	1.26	1.3	1.04	1.0

SOURCE: (Organization for Economic Cooperation and Development, 1989).

The differences between countries and over time are very similar with both measures (Table 7). As can be seen in Table 7, several European countries have an infant mortality rate that is 30-40 percent lower than that of the United States. Smaller countries can be expected to have lower rates because of greater cultural homogeneity, but it may be observed that the rates are also lower for the big European countries. Taking into account the high GDP per capita and the high rate of health expenditures, one would expect the United States to have significantly lower infant and perinatal mortality rates than the Federal Republic of Germany, France, and the United Kingdom. To the extent that the differences between Europe and the United States can be attributed to medical action, the lower mortality rates must have been achieved mainly by preventive measures. The resources for neonatal intensive care and the frequency of cesarian delivery are higher in the United States, but this obviously does not result in a lower infant mortality rate.

My hypothesis is that it is easier to allocate resources to programs like prenatal care and vaccination for children in a more comprehensive system. Considering the relative efficiency of health care services, it is difficult to allocate resources to interventions with dubious value, when even basic services with proven or obvious cost effectiveness are not being provided. The underprovision of such inexpensive but cost-effective services is a serious inefficiency in a health care system.

The commitment to primary health care and prevention in many European countries must be considered in the shaping of the future U.S. health care system. But this policy has not been without its problems, and, in many instances, it has been only a verbal commitment. In other instances, it has resulted in overoptimistic expectations about its ability to solve health problems or even to control escalating health care costs. But there is much to be learned from the mistakes as well as the successes. Focusing on health problems from a population perspective, rather than an individual perspective, gives new insights into the relative efficiency of different interventions. It also indicates that more health services are not always a solution to social problems; rather the solutions to social problems can have a significant impact on health. A comprehensive system enforces this broader perspective.

Regionalization, global budgets, and planning

One important common aspect of European health care systems is regionalization. Typically, regions, rather than the country as a whole, are the basis for the allocation of health resources. However, regionalization is achieved in different ways in each country. In Sweden, for example, the regions (counties) have total responsibility for both the health of the population and the provision of health care. The average population of a region is 350,000 inhabitants, and the decisions about health services

provision are made by elected representatives (community councils) in the region. The financing of services comes from a local proportional income tax.

Similar systems can be found in the other Scandinavian countries of Denmark, Norway, and Finland. However, in Finland, the local communities are the basic regional unit, and in Norway, the regions (fylke) are responsible for hospital care and the local communities for primary care. In Denmark, the responsibility for hospital services, general practitioners, and practicing specialists is decentralized to 16 regions (counties or "amt"), the typical population being 250,000-300,000 inhabitants. Local health and social services, including home care, are run by communities of varying size. The Copenhagen and Frederiksberg communities, in the Copenhagen metropolitan area, have community as well as county obligations.

In contrast, in the United Kingdom, regional authorities are not elected, nor do they have tax powers, nor do the districts beneath them, which are responsible for the provision of hospital care to the locality. Instead, their finances are directly controlled by cash-limited budgets allocated from the center. Since 1977, the allocation of resources among regions has been based on the Resource Allocation Working Party (RAWP) formula, with the objective of securing geographical equity in the availability of resources (Department of Health and Social Security, 1976). Different indicators of need determine the per capita-based funding for the regions. RAWP has been controversial, and there is an extensive literature of criticism and comment (Mays and Bevan, 1987). But after 10 years, the gap has narrowed substantially between the regions receiving the most and the least funds.

Regionalization is also strong in insurance-based systems such as those in Germany, the Netherlands, and Switzerland. In the last country, health care is by law a responsibility for the regions (cantons), some of them very small. Although the majority of financing comes from private and public insurance (Krankenkassen), it is the canton that has the overall responsibility for the provision of health care resources. The cantons also have to underwrite the deficit in public hospitals operated by them. This gives them a strong influence over the allocation of resources.

In the Netherlands, hospitals, whether owned by local communities or lay boards of trustees, operate on a fixed predetermined budget since 1984. The budget is negotiated with the third-party payers. The central government has a strong influence on construction of facilities and acquisition of major medical equipment through licenses, which are issued on the basis of regional and national health sector planning.

The strict planning systems for hospital care in Switzerland and the Netherlands, the two European systems most similar to those of the United States, are the major reason why expenditures are constrained in these countries, and the share of GDP that goes to

Figure 1
Worksheet used to develop a classification system for regionalized health care systems

Aspects of regionalization in European health care systems

Federal country	Yes	No
Typical size of region (millions of inhabitants)	————	
Region governed by elected representatives	Yes	No
Regional tax power	Yes	No
Region is both purchaser and provider	Yes	No
Percent of hospital beds provided by the region	————	
Global budget for total health expenditures	Yes	No
Global budget for hospital expenditures	Yes	No
Percent of total expenditures within global budget	————	
Percent of expenditures on health	————	
Region regulates number and activities of other (private) providers:		
Doctors	Yes	No
Hospitals	Yes	No
Nursing homes	Yes	No
Regional fee negotiations	Yes	No
Central approval of fees	Yes	No
Central wage negotiations	Yes	No
Central regulation of capital investments	Yes	No
Integration with social services	Yes	No

SOURCE: Jönsson, B.: Linköping University, Linköping, Sweden, 1989.

health care is kept below that of the United States. In practice, these countries have global budgets for the most expensive part of health care, hospital services.

In Germany, the hospitals are financed through prospective, hospital-specific, all-inclusive per diems negotiated between the hospital and regional associations of sickness funds. These rates are subject to approval by the State governments, which also must approve and finance capital investments, based on statewide hospital planning. The State governments therefore control the capacity of the hospital system.

In Figure 1, a first attempt to develop a way to classify regionalized health care systems is shown. The first question to be asked is whether regionalization is based on a federal structure of the country as in Canada, Switzerland, and Germany. This aspect is of particular relevance for the United States, being a federal country. In federal countries, the constitution usually states the division of responsibilities in health care between the federation and the individual States. The constitution determines the possibilities and limitations for regionalization. In Switzerland, the constitution clearly states that the cantons forming the federation are responsible for health care within their borders.

The second aspect of regionalization concerns the size of the population in the region, because this determines how regionalization works in practice. Very large regions must be divided into smaller regions in order to find a suitable size to manage health care institutions. An example of this is the Regional Health Authorities in the United Kingdom,

which are divided into districts that provide health services. Very small regions (such as some cantons in Switzerland) must rely heavily on cooperation with other regions for provision of specialized services.

If the region is governed by elected representatives, there is a political process behind the allocation of resources. This is, of course, the case in the federal countries, but also in the Scandinavian countries. However, in the United Kingdom, the members of the RHAs and District Health Authorities (DHAs) are appointed by the government. A system with elected representatives is usually combined with the right to levy regional taxes. But elected representatives and the power to tax do not always go together. In Norway, the regions (fylke) receive 50 percent of their budgets from the central government; once they reach the cap on their own tax power, they cannot spend more than the amount set by the government. In Sweden and Denmark, the regions (landsting and amt, respectively), can finance health care through a proportional income tax.

A region can be both a purchaser and a provider of care. Usually the two functions go together. However, in Germany, the states finance capital costs, but do not themselves provide any services. In Sweden, Denmark, and Switzerland, the regions are also the main providers of hospital services, but there is also a "market" for services, mainly tertiary care, between regions. In the United Kingdom, there is discussion about separating the regions' roles of purchaser and provider. Similar discussion is found in Denmark and Sweden.

In most regionalized systems, the region operates a global budget for health services. Although this is not the case in, for example, Germany, there have been attempts to form a voluntary agreement, negotiated between the different interest groups, to contain costs through a global budget. For a description of the German Health Care Cost Containment Act of 1977, see Stone (1979). In Sweden,the global budget includes all health expenditures except drugs and dental care, but in other countries, such as Switzerland and the Netherlands, it includes only hospital expenditures.

For many regions, health care is their main responsibility. In other instances, they have a wider responsibility for public services and transfer payments. This obviously has implications for the tradeoff between health care and other public expenditures. The percentage of the total budget that comes from central funds can also have significant implications for the relationship between central and regional governments and for total spending on health care, as well as for the allocation of resources to different services. Even in countries in which regions have the power to tax, the central government exercises influence through different types of government grants. In Sweden, the tax equalization plan and transfers from the social insurance system to the counties are of great financial importance for the regional budget.

Another significant aspect of regionalization is the distribution of regulatory power between the central government and the regions. This is done very differently in different countries. Usually the central government regulates fees and capital investments. However, regions can also have important regulatory power. In Sweden, the county councils regulate how many private practitioners are allowed to practice under the health insurance plan and how many patient visits they can have during a year. In Germany, there are regional negotiations of reimbursement rates.

Regionalization is one way of controlling total health care expenditures as well as guaranteeing everyone access to basic and effective health services. Public choice theory tells us that, the larger the population served by a given budget, the more difficult it is to manage that budget. Rent-seeking from different interest groups becomes impossible to handle when the budget serves a country as large as the United States. It is impossible to make rational decisions about allocation of resources based on knowledge of local health needs.

In Europe, it is only the United Kingdom that has for a long time operated a global budget for the whole country. But there the total budget is allocated to the Regional Health Authorities, according to a weighted population formula, and it is the RHAs that determine the allocations within these geographical areas. This global cost containment has obviously been successful, if we look at total health care expenditures and value for money. However, we must not forget that a major reason behind the lower share of GDP allocated to health care in the

United Kingdom, compared with the United States, is the significantly lower GDP per capita.

The major advantage of regionalization is that it provides a forum for discussion about priorities in health care and value for money for different services. It also gives an opportunity to identify the total resources for health care spent on a population and to assess the appropriateness of these expenditures in relation to population needs. Because the need (defined as services with a positive marginal product on health) is for all practical purposes unlimited, a tradeoff between health care and other goods and services has to be made. Regionalization is a way to make this tradeoff more transparent and responsive to local needs. The region also forms the basic unit for planning of facilities and mobilization of resources. It is also an important mechanism for ensuring geographical equity in the availability of services.

Regionalization, freedom of choice, and competition

I have introduced concepts such as regions, priorities, value for money, planning, and global budgets in relation to population needs. Does this not amount to socialized medicine? Without very precisely defining what "socialized medicine" is, I will argue that this is not the case. My main argument is that regionalization can take many different forms and is consistent with different degrees of freedom of choice and competition among providers. The wide variety of European health care systems, all more or less based on the concept of regionalization, shows that regionalization can be combined with different financing systems, different reimbursement systems, different mixes of private and public providers, and different regulatory mechanisms.

A comparison between Sweden and Switzerland can illustrate the different forms that regionalization can take. In Switzerland, ambulatory health care is provided by private practitioners working on a fee-for-service basis. The costs are reimbursed by private or public insurers. The copayment is very small and almost everyone is covered. Physicians can locate where they wish, but there is an incentive plan to stimulate location in remote (mountain) areas. The majority of the hospitals are owned and operated by the cantons. There are also private and community-owned hospitals. The hospitals are reimbursed from the insurance plans on a per diem basis. The public hospitals, which constitute the majority, run deficits that are covered by regional taxes. This provides the raison d'être for a strict planning and budgeting system for hospital services. Doctors in hospitals are salaried but can take private patients both as inpatients and outpatients, and share the revenue for these patients with the hospital. Patients can choose their doctors as well as the hospitals where they are treated.

In Sweden, the county councils are responsible for all health care for a defined population—a county or region. Ambulatory care is delivered in public health centers as well as in outpatient clinics at the hospitals. The number of private practitioners is small, and their activities are highly regulated, both in terms of the number of patients they can treat and the reimbursement their patients can receive from health insurance. There is a small market for private care outside the public reimbursement system. The choices are limited for the patients, who are assigned a specific health center and a hospital and seldom have any influence over which doctor treats them.

The Swiss experience tells us that an insurance-based system with both private and public insurance and total coverage of the population can be combined with a strict planning system for hospital care at the regional level. The strict planning system is a prerequisite for controlling the health care budget funded by the canton. In terms of cost containment, it has been very successful. In dollars (PPP), Sweden and Switzerland spend almost exactly the same amount on health care (Table 3), which is far less than the United States spends, both in absolute terms and in relation to GDP.

The Swedish experience shows that a regional monopoly can be successful in creating access for everyone to health services and in containing costs. The quality of care is also judged to be high. However, there are problems with that type of organization that should not be overlooked and from which we can learn. First, among the people, there is dissatisfaction with not being able to make any choices in health care. But this lack of choice is not inherent in either regionalization or regulation. It can be changed in different ways within the system. Saltman and von Otter (1987) have suggested that opportunities for consumers to choose which health care center to use, which doctor to see, and which hospital to use should be increased. This will, however, have very little impact on efficiency unless the choices have financial consequences for the providers. We still do not know if the budget system can be made flexible enough to accommodate such choices. However, the experiences in the United Kingdom show that strict regulation can be combined with freedom for patients to choose a doctor and hospital. In the United Kingdom, the patient is free to select any general practitioner (GP) and the GP is likewise free to accept the patient or not. GPs are also free to refer patients to consultants of their choice, including those in hospitals outside the region. The GP's income comes partly from capitation and partly from fee for service. In contrast to Sweden, the global regional budget does not include ambulatory care; therefore, the Swedish system can be seen as financially more tightly controlled than the system of the United Kingdom.

Second, there is a problem with incentives for providers working on a fixed budget without competition. One way to improve productivity and efficiency among providers is to separate financing from provision of services in order to create competition. In Sweden, it has been suggested that the purchase of health care should be transferred from the county councils to the local communities (Jönsson and Rehnberg, 1987). The county councils should continue to be primarily providers of hospital services to the local communities. The ideas behind such a division of health care services relate closely to the discussion and research on HMOs and managed competition in the United States during this decade (Enthoven, 1980). In this issue, Culyer's article presents similar ideas for improving internal efficiency in the National Health Service (NHS). The advantage of separating financing from delivery is mainly that public providers must compete with each other and with private providers. One can, of course, question whether local communities can efficiently carry out the two roles as sponsors (Enthoven, 1988) and financers of health care, but it is a first step in creating managed competition in a regionalized system such as those in the United Kingdom and Sweden.

Today, in both Sweden and Switzerland, there is a well-functioning market for specialized (tertiary) care, in which one region buys services from providers in other regions. This gives smaller regions access to high-quality specialized care. For some services, they are buyers, and for others, they are sellers. This division of tasks is created with planning and competition, the latter increasing in importance over time. To an increasing extent, the payments are based on (prospective) prices that have been negotiated using a DRG-type framework. There is no reason why this market could not also be extended to referrals, not only between hospitals, but also between primary care centers and hospitals. Discussion about competition as a way to improve health services has taken place primarily in the United States. However, the reforms being implemented in Europe will provide not only interesting information about the problems of and opportunities for managed competition, but also examples for decentralized experiments in the United States.

Introduction of new medical technology

One important aspect of a health care system is its ability to control the introduction and diffusion of new, and often expensive, medical technologies. The European countries provide good examples of how new medical technology is managed in a comprehensive health care system based on regionalization. Because systems differ, the pattern of introduction and diffusion differs among technologies and countries, providing an interesting variety for study and analysis. Because information about new medical technology is more or less simultaneously available in all industrialized countries, the same opportunities for adoption and diffusion exist in all countries. Differences in rates of adoption and levels of diffusion can be explained primarily by characteristics of the national health care systems, including availability of resources and cultural patterns. The European countries therefore provide a laboratory in which the United States can observe the management of new medical technology.

The introduction of dialysis and transplantation for treatment of end stage renal disease (ESRD) in the 1960s can serve as an example of how the introduction and diffusion of a new technology is managed in European countries compared with the United States. In 1970, the number of treated patients per 1 million of population was about 25 in the United States, which was only one-half the number treated in Denmark, Sweden, and Switzerland, and about the same as in the United Kingdom. Two years later, when the Social Security Act was amended to authorize funding for the treatment of ESRD under Medicare, the rate of treatment was also significantly higher in countries such as Belgium, Finland, France, and the Netherlands than in the United States.

When treatment of ESRD became available, it was obvious that many Americans could not afford it and people were dying, for lack of adequate insurance coverage. There was no way that the new technology could be accommodated within the existing system. A separate reimbursement program had to be enacted to provide equity of access to these costly new technologies. When reimbursement became available, the number of persons treated increased rapidly. By 1975, the treatment rates in the United States were higher than in all but two European countries, and, in 1980, the treatment rate in the United States was the highest in the world (Table 8). In the 1980s, the treatment rate has continued to increase and is now far higher than in most European countries, although Belgium and Switzerland seem to be catching up.

The European countries experienced the same emotional debate about equity, access, and costs, but the situation was different in that the new technology could be accommodated within the existing systems of resource allocation. However, tradeoffs had to be made between this new technology and treatment for other conditions. The need to establish priorities had a significant impact on the choice of technology for treatment of ESRD. Thus, in the United Kingdom, a high proportion of patients was treated with home dialysis. Before the establishment of the Medicare ESRD program, 40 percent of treatment in the United States was home based. Because home dialysis support services furnished by nonphysicians were not covered in the original legislation, physicians had no incentive to steer patients toward this treatment. Therefore, the proportion of patients treated by home dialysis in the United States declined to 12 percent by 1978 (Drucker, Parsons, and Maher, 1986). Also the age distribution of patients shifted, so that the proportion of patients 55 years of age or over increased from 7 percent in 1967 to 45 percent in 1978 (Drucker, Parsons, and Maher, 1986). In 1981-82, the rate of treatment was 82.4 per 1 million of population in the United States, compared with 25.8 on average for the 32 countries in the European Registry (Marine and Simmons, 1986). High-rate countries, such as Belgium and Switzerland, had 44.1 and 44.9, respectively. The share of patients 60 years of age or over at the start of treatment was 26 percent in the 32 countries, compared with 38 percent for the United States. The introduction of reimbursement has obviously shifted the indications for treatment, without any assessment of the marginal costs and benefits.

Another important difference between the United States and Europe is the share of patients treated with transplants. It is well documented that this treatment is the cost-effective alternative when possible. It also gives the patient a better quality of life. The proportion of patients with functional transplants in the United States is difficult to document, but best estimates give a figure of about

Table 8

Number of patients receiving treatment for end stage renal disease: Selected countries, selected years 1970-86

Country	1970	1975	1980	1984	1985	1986
			Rate per 1 million people			
Austria	13	56	134	210	256	294
Belgium[1]	30	103	233	394	333	392
Denmark[1]	56	132	202	252	190	262
Finland	25	71	135	232	253	262
France	26	102	229	286	291	303
Germany	18	88	208	301	305	333
Greece	5	48	119	142	154	225
Iceland[1]	20	42	75	105	67	158
Ireland	20	45	99	161	179	193
Italy	6	81	197	238	263	305
Luxembourg	7	91	178	225	277	383
Netherlands	36	90	186	293	289	318
Norway	9	67	134	201	227	234
Portugal	2	4	28	158	197	269
Spain[1]	4	27	145	284	232	337
Sweden	54	85	178	198	319	283
Switzerland	49	136	260	357	383	405
United Kingdom	23	62	128	200	216	242
United States	25	106	272	393	—	—

[1]Because of changes in reporting and incomplete surveys, some entries do not correctly portray trends.

SOURCE: (Organization for Economic Cooperation and Development, 1989).

Table 9

**Patients under treatment for end stage renal disease with functional transplants:
Selected countries, selected years 1970-86**

Country	1970	1975	1980	1984	1985	1986
			Percent of patients			
Austria	19	33	19	23	24	30
Belgium[1]	34	27	28	36	24	33
Denmark[1]	62	53	47	49	45	48
Finland	42	60	65	65	63	58
France	15	13	13	17	19	31
Germany	7	6	8	14	16	17
Greece	39	16	13	13	9	14
Iceland[1]	25	44	53	—	24	47
Ireland	18	27	43	54	52	47
Italy	2	6	7	5	9	12
Luxembourg	—	10	3	8	13	16
Netherlands	18	25	30	42	41	44
Norway	51	74	66	70	75	78
Portugal	1	3	3	7	9	8
Spain[1]	10	4	8	17	19	23
Sweden	50	48	47	47	57	55
Switzerland	31	35	34	40	42	33
United Kingdom	27	36	44	50	48	50
United States	—	—	—	—	[1]22	—

[1]Because of changes in reporting and incomplete surveys, some entries do not correctly portray trends.

SOURCE: (Organization for Economic Cooperation and Development, 1989).

20 percent of all patients treated for ESRD (Bonair, 1988; Eggers, 1988), which is less than one-half the rate of the Scandinavian countries, the United Kingdom, the Netherlands, and Switzerland (Table 9). Efforts have also been made to provide incentives for more transplants in the United States (Eggers, 1988).

The effect on cost per case is difficult to assess for each system. However, there is reason to believe that the incentives in the United States have had an impact on not only the number of treated cases but also the cost per case. Many European health care systems seem to have performed well, compared with the United States, when we look at both cost and cost effectiveness of treatment for ESRD—that is, they have achieved a lower treatment rate and a higher share of transplants. (Also, for many years during the introduction of the technologies, the rate of treatment was higher in many European countries than it was in the United States.) The higher incidence of treated renal failure in the United States is, of course, not necessarily a bad thing. One could argue that the United States is providing better access to a life-saving technology than are the European countries. But the marginal costs and benefits of the extended indications for intervention are largely unknown, and a comparison with European countries is one way to answer the question. The comparative studies that have been undertaken between the United States and the United Kingdom (Aaron and Schwartz, 1984; Marine and Simmons, 1986), do not give a full account of how new technology is managed in Europe. By looking at a greater number of European countries, a better perspective on the U.S. allocation of resources to new technologies can be achieved.

Extracorporeal shock wave lithotripsy

A more recent example of a new medical technology is extracorporeal shock wave lithotripsy (ESWL) for treatment of kidney stones and lately also gallstones. This technology disintegrates stones through the use of shock waves and does not require an incision. It is an equipment-embodied technology and the equipment cost is several million United States dollars. A single ESWL unit can serve a large population, analogous to the specialized services of a heart surgery center or a burn unit. The cost per treated patient is dependent on the number of patients treated per year. ESWL was developed in Germany,

Table 10

Number of extracorporeal shock wave lithotripsy units in operation: Selected countries, May 1989

Country	Total	Per 1 million inhabitants
	Number of units	
Belgium	11	1.10
Germany	57	0.93
Spain	34	0.88
Italy	48	0.84
Sweden	5	0.60
Ireland	2	0.56
Netherlands	8	0.55
France	29	0.53
Greece	5	0.50
Denmark	2	0.39
Portugal	3	0.30
United Kingdom	12	0.21
United States	225	0.88

SOURCE: Jönsson, B.: Linköping University, Linköping, Sweden, 1989.

and the first patients were treated there in 1980. The lithotriptor was approved for widespread clinical use in the United States by the Food and Drug Administration in December 1984, at which time six experimental sites had lithotriptors (Bloom et al., 1989). By July 1, 1986, there were 84 ESWL units in operation in the United States. At that time, 31 States had at least one unit; there were 11 in California, 6 each in Illinois and Texas, and 5 in North Carolina (Bloom, et al., 1989). In the spring of 1989, the number of lithotriptors had increased to about 225. In relation to the size of the population, it is about the same as in countries such as Belgium, Italy, Germany, Spain, and Switzerland (Table 10). However, there are wide variations among European countries; the United Kingdom has by far the lowest number in relation to the population.

The introduction of ESWL has brought up a number of policy issues relating to the introduction of new medical technology in both the United States and Europe. In the United States, the discussion has centered around the problems of adapting the Medicare payment system to this new technology (Office of Technology Assessment, 1986). Because it is neither "medical" nor "surgical" technology, there is no appropriate DRG to which the treatment can be assigned. If the surgical DRG is used, it will grossly overpay the procedure. If the most appropriate medical DRG is used (324-urinary stones, patient age under 70 years, without complications or comorbidities), it only covers about 60 percent of costs (Cotter et al., 1986). The compromise seems to have been to assign all patients treated with ESWL to DRG 323 (urinary stones, patient age over 69 years, with complications or comorbidities), which comes closer to the estimated costs for the procedure (Cotter et al., 1986). However, it has also been suggested that a special DRG should be established for ESWL.

Unlike the situation for many other technologies, the European countries can provide comparative information on both costs and charges for ESWL. In Table 11, a detailed account of the costs for treating the average patient with ESWL in Sweden in 1985 is shown. These costs (U.S. $3,900) include physician salaries and can be compared with an average of $5,700 in the United States (Bloom et al., 1989). The difference in costs can be studied in detail and can give important lessons about the way this technology is used and managed in the different countries. Even more interesting is to look at how costs vary among different types of patients. In Table 12, the cost per patient for treatment of different sizes of kidney stones is shown. Costs increase with the size of the stone, especially for stones larger than 30 millimeters.

Table 11
Distribution of costs for extracorporeal shock wave lithotripsy (ESWL) treatment, by item: Sweden, 1985

Item	Cost per patient[1]	Percent of total
Total costs	24,826	100
Equipment	5,150	21
Building	283	1
Physician salaries	1,360	6
Other salaries	654	3
Anesthesia	1,972	8
Materials, drugs	3,736	15
Other services	1,039	4
	14,194	57
Adjuvant procedures	515	2
Laboratories:		
Radiology	2,122	9
Chemistry	1,593	6
Intensive care	1,057	4
	4,772	19
Ward:		
Building	449	2
Physician salaries	768	3
Other salaries	1,917	8
Materials, drugs	516	2
Services (excluding laboratory)	1,695	7
	5,345	22

[1]In Swedish kronor.

NOTE: Percents may not add to totals shown because of rounding.

SOURCE: (Carlsson, Jönsson, and Tiselius, 1987).

Table 12
Costs[1] per patient for extracorporeal shock wave lithotripsy (ESWL) for different types of stones, by cost item: Sweden, 1985

Cost item	Size of stone				Ureter stone	Bilateral treatment
	5 mm or less	6-20 mm	21-30 mm	30 mm or more		
Total cost per patient	17,880	20,437	26,689	49,416	17,618	32,707
ESWL treatment	8,879	11,680	14,892	22,766	8,768	17,474
Intensive care unit	900	987	1,074	1,800	900	1,800
Radiology	2,561	2,017	2,365	5,000	2,427	3,658
Clinical chemistry laboratory	1,448	1,466	1,706	2,516	1,458	1,761
Adjuvant procedures	220	230	198	3,045	100	1,100
Recovery	3,872	4,057	6,454	14,568	3,965	7,014
Number of cases	4	84	31	13	15	14

[1]In Swedish kronor.

SOURCE: (Carlsson, Jönsson, and Tiselius, 1987).

Detailed comparisons of costs and charges can give interesting information of relevance in assessing the consequences of the reimbursement system in the United States and can suggest ideas for reform. However, there are also other aspects of health systems that must not be overlooked. The regionalized systems in Europe can provide population-based data on utilization of medical technology that can be used to study the proper indications for as well as the consequences of new medical technology. The role of medical technology assessment in the management of new technology can also be an interesting area for comparison. The European countries do not have a formal approval system for medical devices. Nevertheless, many countries in Europe have performed more comprehensive evaluations, including not only safety and efficacy, but also cost effectiveness and quality of life, of ESWL than have been undertaken in the United States. Such comprehensive evaluations of ESWL for the treatment of gallstones are now under way in both Sweden and the United Kingdom. These assessments form part of the policy for controlling the diffusion of medical technology. In addition, the wide diversity of policies used in the European countries can yield interesting lessons for the management of the same technologies in the United States.

Are health care systems converging?

European health care systems obviously differ from the U.S. system in important aspects. There are also important differences among European systems. One important difference is the open-endedness (that is, the lack of budget restrictions) of the systems. However, the need to contain costs has forced open-ended systems to find different ways to restrict total expenditures for health care. It seems clear that a "free" market cannot solve the basic resource allocation problems in health care: efficiency and equity in health care production and consumption. Public insurance systems, tax subsidies to private insurance, asymmetric information between producers and consumers, and provider monopolies through licensing (doctors) are inherent factors in a health care system that make free competition an ineffective policy; competition has to be "managed."

In the United States, the discussion of managed competition has centered on HMOs and their ability to provide total coverage for health care at a lower cost than traditional fee-for-service arrangements. The jury is still out (see the article by Culyer in this issue), but the discussion has already changed the perception of what is needed to contain costs and increase efficiency in health care. The idea of prospective payment lies behind the development of DRGs to classify patients. This system, developed at Yale University, is as close as one can come to what Oscar Lange (1938) called "market socialism." Hospitals compete against a set of predetermined administrative prices. So far, this payment method has been used only for Medicare-covered inpatient

acute hospital care, but work is under way to extend it to ambulatory care. Another example of how the health care market has changed in the United States is the introduction of medical technology assessment (MTA) as a tool for health policy. The role of MTA in U.S. health policy has been controversial, but it was invented as a response to a need for more information for policymakers—this information will be needed even more in the future. Today, when the era of rapidly expanding health care resources has come to an end, new medical technology is the major dynamic factor in health care. Clearly, future policy will be aimed at control of introduction and diffusion of new medical technology. Medical technology assessment, based on explicit cost-effectiveness and cost-benefit studies, will certainly have a major role in the development of those policies.

The convergence theory implies that planning will play an increasing role in market economies. Developments in the United States during the 1980s cannot accurately be described as increased health care planning. But they certainly represent an increase in public control over the health care system. This can best be understood by looking at the great attraction HMOs, DRGs, and MTA have had for health researchers and policymakers in Europe. These ideas have fit in well with the more comprehensive and planned systems in Europe. They have been seen as a way to increase the role of markets and competition within systems in which traditional planning has proven impotent to adapt to a situation of slower resource growth with continued introduction of new medical technology. In this way we can talk about a convergence of systems.

This convergence creates interesting opportunities for the future. When new ideas, such as HMOs, DRGs, and MTA, are transferred to European countries, it is possible for the United States to learn how they work under different regulatory conditions. How will HMOs work when based on regional, rather than voluntary, participation? How will HMOs that include the elderly work? It has been suggested that the evidence for cost savings from HMOs in the United States is not relevant for Europe, because the majority of HMO members are under 65 years of age. This may be the case, but one hypothesis could be that HMOs will yield even greater savings for the elderly, who have higher consumption rates of care and for whom there are more alternatives for intervention. These questions can be answered, if experimentation on a broad basis can be started in Europe. Changes in the health care systems of the Netherlands and the United Kingdom, based on Enthoven's ideas, are already under way. The first HMO is also about to be started in Switzerland.

The DRG system has been introduced, at least on the research agenda, in most European countries from Sweden in the north to Portugal in the south. There is also a very interesting experiment under way with financial incentives for hospital efficiency in Leningrad, U.S.S.R. (Hakansson et al., 1988). The research and the experiments in Europe will give not only interesting comparative data on DRG groupings, but also information about how, for example, physician costs can be integrated in the DRG payment and how this will change the weights.

Medical technology assessment, including consensus conferences, has also been imported into Europe from the United States. The Netherlands and Sweden have been in the forefront of this movement and have established special government committees for MTA. The European Regional Office for the World Health Organization has a special program for MTA, and introduction of MTA is one of the targets for "Health for All" by the year 2000. Within the European Common Market, a special committee for MTA has been set up within the health service research committee. It seems that today, MTA is more vital and growing in Europe than in the United States. This will, in the longer term, produce important information on medical technologies that are also used in the United States and will give lessons on how MTA can be implemented as part of health policymaking.

Conclusion

The single most important lesson from the European health care systems during the 1980s concerns the role of central government. The European systems have been able to reduce the total costs of health care not so much through central planning and regulation as through global budgets at the regional level. In fact, the role of the central government in health care policy has never been as strong in Europe as is perhaps thought in the United States, and during the 1980s there has been a strong trend toward decentralization. The reason for this is the obvious difficulty in managing such a huge and complicated system from the center. Compared with Europe, the U.S. Federal Government seems to have less control over the totality of the system, at the same time that it is more directly involved in detailed regulation of efficacy, safety, and price setting. Leadership and control of global expenditures and decisions regarding the comprehensiveness of the system must come from the center, but planning and management should be left to the regional level. Decentralization can be combined with internal markets and competition among providers. Planning and markets are not necessarily antithetical; they can work together to create better health services.

Acknowledgments

I am grateful for the helpful comments of A. J. Culyer and Jean-Pierre Poullier.

References

Aaron, H. J., and Schwartz, W. B.: *The Painful Prescription: Rationing Hospital Care*. Washington. Brookings Studies in Social Economics. 1984.

Anderson, O. W.: *Health Care: Can There Be Equity? The United States, Sweden and England*. New York. Wiley, 1972.

Bloom, B. S., Hillman, A. L., Roy, R. B., and Swartz, J. S.: Early patterns of diffusion, organization and use of ESWL. *Scandinavian Journal of Urology and Nephrology* (supplementum 122): 95-102, 1989.

Bonair, A.: *Spridning av medicinsk teknologi*. Report prepared for SBU, The Swedish Council on Technology Assessment in Health Care. Linköping, Sweden. 1988.

Carlsson, P., Jönsson, B., and Tiselius, H. G.: Impact of extracorporeal lithotripsy on patient management: Intermediate results from the Swedish assessment study. *International Journal of Technology Assessment in Health Care* 3(3):405-417, 1987.

Cotter, D. C., Chu, F., Braid, M. J., and Perry, S.: *National Health Services and Practice Patterns Survey: Report on Extracorporeal Shockwave Lithotripsy Operating Costs, Medicare Payments, and Utilization Rates*. Washington, D.C. Institute for Health Policy Analysis, Georgetown University Medical Center. 1986.

Culyer, A. J., Maynard, A., and Williams, A.: Alternative systems of health care provision: An essay on motes and beams. In Olson, M., ed. *A New Approach to the Economics of Health Care*. Washington, D.C. American Enterprise Institute, 1981.

Davis, K.: National health insurance: A proposal. *American Economic Review* 79(4):349-352, 1989.

Department of Health and Social Security: Sharing Resources for Health. Report of the Resource Allocation Working Party. London. Her Majesty's Stationery Office, 1976.

Drukker, W., Parsons, F. M., and Maher, J. F., eds.: *Replacement of Renal Function by Dialysis: A Textbook of Dialysis*. Martinus Nijhoff Publishers, 1986.

Eggers, P. W.: Effect of transplantation on the Medicare end-stage renal disease program. *New England Journal of Medicine* 318(4):223-229, 1988.

Enthoven, A.: *Health Plan: The Only Practical Solution to the Soaring Costs of Medical Care*. Reading, Mass. Addison-Wesley, 1980.

Enthoven, A.: Managed competition: An agenda for action. *Health Affairs*, pp. 25-47, Summer 1988.

Fries, J. F.: Aging, natural death and the compression of morbidity. *New England Journal of Medicine* 303:130-135, 1980.

Gerdtham, U., Andersson, F., Sögaard, J., and Jönsson, B.: *Econometric Analysis of Health Care Expenditures*. Report 1988:9. Linköping, Sweden. Center for Medical Technology Assessment, Linköping University, 1988.

Gygi, P., and Frei, A.: *The Swiss Health Care System*. Basle. G. Krebs and Co., 1986.

Hakansson, S., Majnoni d'Intignano, B., Roberts, J., and Zollner, H.: The Leningrad Experiment in Health Care Management. World Health Organization Report SSR/MPN 501. Copenhagen. 1988.

Henke, K.: What can Americans learn from the German health insurance system? *Social Science* 55:134-137, 1980.

Jönsson, B., and Rehnberg, C.: *Effektivare sjukvård*. Stockholm. Almqvist & Wiksell, 1987.

Kasper, J. D.: *Perspectives on Health Care: United States, 1980.* National Medical Care Utilization and Expenditure Survey. Series B, Descriptive Report No. 14. Office of Research and Demonstrations, Health Care Financing Administration. Washington. U.S. Government Printing Office, Sept. 1986.

Lange, O.: On the economic theory of socialism. In Lipincott, B. E., ed. *On the Economic Theory of Socialism.* Minneapolis. University of Minnesota Press, 1938.

Le Grand, J., and Rabin, M.: Trends in British health inequality, 1931-83. In Culyer, A. J., and Jönsson, B., eds. *Public and Private Health Services.* London. Basil Blackwell, 1986.

Lembcke, P. A.: Hospital efficiency—A lesson from Sweden. *Hospitals* 33:34-38, 1959.

Marine, S. K., and Simmons, R. G.: Policies regarding treatment of end-stage renal disease in the United States and United Kingdom. *International Journal of Technology Assessment in Health Care* 2(2):253-274, 1986.

Mays, N., and Bevan, G.: Resource Allocation in the Health Service. Occasional Papers on Social Administration No. 81. London. Bedford Square Press, 1987.

Navarro, V.: *National and Regional Health Planning in Sweden.* DHEW Pub. No. 74-240. Washington. U.S. Government Printing Office, 1974.

Organization for Economic Cooperation and Development: *Financing and Delivering of Health Care: A Comparative Analysis of OECD Countries.* Social Policy Studies No. 4. Paris. 1987.

Organization for Economic Cooperation and Development: Health Data File. Paris. Directorate for Social Affairs, Manpower, and Education, 1989.

Office of Technology Assessment, U.S. Congress: *Effects of Federal Policies on Extracorporeal Shock Wave Lithotripsy.* Pub. No. OTA-HCS-36. Washington. U.S. Government Printing Office, 1986.

Parkin, D.: Comparing health service efficiency across countries. *Oxford Review of Economic Policy* 5(7):75-88, Spring 1989.

Reinhardt, U. E.: Health insurance and cost containment policies: The experience abroad. In Olson, M., ed. *A New Approach to the Economics of Health.* Washington. American Enterprise Institute, 1981.

Rosenthal, M.: Beyond equity? Swedish health policy and the private sector. *The Milbank Quarterly* 64 (supplement 1):34-55, 1986.

Rosenthal, M.: *Dealing with Medical Malpractice: The British and Swedish Experience.* London. Tavistock, 1987.

Rutten, F.: Health policy in the Netherlands. In McLachland, G., and Maynard, A., eds. *The Public/Private Mix for Health.* Abingdon, United Kingdom. The Nuffield Provincial Hospitals Trust, 1982.

Saltman, R. B., and von Otter, C.: Re-vitalizing public health care systems: A proposal for public competition in Sweden. *Health Policy,* pp. 21-40, 1987.

Stone, D. A.: Health care cost containment in West Germany. *Journal of Health Politics, Policy and Law* 4:176-199, 1979.

Stahl, I.: Can equality and efficiency be combined? The experience of the planned Swedish health care system. In Olson, M., ed. *A New Approach to the Economics of Health Care.* Washington. American Enterprise Institute, 1981.

van de Ven, W.P.M.M.: A Future for Competitive Health Care in the Netherlands. NHS White Occasional Paper No. 9. York, United Kingdom. Center for Health Economics, University of York, 1989.

Waaler, H. T., and Sterky, G.: What is the best indicator of health care? *World Health Forum* 5:276-279, 1984.

World Health Organization: *Development of Indicators for Monitoring Progress Towards Health for All by the Year 2000.* Health for All Series, No. 4. Geneva, 1981.

Respondents:

Klaus-Dirk Henke

The Federal Republic of Germany (hereafter called Germany) proves that one can achieve universal enrollment and comprehensive insurance coverage without having a form of socialized medicine. In addition—and this is a European challenge to the United States—medical care is provided to everyone, regardless of income, social status, or residence. This is accepted as a major goal of national health insurance in Germany and other European countries.

The sickness fund system, which covers approximately 90 percent of the population, is decentralized and self-governed by autonomous administrations. There are no government agencies; the funds are almost completely independent of the

Reprint requests: Professor Klaus-Dirk Henke, Universität Hannover, Institut für Volkswirtschaftslehre, Wunstorferstrasse 14, D-3000 Hannover, Bundesrepublik Deutschland.

Federal Government and the States (Länder). Federal law merely requires that persons with incomes below a certain level receive mandatory health insurance coverage and that health care be sufficient and effective according to the standards of medical practice. This means that the organization of the sickness funds and the medical associations make their negotiations in the fields of hospital and ambulatory care, dental care, medical appliances, etc., in principal without government interference. This mixture of Federal control and decentralized administration is typical of the European countries, as Jönsson has written.

The statutory insurance plan, with the underlying principle of self-government, is administered by some 1,150 different funds (local sickness funds, industrial funds, crafts funds, rural funds, sailors' fund, miners' fund, blue-collar-workers' funds, and white-collar-workers' funds). The different types of sickness funds vary as to the number of individual member funds. In 1988, almost 24 percent of all funds were local sickness funds, with 46 percent of the mandatorily insured. At the same time, the industrial funds, comprising more than 60 percent of all funds, covered only approximately 11.5 percent of the population insured with the sickness fund system.

The funds are governed by a board of directors and an assembly of representatives from both the insured employees and their employers. The payroll tax that finances the system is split equally between the employees and employers. The payroll tax base consists mainly of wages, salaries, and lately also pensions. Thus the payroll taxes are totally independent of individual, medical, and social risks of the insured and provide coverage for the insured and (nonworking) family dependents. In case of unemployment, old age, disability, or poverty, special provisions are made for paying contributions. Either other branches of the social security system (old age fund, unemployment fund, etc.) or the Federal/regional government pays the contribution fees. In Germany, the old age fund provides a transfer to the statutory insurance fund system, and the unemployment fund pays the fees in case of unemployment. The unemployed, disabled, or aged are covered within their fund, and the fund is compensated for the fees.

The tax base for the payroll tax is defined by the Health Insurance Law and does not correspond to the broader concept of income used for taxing personal income. Copayments (user charges) under statutory health insurance are limited to a few items, such as dentures, eyeglasses, and prescription drugs. There is also a small daily charge for the first 14 days in a hospital, and a daily charge for inpatient rehabilitation treatment. Experts estimate the total of copayments to be only about 5 percent of total health care expenditures of the statutory sickness funds. This percentage will rise in the near future as a consequence of the 1989 health reform law, one of the major objectives of which is the stability of the payroll tax rate, which is presently at a level of almost 13 percent. The philosophy behind payroll tax stability is to steer the health care sector according to the revenue available and thus hold down labor costs. The current payroll tax rate, which may (from an American perspective) seem incredibly high, finances all the benefits under the plan that are centrally defined, with only little freedom for the funds to add certain services.

The sickness fund plan

The insured population is limited by residence and occupation in its freedom to choose a sickness fund. Approximately 50 percent of the individuals may choose their own health insurance, but this choice does not mean that the benefit packages differ much. The benefits (services) under statutory health insurance in Germany are almost the same for all covered persons and include:

- Free ambulatory care and free (unlimited) hospital care.
- Freedom to choose any general practitioner or specialist (including dentists) registered with the sickness fund.
- Preventive care.
- Family planning.
- Medical services when needed for rehabilitation.
- Maternity benefits (free pregnancy tests, free ambulatory and hospital treatment, midwife care, cash benefits, and household help if the pregnant woman has children under 8 years of age or a disabled child).

Legal maternity leave extends from 6 weeks prior to 8 weeks after confinement. Moreover, the mother can choose to stay at home for 6 months after confinement, with a small monthly salary paid by the employer.

Upon expiration of the continued payment period (generally 6 weeks, during which the employer continues to pay one's salary), an employed person insured by statutory health insurance receives, when he or she is unfit for work, sick benefits (80 percent of the normal wage or salary) for a period of up to 78 weeks (within any 3-year period). When this period expires, the beneficiary is entitled to a pension based on disability or to social assistance (welfare payments). With the new health insurance law, benefits for people who care for the elderly, new services in prevention, and quality assurance are included under the sickness fund plan. At the same time, certain services are reduced (e.g., burial allowances, cash subsidies for dentures).

The range of benefits is extended by a certain degree of competition among the various sickness funds, which may provide extended medical services. The Health Insurance Law requires that medical care be "sufficient and effective according to the standards of medical practice." With only the qualification that it be "necessary," the built-in tendency for expansion of benefits is further strengthened in the system. Furthermore, adjudication of insurance claims is handled by a system of special courts (Sozialgerichte), which are generally inclined toward a generous interpretation of the claimants' rights.

At present there is a lively political and academic debate about the various risk structures of the different funds. With regard to age, sex, number of family dependents, and payroll tax base, there are significant differences that cause unfair competition among the funds. Various solutions for balancing these risk structures are in the center of the discussion and are considered a major subject for further health care reforms. A balanced risk structure would offer a basis for persons to choose not to participate in the system and to choose from a variety of health plans with a minimum level of protection. At present, only persons with incomes above a certain income level (54,900 Deutsch marks in 1989, which is roughly equal to the average annual employee compensation) may join a private health insurance plan. If one's income again falls below the (dynamic) income level, he or she may stay in the private plan or go back to the statutory health insurance plan.

In addition to the statutory health insurance system, there is a small public health service, administered and financed on a local basis, and a factory-based physician service, organized and paid for by the employers, in large companies.

Health care for the mentally ill is considered to be poor. Care for the elderly in nursing homes is not included under public or private health insurance plans and is financed by local welfare funds, if individual incomes are insufficient to cover the nursing home bill.

Redistributive effects

Benefits from private health insurance are, to a certain degree, equivalent to those already described, except that private insurers offer a variety of plans with copayments. But one must keep in mind the different redistributive effects of an income-related financing system and a risk-oriented premium system. According to the provision of benefits and income-related financing, there are not only risk-related redistributive effects between age and sex groups but also between:

• Single-person households or couples without children, and families.
• Persons with differing incomes.
• Retired persons and employed persons.

These and other processes of income redistribution through the statutory sickness fund system are known on a qualitative level but are largely unknown quantitatively. This is particularly true when considered from a life-cycle perspective, rather than a cross-sectional-analysis view. In private health insurance plans, these effects are restricted to distributive effects within the age cohort in question. These effects play a significant role in the European context and are not particularly dealt with in Jönsson's article. The sickness fund system is a significant instrument of income redistribution. Politicians must decide whether they want this redistribution restricted to the population involved or to the total population through the tax transfer system. Many experts already consider the social security system in Europe to be part of the overall transfer system.

Lack of cost-consciousness

A negative feature of German national health insurance is the absence of cost consciousness among physicians and patients. A major cause could be that there is no direct economic relationship between the two. The basis of demand for health services is the sickness voucher that each insured person receives on request from the sickness fund for each calendar quarter. Providers keep a record of the services rendered on the sickness voucher, which is normally not signed by the patient. The patients insured by the statutory health insurance fund are not given an invoice for their medical treatment either. Office-based physicians receive their reimbursement quarterly from the various statutory health insurance funds to which their patients belong and by way of the regionalphysicians' association (Figure 1). Because of

this institutional setting and because copayments still play a minor role, cost consciousness on the part of patients and physicians is severely underdeveloped. This may lead to both fiscal illusions and an abuse of the system by both parties. Patients may insist on overtreatment or certain types of services. Doctors, in turn, are stimulated to provide these services by the fee-for-service system, which induces them to see as many patients as possible and to provide as many services as possible in a given time span. A better understanding of costs and benefits could be achieved in Germany if health insurance were changed from a system of benefits in kind to a cost-reimbursement system, in which the patient pays the medical bill first, then is reimbursed by the sickness fund. This system, although difficult to introduce completely, would then facilitate the introduction of certain types of coinsurance. At present, expenditure targets and other cost-control mechanisms are being installed or intensively discussed for the different sectors (pharmaceutical, inpatient, or outpatient care, etc.).

Cost containment

Health care expenditures could be reduced in many ways. For example, many routine physician activities could be handled by paraprofessionals, thus saving money. Such activities include renewing prescriptions and issuing certificates of illness, which are needed by patients to receive their sickness allowances. More and better medical knowledge, healthier life styles, risk rating, and more concern for medical costs must not be ignored. Programs to better inform and educate patients are still in their infancy and call for further debate and vision. Furthermore, the power of the sickness funds must be increased to make them more effective when negotiating with the physician associations.

In 1977, a new instrument of health policy was established, called Concerted Action in Health Care, bringing together the main participants in the health care system, i.e., representatives of health services providers, health insurance funds, employers, trade unions, and State and Federal governments. Concerted Action deals primarily with managing the expenditures of the statutory health insurance funds. Its participants will develop recommendations to improve efficacy and efficiency in health care. On the basis of the findings of Concerted Action, the providers and funds make their negotiations and contracts.

Since 1986, a board of (medical and economic) advisers to Concerted Action in Health Care provides in its annual reports medical and economic guidelines on which Concerted Action can base its various recommendations. Concerted Action is the major forum in which the various health care participants meet publicly to decide upon the further development of the health care system. In particular, the group discusses the allocation of financial resources of the statutory health insurance funds for the various types of services.

Figure 1
Flow of funds and sickness vouchers in ambulatory care: Federal Republic of Germany

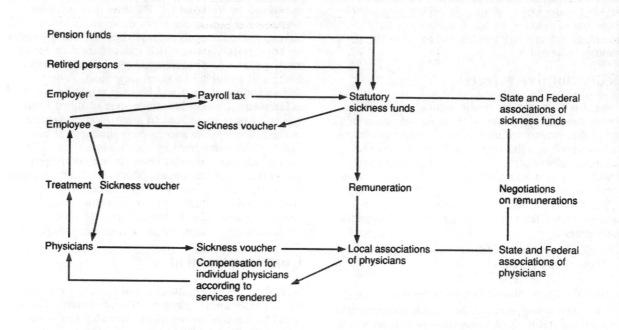

NOTES: The sickness voucher that insured persons receive on request from their sickness funds each calendar quarter is the basis for their demand for covered services. The assocation of physicians registered with the statutory health insurance fund has to guarantee sufficient medical service everywhere.

SOURCE: Henke, K. D.: Universität Hannover, Hannover, Federal Republic of Germany, 1989.

To realize a constant payroll tax rate, expenditures for the various types of health services may, on average, increase only by the rate of growth of the payroll tax base. This economic guideline should, in fact, leave enough room for the expenditure categories to increase by different rates, according to necessary changes in the treatment mix. But there is still the question of who will establish health care priorities and by what means these priorities will be set. With payroll tax rate stability being a major objective, a permanent change of emphasis from unnecessary to indispensable health services is called for. In making this change, the right incentives are important, if one does not want the government or parliament to define health care priorities. In addition, it is necessary to discuss in more detail the development of and the differing pricing mechanisms in the various health care fields (e.g., dental, inpatient, outpatient, pharmaceutical). Otherwise, it is impossible to find ways to equalize—as the economists would say—the marginal utility of health care expenditures by the statutory health insurance system. So far, there are no evaluative studies concerning the effectiveness of these cost-containment efforts.

Summary

In case the majority of Americans want more universal and comprehensive insurance coverage, while avoiding socialized medicine (in either provision or financing of care), the German, Dutch, French, and other European health care systems offer valuable lessons. Their experiences prove that federally mandated systems need not include federal administration of the system. At the same time, federal leadership is required to encourage competition. International health services research is needed to provide the necessary data, including better and more up-to-date information on current health care reforms in Europe.

Uwe E. Reinhardt

In this commentary, I should like to summarize my understanding of Jönsson's article and complement his remarks with some additional perspectives. To provide a backdrop for my remarks, I begin with a bird's-eye view of the fiscal relationships in modern health care. Next, I employ a compact menu of alternative cost-control policies to highlight the differences between the European and the American approaches to that task, relying on both Jönsson's and my own insights into European health systems. Finally, I comment on the "convergence theory" proposed by Jönsson and add another convergence theory of my own.

I should mention at the outset that I have enjoyed reading Jönsson's instructive paper and that I have gained valuable new insights from it.

Economic relationships in health care

At the highest level of abstraction, the economic relationships embedded in the delivery of health care

Reprint requests: Uwe E. Reinhardt, Ph.D., Woodrow Wilson School of Public and International Affairs, Princeton University, Princeton, New Jersey 08544.

can be distilled into three distinct nexuses, as shown in Figure 1.

In nexus A, a third-party payer—either a private insurance carrier or a government—shoulders the financial risks of illness the patient would otherwise face, in exchange for a transfer of money. At one extreme, this transfer takes the form of "actuarially fair" insurance premiums that reflect the insured's own health status as best as it can be determined by the insurer, as would be the case for an individually purchased health insurance policy bought from a commercial carrier. At the other extreme, the transfer takes the form of taxes or premiums that are totally divorced from the insured's health status and based strictly on ability to pay.

All of the European health insurance systems are based on the latter extreme for the great bulk of their populations, because Europeans tend to view actuarially fair health insurance premiums as manifestly unfair and believe that contributions to health insurance should be based on ability to pay. Most Americans probably abhor actuarially fair health insurance premiums as well. Indeed, the bulk of Americans are covered either by tax-financed government programs or by private group policies that socialize health insurance, at least within the community of a single business firm.

Figure 1
Economic relationships embedded in the delivery of health care

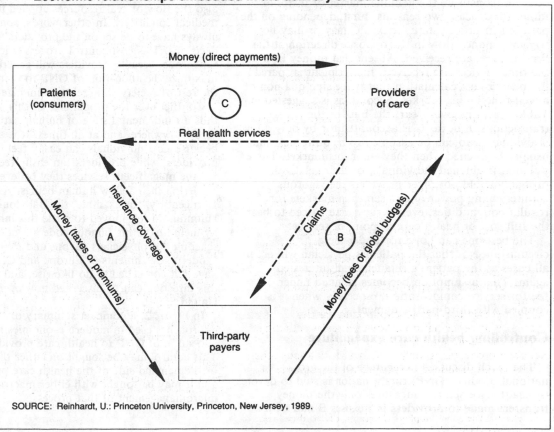

SOURCE: Reinhardt, U.: Princeton University, Princeton, New Jersey, 1989.

Table 1

Distribution of health expenditures, by magnitude of expenditures: United States, selected years, 1970-80

Percent of population ranked by expenditures	1970	1977	1980
Top 1 percent	26	27	29
Top 2 percent	35	38	39
Top 5 percent	50	55	55
Top 10 percent	66	70	70
Top 30 percent	88	90	90
Top 50 percent	96	97	96
Bottom 50 percent	4	3	4

SOURCE: (Berk, Monheit, and Hagan, 1988).

In nexus B of Figure 1, the third-party payer transfers money to providers under a variety of distinct compensation methods. These methods may range all the way from piece-rate compensation (triggering a money flow for each distinct service or supply a provider reports to have delivered to a patient) to prepaid compensation in the form of capitation or salaries for physicians or global budgets for inpatient facilities. One finds all of these methods used in the European health systems.

Finally, in nexus C of Figure 1, health services and supplies are transferred from individual providers of health care to individual patients. Nexus C represents what economists call the "market" for health care (services and supplies). In fact, however, that nexus does not constitute the genuine market of textbook fame, for at least two reasons. First, depending on the patient's insurance status, nexus C may or may not trigger a money flow in the opposite direction at the time services are received. Absent that money flow at the time services are received, the recipient is spared the benefit-cost calculation that is the sine qua non of a well-functioning market. Second, as is suggested in Table 1, in any given year, the bulk of the transactions in nexus C is accounted for by only a few individuals who can be assumed to be quite sick and usually frightened when they enter this market. These sick and frightened individuals, or their relatives, probably could not offer providers the vigorous countervailing power one observes in markets for regular commodities, even if they were forced to bear the full cost of health care at point of service.

The best one can hope for under these circumstances is that the patient's physician will act in all cases as the patient's financially disinterested agent. That assumption becomes strained under fee-for-service compensation, especially when it is coupled with third-party payment.

Controlling health care expenditure

The much-discussed percentage of the gross national product (GNP) that a nation is said to devote to health care actually measures only the money transfers made to providers in nexuses B and C; it does not reveal what real resources actually flowed to patients in return for this money transfer. Strictly speaking, that percentage also includes whatever funds the third-party payers retained as income or to cover administrative expenses. Furthermore, it includes certain expenditures (e.g., the construction of certain types of facilities or spending on basic medical research) not factored into the payments made directly to the providers of health care. Even within an American city, one finds vast differences in the money transfers made to doctors and hospitals for well-defined standard medical procedures, and one observes similar variation across national borders.

There is, then, considerable leeway in the amount of GNP that providers can extract from the rest of society per unit of health service and overall. American readers, for example, should be intrigued by Jönsson's suggestion that the amount of GNP transferred to American providers per patient treated with extracorporeal shock wave lithotripsy (ESWL) appears to be about 50 percent higher than the amount of GNP per patient that Swedes transfer to their providers of ESWL. To be sure, Jönsson's is a very rough estimate. Even so, he is correct in asserting that much could be learned by Americans from Europe in the use and pricing of new medical technologies.

To control the allocation of GNP to providers, the rest of society must somehow control not only the amount of money providers may extract from society per unit of real resource transferred to patients, but also the flow of real resources applied to given medical conditions. In other words, some limits will always have to be set on the providers' clinical decisions. This cost-control process is inherently rancorous, because providers will generally seek to maximize the allocation of GNP to themselves, and the rest of society will seek to minimize it.

Conflict over the proper size of this allocation is thus a fundamental state of human nature in health care everywhere, and at all times. It is all the more so because sick individuals can easily feel exploited by providers, while providers can easily feel underpaid for the magnificent services they believe they are rendering their fellow human beings. As early as the 18th century, for example, the Babylonian King Hammurabi felt moved to settle this inherent conflict by including in his famous code a binding fee schedule for physicians (Lyons and Petrucelli, 1978). Modern governments in Europe and Canada typically have felt compelled to do likewise, and a stirring in this direction can be discerned now even in the United States.

In Figure 2, a compact summary of the various approaches used in modern economies to control the allocation of GNP to health care providers is shown. This control may be sought on either the supply side or the demand side of the health care process, and it may be sought with either macro- or micromanagement of that process.

Figure 2

Alternative cost-containment strategies in health care

Target	Micromanagement	Macromanagement
Supply-side strategies	• Encouragement of efficiency in the production of medical treatments through economic incentives, for example, diagnosis-related groups or capitation. • Legal constraints on the ownership of health care facilities.	• Regional planning designed to limit the physical capacity of the health system and to ensure its desired distribution among regions and social classes.
Demand-side strategies	• Conversion of patients to consumers through cost sharing. • Hands-on supervision of decisions of doctors and their patients (managed care).	• Predetermined global budgets for hospitals and expenditure caps for physicians.
Strategies aimed at the market as a whole		• Price controls.

SOURCE: Reinhardt, U.: Princeton University, Princeton, New Jersey, 1989.

European macromanagement

As Jönsson shows, most European nations tend to emphasize macromanagement in the control of their health systems. They seek to guide their health systems not primarily through the use of fine-tuned financial incentives aimed at providers and patients but instead through direct, regulatory edict.

The supply side of European health systems is typically managed with explicit regional planning, designed to distribute health care equitably among regions and social classes. In addition, there are usually strict limits on the overall physical capacity of at least the hospital sector, designed to control the flow of real resources into health care.

Because the supply-side regulations favored in Europe inevitably create provider monopolies, these regulations are accompanied on the demand side by strong controls on the compensation of providers. The European nations achieve these demand-side controls by concentrating the flow of money from third-party payers to providers (nexus B in Figure 1) into one or more large pipes, the monetary throughput of which can easily be controlled with the turn of one or more powerful valves. These valves are operated either by a government (e.g., in the United Kingdom and the Scandinavian countries) or by regional associations of private health insurers endowed by statute with quasi-governmental powers to operate all-payer systems that negotiate binding contracts with regional associations of providers as in, for example, the system of the Federal Republic of Germany (hereafter called Germany).

Usually, the individual European patient is not viewed as a potent agent of cost control—certainly not in the case of serious illness. Indeed, in many European countries (the Scandinavian countries, the United Kingdom, Germany, and Italy), nexus C, between patients and providers, does not involve a money flow at all.

Where European providers are compensated on a fee-for-service basis, their prices are typically subject to binding price ceilings. In such cases, the utilization of services is usually monitored by third-party payers through retrospective statistical profiles of individual providers, who may face financial penalties if they deviate significantly from the average. Because it is so difficult to effectively control the volume of health services through retrospective utilization review, however, the demand side in European health care is frequently subject also to fixed overall budget constraints. This approach is natural where the public sector actually owns the bulk of health care facilities (e.g., in the United Kingdom and the Scandinavian countries). But such overall budget caps are now being used also in countries dominated by private providers. In Germany, for example, the individual physician in ambulatory practice is compensated on a fee-for-service basis, but subject to a global expenditure cap for all physicians in a region (the state). If total billings by physicians exceed the global budget, fees are later reduced commensurately. (Inpatient physician services are rendered by salaried physicians employed by the hospital and thus are not affected by this cap.)

Americans who look to European health systems as potential models for the United States learn from Jönsson's article that many Europeans are now actually somewhat disillusioned with the heavy-handed fiscal and physical controls on their health systems.

To be sure, they have been successful in stemming the flow of money to providers. Throughout the 1980s, most of these systems have succeeded in maintaining the percentage of GNP going to health care at a relatively constant level, ranging between 6 and 9 percent across Europe. At the same time, health spending in the United States rose from 9.1 percent of the GNP in 1980 to 11.4 percent in 1987. On the other hand, the regulatory strictures in Europe often limit the freedom of choice available to patients and, in particular, the amenities accompanying the delivery of care.

For many years now, European health policy analysts have scouted the American landscape to learn which of the many new economic arrangements developed and practiced here might be grafted onto the European systems. As Jönsson notes, attempts are under way now to insert such American inventions as diagnosis-related groups (DRGs) and health maintenance organizations into the regulatory European systems. How these American inventions perform within the more highly regulated European structures, suggests Jönsson, will furnish a valuable object lesson for Americans, who are beginning to question their entrepreneurial, market-driven health system and to reexamine their traditional aversion to regulation.

American micromanagement

Throughout their history, Americans have been fearful of concentrating economic power in the hands of a few who might be either corrupt, or inept, or both. Consequently, Americans have traditionally looked askance at regulatory macromanagement of their health care system. Instead of concentrating the flow of money to providers into one or a few major pipes, the American health system lets these funds flow through a myriad of small, uncoordinated conduits coming directly from patients (nexus C in Figure 1) and from literally thousands of third-party payers, including governments at all levels, business firms, insurance companies, labor unions, and countless private, voluntary agencies (nexus B).

The global health care budgets imposed in Europe can easily be kept too tight, thereby withholding from the citizenry health services that they might wish to procure and to finance. Such mistakes are unlikely in the pluralistic American system, where any attempt on the part of one third-party payer to tighten the valve under that payer's control would quickly result in loss of access to health care for patients insured by the payer. An individual payer—even one as large as a nationwide commercial insurer or General Motors—will therefore always think twice before attempting rigorous cost-control over providers, even if the payers believe they are paying too much for too many services and supporting vast excess capacity in the system.

And therein, of course, lies one reason for this Nation's extraordinarily high health care expenditures. For better or for worse, our health system is designed to render patients and third-party payers relatively impotent in the market for health services. This then vastly enhances the GNP share that providers can receive, not only per year but also per unit of health care delivered. Where European (and Canadian) providers have for years chafed under the yoke of a monopsonistic health care market—leaving the rest of society luxuriating in relatively low health care expenditures—their American counterparts have been able to luxuriate in a system over whose financial flows they have wielded substantial control through the principle of "divide and rule"—leaving the rest of American society to chafe under the yoke of seemingly uncontrollable health expenditures.

In seeking control over their ever-rising health care costs, Americans have meandered back and forth between advocacy of government regulation and espousal of free-market principles (Altman and Rodwin, 1988). During the 1960s and 1970s, for example, American health policy tended to move toward more regulation, which went so far as to embrace, during the mid-1970s, some feeble and therefore unsuccessful attempts at regional planning. During the early 1980s, Americans had tired of regulation—without really having tried it—and embraced with enthusiasm the so-called pro-competitive market approach. At this time, the Nation appears to be tiring of that approach as well—once again, without really having tried it—and the 1990s are likely to witness a reversion to various forms of regulation.

The so-called pro-competitive strategy of the 1980s was based on the thesis that a set of carefully crafted financial incentives could efficiently and optimally allocate real health care resources among patients and could also determine the proper allocation of GNP to providers. These incentives were to be aimed at both the supply side and the demand side of the health care market. The effectiveness of that approach, in terms of its stated objectives, remains a matter of controversy.

Micromanagement of the supply side

Global constraints on the supply side, so common in Europe and briefly espoused during the 1970s even in the United States, are anathema to the new American "market strategy." On the contrary, that strategy openly invites the Nation's profit-seeking entrepreneurs to find in health care a new economic frontier. In that respect, the strategy certainly has been successful. It has drawn into health care not only vigorous entrepreneurship in the development of new health care products and delivery systems but also new legions of management, marketing, and financial consultants needed to help both payers and providers cope with the turmoil and complexity of the new market environment.

The market strategy did call, on the supply side, for paying providers in a manner that would induce them to minimize the real-resource flow to patients per episode of illness. Thus, prepaid capitation for

Table 2

Percent of family health expenditures paid for out of pocket, by type of service: United States, 1977

Type of service	Percent paid out of pocket
Outpatient physician services	49
Inpatient physician services	22
Outpatient hospital care	21
Inpatient hospital care	9
Dental care	72
Prescribed medicine	73
Other	60

SOURCE: Kasper, J. A., Rossiter, L. F., and Wilson, R.: A summary of expenditures and sources of payment for personal health services from the National Medical Expenditure Survey. Data Preview No. 24. National Center for Health Services Research and Health Care Technology Assessment. Public Health Service. Rockville, Md. May 19, 1987.

comprehensive health care, in place of fee-for-service compensation, became the ideal among both private and public payers. For its part, the Medicare program switched from paying hospitals retrospectively for reported actual costs to paying them predetermined global fees per medical case, based on the assigned DRG. One may think of it as prepaid capitation per inpatient medical case.

Micromanagement on the demand side

Initially, the market strategy envisaged that the search for health care mammon on the part of the newly invigorated health care entrepreneurs (doctors and hospitals now exuberantly among them) could readily be controlled by a resuscitated demand side. Fundamental to this demand-side strategy was the conversion of the American patient into the genuine consumer of textbook fame. This conversion was to be achieved by rolling back the patient's insurance coverage, which, however, had never been nearly as complete in the United States as it has long been elsewhere, even in the mid-1970s, the heyday of America's Great Society programs (Table 2).

Furthermore, as was shown in Table 1, in any given year, the bulk of all health expenditures are made in the names of a relative few, probably fairly sick, individuals. The belief that overall health care expenditures can be effectively controlled by these sick human beings at the nexus between patients and providers (nexus C in Figure 1) seems to be uniquely American and, even within the United States, uniquely incident upon the economics profession, whence the idea originated (e.g., Baumol, 1988[1]).

To bolster patients in their role as consumers of health care, they (and third-party payers paying on their behalf) were to be equipped with reliable information on the cost and quality of services produced by individual, competing providers in a given market area. In practice, of course, that tactic represents a monumental analytic task, for the typical provider represents a multiproduct firm whose quality and cost are not easily captured in readable, one-dimensional index numbers that can be meaningfully compared across providers.

Remarkably, it was not deemed necessary under the market strategy to gather patients and third-party payers into organized huddles to coordinate their defensive tactics—for example, to form all-payer systems in which all payers in a market jointly negotiate single compensation rates with providers (on, say, the German mode). On the contrary, it was thought that the strategy would work best if each payer, large or small, were left to fend for him- or herself in a genuine market free-for-all. Furthermore, it was believed that, singly and uncoordinated, payers (individual patients among them) could at long last turn the tables on providers, by dividing and ruling them with genuine price competition.

The convergence of health systems

Oddly, just as many Europeans apparently have begun looking longingly at this novel American market approach, the American public itself appears to have become rather disillusioned with that very strategy. For, whatever that strategy may have achieved so far, it has not reduced the money flow to providers; it has increased that flow, even after adjustment for general price inflation (Fuchs, 1988). Furthermore, by commercializing the entire process of health care more fully than ever before, the strategy has served to worsen the plight of the estimated 31 to 37 million Americans with no health insurance coverage altogether, who find it ever more difficult to secure charity care from providers increasingly focused on their bottom line.

A problem with assessing the new market strategy has been that so little of it has actually found its way from the blueprint to actual practice, which speaks volumes on the practicality of the entire notion. It is truly remarkable, for example, that the Reagan Administration, always the most vocal champion of deregulation and markets, actually operated the health programs under its purview with the most regulatory

---

[1]In his testimony, commissioned by the American Medical Association and presented before the Physician Payment Review Commission (which advises Congress on payments of physicians by the Federal Medicare program), noted economist William Baumol warned the commission against the imposition of ceilings on the fees physicians may charge the aged over and above those approved by Medicare. He recommended instead that they increase cost sharing borne by the aged at the point of service, although the aged already pay for the first hospital day in a stay, 20 percent of approved physician fees (and whatever extra charges the physician may bill the patient), and virtually all prescription drugs. For the

poor aged, these out-of-pocket expenses amount to an average of 20 percent of disposable income. "Such enhanced user sharing arrangements," Baumol suggested, "would provide a greater incentive for patients to shop around, to provide demand-side pressures that impede excessive charges, and would also help to curb unnecessary use of medical facilities." Baumol's testimony, endorsed in writing by 10 prominent economists—several Nobel Laureates among them—suggests a remarkable faith in the ability of frail, elderly persons struck by illness to function as vigilant, rational health care shoppers, capable of disciplining wayward doctors and hospitals.

regimen ever in American health care. In principle, the DRG system for hospitals is but a relative value scale for inpatient care, the monetary point value of which could have been determined either by negotiation with hospitals or even by competitive bid. Instead, however, the Medicare program has so far implemented the DRGs in a manner more reminiscent of price controls imposed by central governments behind the Iron Curtain: Year after year, the DRG rates have been set unilaterally by the Federal Government on a take-it-or-leave-it basis. Payments by Medicare to physicians have also been subject to unilaterally set price ceilings throughout much of the 1980s.

Nor has the supply side of the American health care market ultimately remained as free of direct regulation as certainly the providers of health care once hoped it would be. To control the flow of health services from providers to patients—a flow that the new health care consumers seem either unwilling or unable to control—both public and private third-party payers increasingly intervene directly in the individual physician-patient encounter. This is done by means of what is called "managed care," that is, by prospective, concurrent, and retrospective reviews by outside monitors of individual medical treatments. (I consider the peer review organizations to be a form of managed care.) Although European health systems relying on fee-for-service compensation do employ retrospective statistical profiles of individual providers (notably physicians), the direct outside interventions into individual medical treatments now increasingly common in the United States are as yet unknown in Europe. The proponents of the American market strategy may well conceive of these interventions as normal features of a market. American physicians and hospitals, however, decry them as nettlesome private and public regulation of their professional domain, which, of course, they are.

In the meantime, American patients, providers, and third-party payers alike are beginning to appreciate that the American style of micromanagement visits upon all of them a vexatious and costly paper war that can be handled only with the help of specialized paper-war consultants. The cost of this paper war alone, relative to the much simpler Canadian and European health systems, has been estimated to amount to some 8 percent of total national health expenditures, which would be about $48 billion in 1988 (Himmelstein and Woolhandler, 1986). That figure, however, does not even include an imputed value for the time patients spend choosing among competing insurers and claiming reimbursement from insurers.

In a recent nationwide survey, about 90 percent of those surveyed felt that the American health system requires "fundamental change or a complete rebuilding," and, remarkably, more than 60 percent professed an outright preference for the Canadian health system (Blendon, 1989). Although it is never quite clear just what one such survey really portends, it is, as noted, a safe bet that the United States will

embrace a more regulatory approach during the decade ahead. Indeed, the Government is likely to be encouraged in this direction by American businesses, which now finance, through employer-paid health insurance coverage, more than one-third of the national health bill and which now find themselves at a loss over how to control that ever-growing drain on their treasuries.

It is therefore quite possible, as Jönsson implies, that the American and European health systems may eventually converge onto a common middle ground. If so, these systems might learn from one another as they stumble along the path toward convergence.

Just what that common ground might ultimately look like remains anyone's guess. Perhaps it will closely resemble the type of arrangement first envisaged by Alain Enthoven in his *Health Plan* (Enthoven, 1980 and 1989). That approach abandons the peculiar idea that health care costs can be effectively controlled by the sick and anxious individuals facing providers in nexus C of Figure 1. Instead, Enthoven envisages a two-stage process. In nexus A of Figure 1, well-informed, healthy individuals choose among competing, managed-health-care plans, offered to them by so-called sponsors, which may be either a government or a private business entity. In nexus B, these sponsors procure health care from the competing, managed-care systems, typically health maintenance organizations or other delivery systems that control both prices and utilization. Were such a system introduced in Europe, it would in effect replace the current system of highly centralized regulation with a more decentralized set of smaller, private regulators, among which prospective patients choose when they are still healthy. After all, managed care, even if administered by private plans, is nevertheless direct regulation of doctors and hospitals.

If the American and European health systems did converge toward this form of pluralistic, private regulation of health care providers, one must wonder what would happen to their respective class structures. Would the private regulators specialize by income class? That is, would the quality and amenities of the care offered by the competing managed-care plans vary by income class? Would plans offering few amenities and harsh regulation of providers be reserved mainly for low-income subscribers and plans approximating the more open-ended style of traditional fee-for-service medicine attract mainly high-income groups?

Convergence toward two-tier health care

American critics of European health care frequently decry it as two-class medicine—so-called socialized medicine for the poor and private medicine for the rich. Conversely, European critics of American health care frequently depict it as leaning toward Social Darwinism.

Both visions contain kernels of truth.

Broadly speaking, in the current European health systems, about 90 percent or so of the population share a one-tier health system. That system may couple privately owned production of health care with socialized insurance (for example, France and Germany), or it may couple socialized insurance with public ownership of substantially all production of care (e.g., the Scandinavian countries and the United Kingdom). Typically, an affluent and highly mobile 5 to 10 percent of families in these countries are permitted to opt out of the public plan in favor of private health insurance. They procure health care on what they believe to be superior terms either in their own country or abroad. In this sense, the typical European health care system does represent two-class medicine.

By contrast, Americans in the top 80-85 percent or so of the Nation's income distribution have access to what is called mainstream American medicine. But, as Rosemary Stevens demonstrates in her fascinating recent book, *In Sickness and in Wealth* (1989), even this mainstream system has always reserved special treatment and accommodations for the high upper income groups. Millions of low-income uninsured or underinsured Americans, however, are left merely to nibble at the fringes of this mainstream system. When illness strikes, they approach that system in the role of health care beggars in search of charity care. They may receive such care from kindly providers within the mainstream system. Alternatively, they may be relegated to sorely underfunded and overcrowded government hospitals, sometimes in the perilous process of "dumping," in which barely stabilized patients are transferred from mainstream facilities to government-owned hospitals. In some instances, such individuals are left out of the health system altogether, as countless disturbing vignettes in the daily media and some more formal surveys (Robert Wood Johnson Foundation, 1987; Blendon, 1989) suggest. At its worst, then, the American health system does seem to slouch toward Social Darwinism.

It is well known that, even after all transfer programs, America's poor have become poorer during the 1980s and the rich have become richer. It therefore can be doubted that, in the face of this dispersion of the income distribution, the United States will ever move all of its citizens into the one-class health care system the Nation has long espoused as the ideal, but has never attained so far. America's growing number of well-to-do individuals are unlikely to finance for the Nation's poor quite the quality of health care they demand for themselves. Thus, even after the convergence postulated by Jönsson, the American health system is likely to remain tiered by income class. However, with some vision and effort, the bottom tier of a future American health system could be made vastly superior to today's much-neglected bottom tier.

The question is whether the European nations can avoid a similar trend toward multiclass health care for the bottom 90 percent of their populations, who now do share a genuine one-class health system. It may be hypothesized that the continued development of the global economy will disperse the income distributions in Europe as it has in the United States. In this newly emerging global economy, individuals endowed with either financial or human capital (i.e., education) are likely to see their relative income position improve. At the same time, the elimination of national boundaries in international trade is likely to rob low-skilled European workers of the protection they have hitherto enjoyed. They may see their real income erode, as they are forced to compete with more abundant, cheaper, unskilled labor elsewhere on the globe.

If European income distributions were to drift apart in this way, the upper-middle income classes in these nations, too, might become unwilling to finance for low-income families quite the health care they seek for themselves—health care with the technical sophistication and often luxurious settings they can witness on their visits to the United States. In fact, the yearning among some European health policy analysts for "more market" on the American model may well betray a yearning for just such tiering by income class. (I should mention that Jönsson's article does not lead one to count him among this group.)

It remains to be seen whether the *Principle of Solidarity* that has for so long now driven European health policy for all but a small, upper-income elite can survive these yearnings for more systematic tiering by income class. At the very least, one would expect the still-tiny private health insurance markets in these countries to grow in size. Perhaps the future evolution of the European health systems will teach Americans that the lack of social solidarity typically ascribed to American health care—and most assuredly typical of American education and jurisprudence—is actually the more natural long-run state of nature.

References

Altman, S. A., and Rodwin, M. A.: Halfway competitive markets and ineffective regulation. *Journal of Health Politics, Policy and Law* 13(2):323-329, 1988.

Baumol, W. J.: Price Controls for Medical Services and the Medical Needs of the Nation's Elderly. Paper commissioned by the American Medical Association and presented to the Physician Payment Review Commission. Mar. 18, 1988.

Berk, M. L., Monheit, A. C., and Hagan, M. M.: How the U.S. spent its health care dollar: 1929-80. *Health Affairs* 7(4):46-60, Fall 1988.

Blendon, R. J.: Three systems: A comparative study. *Health Management Quarterly* 9(1):2-10, 1989.

Enthoven, A. C.: *Health Plan*. Reading, Mass. Addison-Wesley, 1980.

Enthoven, A. C., and Kronick, R.: A consumer-choice health plan for the 1990s. *New England Journal of Medicine* 320(1):29-37, Jan. 5, 1989, and 320(2):94-101, Jan. 12, 1989.

Fuchs, V.: The competition revolution. *Health Affairs* 7(3):5-24, 1988.

Himmelstein, D. U., and Woolhandler, S.: Cost without benefit: Administrative waste in U.S. health care. *New England Journal of Medicine* 314(7):441-445, 1986.

Lyons, A. S., and Petrucelli, R.: *Medicine.* New York. Harry N. Abrams, 1978.

Robert Wood Johnson Foundation: *Access to Health Care in the United States: Results of a 1986 Survey.* Special Report No. 2. Princeton, New Jersey. Robert Wood Johnson Foundation, 1987.

Stevens, R.: *In Sickness and in Wealth: American Hospitals in the Twentieth Century.* New York. Basic Books, 1989.

Karen Davis

Introduction

Jönsson makes a compelling case for the importance of international comparisons of health care systems. Increasingly, health systems in industrialized nations around the world are facing similar problems. The diversity of solutions attempted by different countries yields fertile ground for learning from the ideas and experience of others. Worldwide improvements in communication, information technology, and transportation are converting the world into a global village. Increasingly, nations are realizing that health problems do not recognize national boundaries, regardless of whether the problem is acquired immunodeficiency syndrome (AIDS), drug addiction, or the aging of the population.

In the United States, there is a new interest in learning from the experience of health systems in other countries. In part, this interest is stimulated by new information and data bases that make investigation of other experiences possible. In part, it is a reflection of growing discontent with rapidly rising health expenditures in the United States, coupled with the persistent gaps in health insurance coverage and barriers to access to health care. More fundamentally, it is linked to growing uneasiness about the future of the U.S. economy, and its ability to maintain international competitiveness and a standard of living that has been the highest in the world.

This new interest in international experience does not mean that the United States is likely to adopt the health system of any other country in total. Instead, the United States is likely to continue to shape its health system based on the historical, political, cultural, and economic forces that have shaped it in the past. Research and analysis of the merits of other systems, however, can identify features that show promise of being incorporated in the U.S. health system.

Considerable barriers to capitalizing on the experience of other nations, however, exist. Funding for cross-national studies is extremely limited. Exchange programs to help scholars learn about other systems through indepth exposure are rare. Some of

Reprint requests: Karen Davis, Ph.D., School of Hygiene and Public Health, The Johns Hopkins University, 624 N. Broadway, Baltimore, Maryland 21205.

the aspects of European health system performance that show the greatest promise for adaptation to the American health system are highlighted in this article, and I offer suggestions for some steps that could be taken to facilitate building on this experience.

Comparative performance of health systems

Jönsson joins others (Schieber and Poullier, 1988) in questioning the performance of the U.S. health system. He notes that the United States has higher health expenditures as a percent of gross domestic product (GDP) than do all European countries. Further, he finds that this higher share of economic resources devoted to the health sector cannot be totally explained by the greater prosperity of the United States and the tendency of countries to devote disproportionately more resources to health as per capita income grows.

The growing evidence on the comparative costliness of the U.S. system in the face of inferior health performance shatters many myths that have long been held by policy officials and health professionals. Recent polls have shown that the U.S. public is also more highly critical of its system than are citizens of other countries (Blendon, 1989).

The evidence on the high cost and inferior performance of the U.S. health system strikes at a number of widely held beliefs. It has been argued in the United States that universal health insurance coverage, although desirable on humane grounds, is too costly and would be inherently inflationary. The ability of nearly all other industrialized nations to cover their entire populations with very little patient cost sharing, while devoting a smaller fraction of GDP to health, counters this view rather forcefully.

Perhaps even more disturbing is the fact that health spending continues to increase as a share of GDP in the United States but stabilized during the 1980s in other industrialized nations (Figure 1). In 1970, the United States and Canada each spent 8 percent of their respective GDPs on health care. In 1986, the U.S. share had risen to 11 percent, but Canada's remains at 8.5 percent (Evans, 1989).

This experience argues convincingly that greater reliance on market forces and competition among health systems in the 1980's have not improved U.S. health system performance. Instead, it appears to have worsened relative to other nations that have instituted a stronger governmental role in the

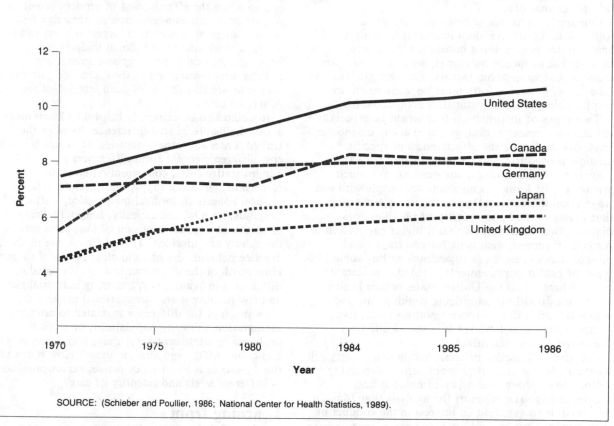

Figure 1
Total health expenditures as a percent of gross domestic product: Selected countries, selected years 1970-86

SOURCE: (Schieber and Poullier, 1986; National Center for Health Statistics, 1989).

establishment of hospital budgets and physician payment rates.

The better health performance of European countries also strikes at the widely held view in the United States that the U.S. health system is the best in the world. Americans are increasingly troubled by the failure of the United States to insure 15-20 percent of the population, by the inadequate care provided to many disadvantaged groups of the population, and by the serious financial burdens inflicted on those with inadequate health insurance coverage who are unfortunate enough to have a serious illness (Davis, 1989; Blendon, 1989).

Health performance

Jönsson points to the high rate of infant mortality in the United States as "proof" that the U.S. health system is not obtaining value for its money. He argues that this health indicator is an especially sensitive indicator of the adequacy of the medical care system.

Other indicators of health performance are equally troubling. The U.S. lags behind other industrialized nations in life expectancy at birth and in mortality rates from chronic conditions (National Center for Health Statistics, 1989; World Health Organization, 1984).

One difficulty in learning from European countries how to improve health performance in the United States is the absence of sophisticated studies that sort out the multiple determinants of health outcomes. Some portion of the inferior U.S. performance, particularly infant mortality rates, would appear to be linked to social and economic factors, as well as to those that are specific to the health system. For example, the United States has a higher poverty rate among children than do European countries (Sawhill, 1988). About one-fourth of all infants and one-half of all black babies are born to unwed mothers (National Center for Health Statistics, 1989). Drug addiction and alcohol abuse are epidemic in some communities. HIV (human immunodeficiency virus) infection is a growing problem in infants born to minority women.

Another difficulty in making cross-national comparisons is the difference in populations. The U.S. population, often referred to as a "melting pot," cannot be readily compared with those of Iceland or Japan, with their much more homogeneous populations. Poor birth outcomes are particularly high among minority populations, including black Americans, Hispanic Americans, and native American Indians. The United States has a large immigrant population, both legal and undocumented, which

113

contributes to unusually high rates of health problems in some communities. The degree to which poor health outcomes reflect social causes versus the inadequacy of the health system or insurance coverage is hard to quantify.

One useful step would be to conduct more sophisticated cross-national multivariate analyses of health outcomes, holding constant for the many factors that influence outcomes, such as poverty and other sociodemographic factors. For such analysis to take place, greater efforts must be made to ensure the comparability of health statistics across countries.

Two types of information that would be especially valuable are research disaggregated at the diagnostic level and studies of the effectiveness of specific medical procedures and patterns of care for various diagnoses. Jönsson notes, for example, the much greater use of kidney transplants for people with end stage renal disease in other countries—a technology that offers much better quality of life than does dialysis. But he also notes that a higher proportion of Americans receive treatment for end stage renal disease. Does greater use of technology buy some types of health improvements, even at considerable cost? Where could the United States reduce health expenditures without sacrificing health gains, and where should it devote more resources to achieve greater health benefits? What is the payoff for preventive health activities?

Clearly, U.S. policy officials and health experts will want to know a great deal more before identifying actions to improve health performance in the United States. The value of the analysis that Jönsson sets forth is to generate an interest in the conduct of such studies.

Cost performance

Perhaps the most convincing argument that the United States needs to examine more carefully the experience of other industrialized nations is the fact that the U.S. health system is the most expensive in the world—and that this disparity is growing greater, not smaller.

Jönsson argues that many European countries have achieved their superior cost performance through regionalization and establishment of global health budgets by government at either the central or local level. The share of the health system financed by the public sector is much higher in European countries. Many countries rely on public provision of services through government-owned hospitals and salaried physicians. Even those countries with private hospitals and private physicians impose strict controls on budgets, fees, and capital expansion.

Although this evidence is compelling, there is little likelihood that the United States will embrace such an extensive role for the public sector. Resistance to higher taxes makes it unlikely that the United States will markedly increase the share of health expenditures financed publicly. Any massive switch to a public system of providing health services would also be strongly resisted by health care providers.

The aspects of the European health experience of greatest interest to U.S. policy officials and experts are the methods used to pay hospitals and physicians and to assess the effectiveness of services provided. Approaches such as negotiation of physician fees, establishment of expenditure targets for physician services, determination of global budgets for hospitals, medical technology assessment, and effectiveness research on medical practice patterns and protocols are all subjects of keen interest on the American scene.

It would also be extremely helpful to know more about the nature of cost differences between the United States and other countries. How much of the cost difference comes from differences in administrative costs, compensation levels of physicians, physician supply and specialty mix, medical education, medical malpractice, staffing of hospitals, hospital bed capacity, hospital admissions or length of stay, or provision of long-term care to the elderly and disabled? How different are medical practice patterns, use of technology, rates of surgery? How much of the difference in costs is related to differences in health risks, including industrialization and environmental and occupational health risks? How much of the difference is related to poverty, immigration, minority populations, or to such problems as adolescent pregnancy, homelessness, drug addiction, AIDS, and alcohol abuse? How much of the difference is inefficiency per se, versus provision of different levels and intensity of care?

Learning from each other's experiences

Although the United States could learn a great deal from the experience of other countries, a number of barriers stand in the way of this cross-national transfer. First, comparable data on health expenditures, health statistics, and other aspects of the health systems of industrialized nations are still in a quite formative stage. Much more needs to be done to standardize definitions and reporting practices to establish comparable, timely, cross-national data bases. Recently, the Organization for Economic Cooperation and Development (OECD) has begun to compile comparable health expenditure data, and the World Health Organization Regional Office for Europe (WHO-EURO) is compiling comparable health statistics on a wide variety of health outcome measures. These efforts should be continued and strengthened. Timely publication and extensive dissemination of such data are essential.

But much of the requisite research requires more disaggregated data than are available from these sources. Greater efforts should be made to conduct studies at the individual patient level, with cross-national comparison of treatment patterns, health outcomes, and costs. The very nature of financing health systems in European countries often makes it difficult to estimate the costs of caring for an individual patient. Methodologies and data systems for making comparative cost comparisons at the individual patient level need to be developed.

A second barrier to the conduct of this research relates to the nature of funding research. European universities are predominantly public. Research is carried out by publicly funded research institutions, universities, or government agencies. This creates pressure to focus on controlled, nationally oriented research agendas. In the United States, health services researchers are frequently based at private universities or organizations, competing for limited research dollars from governmental agencies and private foundations to conduct investigations. Research funding for international comparisons has been severely limited—both by private foundations and by governmental agencies—leading to greater concentration on research within the U.S. system.

Third, the exchange of information across geographic boundaries remains a significant barrier to useful cross-national comparisons. International conferences to share research findings and learn about policy developments are limited. International professional associations are not well developed. Language can be a barrier to learning about significant developments in other countries. Professional journals reporting on cross-national research are not numerous.

Finally, there are few collaborative relationships among research groups in different countries. Developing data bases and research on comparable patient populations in different countries have not been pursued on any significant scale. Exchange programs for scholars to learn about other systems are also extremely limited.

Although these barriers are significant, they are amenable to change. The growing recognition that health services research is essential to improving performance of the U.S. health system is leading to greater support for research funding. The growing concern about U.S. competitiveness generally and the inferior performance of the U.S. health system specifically should continue to lend support to interest in learning from experiences around the world. Developments in data and research sophistication open up new avenues for investigation that should be of tremendous appeal to a growing number of researchers.

One of the most important steps that could be taken is the institution of funding by governmental agencies and private foundations in the United States focused specifically on helping the United States learn from the experiences of other nations. Quite recently, there has been more interest in the United States in learning from the Canadian health system experience (Moloney and Paul, 1989). However, much more extensive efforts are required to draw effectively on the experience of Canada as well as of other nations.

The opportunity to learn from "natural experiments" taking place around the world has great promise. As each country grapples with ensuring good health for its people in the face of economic constraints, the demand for cross-national information is heightened. Fortunately, a growing body of trained researchers with the tools and data to facilitate such research provides a unique opportunity to capitalize on this development. The end result should be growing international cooperation and collaboration dedicated to achieving the World Health Organization goal of health for all people.

References

Blendon, R. J.: Three systems: A comparative study. *Health Management Quarterly* XI(1):2-10, First Quarter, 1989.

Davis, K.: National health insurance: A proposal. *American Economic Review* 79(2):349-352, May 1989.

Evans, R. G., Lomas, J., Barer, M., et al.: Controlling health expenditures: The Canadian reality. *New England Journal of Medicine* 320(9):571-577, 1989.

Moloney, T. W., and Paul, B.: A new financial framework: Lessons from Canada. *Health Affairs* 148-159, Summer 1989.

National Center for Health Statistics: *Health, United States, 1988.* DHHS Pub. No. (PHS) 89-1232. Public Health Service. Washington. U.S. Government Printing Office, 1989.

Sawhill, I. V.: *Children in Poverty.* Washington, D.C. The Urban Institute, 1988.

Schieber, G., and Poullier, J. P.: Data watch: International health spending. *Health Affairs* 5(4):111-122, 1986.

Schieber, G. J., and Poullier, J. P.: International health spending and utilization trends. *Health Affairs* 7(4):105-112, Fall, 1988.

World Health Organization: *Country Reports.* Regional Office for Europe, 1984.

Jack A. Meyer

Introduction

The article by Bengt Jönsson is a useful reminder that different health care systems can learn a great deal from each other. Jönsson properly reminds us that our stereotypes of different systems, corresponding to purely market or purely regulatory regimes, are overdrawn. The U.S. system has many regulatory features, and various models of national health insurance incorporate certain marketlike incentives.

I also agree with what Jönsson calls "the convergence theory," in which planning will play an increasing role in market systems, and market-based

Reprint requests: Jack A. Meyer, Ph.D., New Directions for Policy, Suite 400, 1101 Vermont Avenue, NW, Washington, D.C. 20005.

incentives will play an increasing role in planned systems.

I have a somewhat different view than Jönsson has about the importance of the distinction between central planning and planning conducted at the regional or local level. He is correct in pointing out that many observers in the United States do not understand how localized the decisionmaking is in many European health care systems. But I believe his heavy emphasis on clarifying the locus of decisionmaking obscures more important distinctions.

I also have a different perspective on the apparent gaps between the United States and Sweden (or other Organization for Economic Cooperation and Development [OECD] nations) with regard to health care costs and access. I would like to point out these differences, without detracting from my general agreement with many of the specific points made in Jönsson's article.

Most papers that compare the U.S. health system with other developed countries' systems contain a familiar litany of aggregate facts that are, admittedly, rather embarrassing to the United States. For example, in 1987, U.S. health care spending as a share of gross domestic product (GDP) was 11.2 percent, compared with 9.0 percent in Sweden and 7.3 percent for the OECD countries as a group (Schieber and Poullier, 1989). This gap is probably a little wider now, as U.S. health care costs may approach 12 percent of GNP in 1990.

The United States also has more than 30 million people without health insurance, and life expectancy is about 2 years less in the United States than in Sweden. Meanwhile, the infant mortality rate among white babies in the United States is about twice as high as Sweden's infant mortality rate, and the rate among black infants in the United States is more than three times as high as the Swedish aggregate rate. Jönsson mentions some of these facts.

Most analyses of international differences that involve the United States either stop here or go on to point out that the U.S. public share of health spending (about 40 percent) is well below the OECD average of 76 percent, with the implication that this is the reason that we are the "outlier" with respect to cost and access.

This type of analysis is superficial and misleading. We must dig deeper and explore some tough tradeoffs to get a feeling for intercountry differences. And when we do, we will come face to face with major gaps in our knowledge.

The source of the difference

What makes the U.S. health care system more expensive than those of other countries? Some surprising facts are beginning to emerge. First, the cause is not excessive utilization of services. It is sometimes said (though not by Jönsson) that Americans are hypochondriacs and that this partially explains our cost escalation. If Americans are hypochondriacs, the citizens of most other countries are worse. Cross-country comparisons of utilization make it clear that virtually every measure of utilization is lower in the United States than in other industrialized countries. As Schieber and Poullier (1988), referring to data on international differences in length of hospital stays, note in a recent article, ". . . the U.S. average lengths-of-stay for most DRGs are shorter and those for Switzerland are longer than those of other countries."

For example, in each of 12 DRG categories presented by Schieber and Poullier, length of stay is longer in Sweden than it is in the United States, and it is longer (often by a wide margin) in Switzerland than it is in Sweden. For example, in the case of cerebrovascular disorders, mean length of stay is 12.0 days in the United States, 18.8 days in Sweden, and 29.9 days in Switzerland. Jönsson describes "a strict planning and budgeting system for hospital services" in Swiss cantons. Whatever successes these planners are having, they are not reflected in hospital length of stay.

Moreover, the international differences cannot be explained by the demographics of aging. About 12 percent of the U.S. population is 65 years of age or over today, and about 17 percent of the Swedish population is in this age group. Yet, per capita health spending in the United States was $2,051 in 1987, 66 percent higher than Sweden's figure of $1,233 (Schieber and Poullier, 1988).

What is it then? The major factor that seems to explain the intercountry cost differences is that the United States employs many more people in the health care system and, generally speaking, pays them more. This well-paid army of workers includes not only doctors and nurses but also thousands more people in the United States than in other countries who sell insurance and administer claims. These are the U.S. "health care workers" who are not employed in the business of actually delivering health care.

About 22 percent of U.S. health spending involves administrative costs, and it has been estimated that the United States could achieve an 8- to 10-percent reduction in total health spending just from administrative cost savings if it were to adopt a national health insurance plan (Himmelstein and Woolhandler, 1986).

Thus, the explanation of U.S. "extra costs" lies largely in a combination of greater resource intensity per unit of service delivered, higher salaries for health care workers, and higher administrative costs. The greater resource intensity is not just people; it is also technology.

One more factor is worth mentioning. The U.S. malpractice system is probably adding more to costs than corresponding systems in other countries. Although reliable data are hard to find on this point, the U.S. system seems much more plaintiff- or consumer-oriented than other systems. In part, this may reflect the more fully developed social insurance systems in other OECD countries. But it also reflects the tendency in those countries not to pile huge awards from the judicial system on top of social insurance compensation, as often occurs in the United States.

Indeed, the U.S. malpractice system has both compensation and deterrence objectives. "Collateral source offsets," or the reduction of jury awards to reflect compensation received from other sources such as workers' compensation or disability insurance, are generally disallowed. If the United States is overcompensating some people in an effort to deter dangerous behavior, other countries, in their effort to focus on adequate compensation alone, may be leaving consumers vulnerable to risky behavior. This demonstrates the value of Jönsson's call for different types of systems learning from each other and possibly converging.

Is this all waste?

The really important question is this: What, if anything, does the United States receive for this extra spending? In answering this question, many observers are too quick to assume that the United States receives nothing for it. By contrast, some who are defensive (or naive) about the U.S. system assume that, if Americans are paying more, they must be getting proportionately more in quality.

We know that Americans are not receiving longer lives from the extra 4 percentage points of GDP relative to the OECD average. But is this the end of the story? I think not.

The troubling but honest answer to my question is that we really do not know what we are receiving. In my view, the "premium" we are paying is not pure fat, and it is not pure lean—it is some of each. But it is hard to tell which is which.

My hypothesis is that highly skilled people, and more of them, along with highly sophisticated technology, and more of it, do make some difference in health care outcomes, even though it is not reflected in the life expectancy of the population. The additional human and physical capital per health care encounter that is built into the U.S. system may lead to more comfortable lives, even though not to longer lives.

The real problem is that we lack good health status and health outcome measures. There is a lot that we still do not know about the medical efficacy, much less the cost effectiveness, of many procedures. Vigorous debates—usually uninformed by reliable data from controlled trials—rage on about the effectiveness of hysterectomies, prostatectomies, coronary artery bypass surgery, and other surgeries, along with uncertainty about the number of tests and prescription drugs given to the population.

Picking up on one of Jönsson's themes involving the sharing and testing of ideas across nations, this may be an area in which other OECD nations have something to learn from the United States. Work is well under way in the United States, even though still in embryonic form, to measure and quantify health care outcomes and to profile and rank providers according to their relative effectiveness.

This knowledge is developing rapidly in both the public and private sectors. It may help us move away from the tendency to judge performance of health care systems on the basis of inputs. Judging by the amount of input, the United States clearly appears wasteful. It uses more inputs and pays a higher price for them. What it will look like as we begin to measure value—output or outcome received for any given input—remains unclear. Cross-country comparisons such as Jönsson's would be improved by taking this distinction into account.

The most interesting development in the U.S. health system today is that buyers of care—public and private—are beginning to question outcome for the first time. What most observers of international trends neglect to consider is that it is not the share of the U.S. health care system that is public or private that matters with respect to costs being out of control. Costs have been out of control in both sectors in the United States and for the same reason: Both public and private buyers did not know what they were buying and failed to confront the power of organized medicine with respect to both the price and quantity of services rendered.

Buyers in the United States are now beginning to move beyond the question of "How much does it cost?" to the question of "What happened when you did it?" and "Was it necessary in the first place?" Undoubtedly, these questions are being asked elsewhere. But the technology for answering the questions is developing rapidly in the United States and could be of use around the world, under the kind of cross-fertilization patterns that Jönsson envisions.

In my view, Jönsson's article is a bit too optimistic about the importance of decentralization of decisionmaking in Sweden and other countries. All those decentralized decisions are still playing out against centrally imposed rules and, in many cases, centrally determined overall budget constraints.

The important challenge that all countries now face in health care is not so much how to organize or reorganize the decisionmaking between central and local bodies or even how authority is allocated between public and private sectors within the buyer side. In my view, these are yesterday's debates. The critical challenge today is how to strengthen the buyer side of the market—irrespective of its organization—so that it has both the information it needs and the political will to confront organized medicine on behalf of consumers.

We spend too much time arguing about the relative merits of consumers giving money to private insurance companies in the form of premiums as opposed to giving the money to government (local or national) in the form of taxes. This is not the critical distinction. The most important factor is what the recipient of the money, the third-party payer (public or private), does with it and what pressure that third-party payer brings to bear on the provider community.

It is not being public rather than private that makes a difference in getting better value for the money. It is the knowledge of performance, value, and

117

effectiveness, and the willingness to use it, that matter. We must learn how to pick and choose among providers on the basis of their demonstrated performance as well as their cost. This becomes the preferable alternative to what too often masquerades as cost control—picking and choosing among consumers on the basis of income or health risk.

The most dangerous trend in health care today is the tendency to avoid developing carefully researched and carefully adjusted mechanisms for measuring value and outcome, with the attendant result that costs are "controlled" by controlling consumers— usually on some basis that bears no resemblance to ethically supportable criteria.

I do not count myself among those who believe that the United States is the only country that has fallen into the trap of trying to control costs by placing limits on consumers. Nor is it the only country to postpone developing the alternative to restricting consumers: finding out what is good medicine and bad medicine and steering business to those who practice the former and away from those who practice the latter.

The sad fact is that the United States limits consumers in one way and other countries limit them in another. The United States has a long and indefensible history of limiting access by permitting large numbers of people to be uninsured, which forces them to underconsume, or actually forego, helpful primary and preventive care. To this old story is now being added a new, equally troubling one. People are now being jettisoned from the U.S. health care system because they are high-risk patients—they have preexisting health conditions that make them more likely candidates for large outlays.

Providers and insurers are competing on the basis of good health risks in the United States because they are not yet being forced to compete on the basis of good performance. But this is beginning to change.

The United States will move—in its own pluralistic, fragmented way—toward broader coverage and tougher cost controls that bear down on providers. Thus, we see one piece of Jönsson's convergence theory.

Other countries would never dare deny insurance coverage to large numbers of people. But in most of those countries, health care is rationed on another basis: waiting times and influence. Everyone is covered all right, but not everyone is served on a timely basis. And it is not always medical considerations that determine who moves to the head of the queue. This is the central embarrassment of the national health plans, one that is every bit as indefensible as the source of embarrassment to the United States.

Thus, I reject Jönsson's contention that "It is obvious that the moral bases or values on which health care systems are based differ between the United States and European countries."

The national health plans, as Jönsson points out, are moving to correct their problems, often using a mix of market and regulatory approaches, just as a blend of the two is also found in the United States. This is the other arm of his convergence theory.

In this author's view, if both systems share their successes and learning—as Jönsson calls for—and go to work on their respective embarrassments, both access to health care and cost control would be improved.

References

Himmelstein, D., and Woolhandler, S.: Cost without benefit. *New England Journal of Medicine* 314(7):441, 1986.

Schieber, G., and Poullier, J. P.: Data watch. *Health Affairs* 7(4):105-112, Fall 1988.

Schieber, G., and Poullier, J. P.: Data watch. *Health Affairs* 8(3):169-177, Fall 1989.

Compendium

Health care expenditure and other data

This international compendium from the Organization for Economic Cooperation and Development Secretariat contains available data for the 24 Member countries for 1960 through 1987. The Federal Republic of Germany is listed as Germany. Tables are presented for expenditure on health, health care pricing trends, social protection and public participation, utilization of medical services and available personnel resources, selected variations in common medical care practice, selected health status indicators, and demographic and general economic background data.

There may be some inconsistencies between the data presented in the articles in this issue and those in this data compendium. The articles were based on earlier versions of the Health Data File. As a result, revisions to the data in a number of countries, including Canada, France, Germany, and Italy, are not reflected in the articles. However, the changes are relatively minor and do not affect the results presented in the articles in any substantive way.

Health data file: Overview and methodology

by Jean-Pierre Poullier

Reliable information is essential for rational policymaking. Unfortunately, in many countries, health policies have been framed without the help of systems of national health accounts. Even now, the public debates on health policy in many of the industrialized countries are conducted in terms of partial information (i.e., the division between the private and public shares in the financing of health care is based on hazy concepts and the health accounting framework is typically fragmentary). Moreover, even where these shortcomings do not apply, the dearth of outcome indicators considerably hampers analyses of the overall performance of health systems as well as the effects of particular policy interventions.

Although the simple availability of reliable information does not necessarily lead to appropriate clinical or service delivery decisions, in most areas of public policy, reliable information is an essential ingredient in improving the policymaking process. Few policies, particularly those pertaining to social programs, are framed in an international context. Mainly this is because of the intrinsically national nature of social systems and the dearth of valid, internationally comparable data.

Statistical systems are regularly modified to adapt to the requirements of a changing environment, incorporate new data sources, monitor a wider territory, and facilitate interpenetration with other, related statistical data. Such changes are typically generated by a domestic process; rarely are they triggered at the international level. A community of countries may, however, decide to embark on a new generation of concepts and methods to elaborate, for example, national income and product

Reprint requests: Jean-Pierre Poullier, Organization for Economic Cooperation and Development, 2 rue André-Pascal, 75775 Paris Cedex 16, France.

accounts or employment statistics. The publication *Measuring Health Care 1960-1983: Expenditure, Costs and Performance* by the Organization for Economic Cooperation and Development (OECD) in 1985 triggered such a process of reevaluation of accepted health information and accounting standards in many countries. A sizable number of statistical series have been substantially revised during the past decade to correspond to more exacting standards. For example, in their 1988 national review of progress toward the World Health Organization (WHO) objective "Health for All by the Year 2000," the Danish authorities stressed the importance they attach to the OECD statistical work (and its impact on their welfare-state development) "whose compilation and processing of data, especially concerning health economics and health activities, is considered as a necessary supplement to the WHO activities in these fields." However, the process of revision of accounting standards in OECD countries is far from finished and is likely to be continued in the early 1990s.

Three main approaches[1] to compiling and processing official data at the international level can be identified:

- An international (or related) agency fully finances a survey and, thus, controls its variables. Identical questions, common concepts and definitions, and single processing are employed.
- Agencies from various countries determine that an area is worth a cooperative effort, work together to harmonize concepts and definitions, and supply the corresponding time series to a single compilation unit.
- An analyst attempts to "massage" data from various countries, using as closely comparable units as can be obtained from the information readily accessible.

[1] A more elaborate discussion of these approaches can be found in "OECD experiences with the initiation and coordination of health indicator systems, with special emphasis on interinstitutional coordination and comparability" in *Indicators and Trends in Health and Health Care*, D. Schwefel, ed., Berlin-Heidelberg, Federal Republic of Germany, Springer Verlag, 1987.

The first approach is the surest way to attain fuller cross-national comparability. However, it is only rarely used because it is the costliest in money terms. The second is the most classic method, but it requires years to implement because numerous meetings are necessary to agree on boundaries, classification principles, accounting units, compilation lead-times, etc. The third approach is the least precise because judgments are made by the compiler only. However, with this approach, several years are saved and costly experts' meetings are avoided. Although the learning curve inherent in this approach leads to considerably improved data in later editions, the enhancement process is constrained by the ability of a single investigator to perceive the intricacies of complex systems pertaining to many countries and by inherent difficulties in gaining access to the building blocks of the statistical series to be compared.

Sooner or later, the second approach becomes unavoidable. However, the OECD Health Data File belongs to the third group. Thus, it should be viewed with a knowledge of the weaknesses inherent in such an approach. Its current strength lies in the lack of an alternative.

Data systems are intellectual constructs. As such, they are designed to summarize behavioral relationships that are empirically complex and often not well understood. Statistical systems are thus regularly challenged by their users (and even internally by their producers) for inadequacies in the reductionism employed. Therefore, an international compilation cannot be superior to its national constituent parts.

Because data originate from several sources in each country, and those sources are not necessarily consistent with one another, the Health Data File is fraught with international inconsistencies, gaps in coverage, and definitional heterogeneity. However, in international health comparisons, the tradeoff of precision for timely accessibility of the data is a difficult but necessary one.

The OECD Health Data File is designed to facilitate the identification of trends rather than detailed policy prescriptions, provided that the series exhibited is qualified and the data are used with a certain level of caution. Space limitations preclude adding numerous footnotes to the tables, and the qualifications stated in this overview only briefly address sources and methods. More detailed information on sources and methods that would provide a better understanding of the data being compared are presented in *Measuring Health Care*.

The 67 tables presented in this compendium are a subset of the more than 400 tables being worked on at the OECD as part of the Health Data File. They reflect the October 1989 status of the process initiated with *Measuring Health Care* in 1985. Great care has been taken to present as many continuous time series as possible, but breaks are unavoidable. The cost to statistical offices of revising past data in all series after a benchmark revision is often prohibitive.

As is usual with data from statistical systems, the estimates for the last year (mostly 1987) are provisional, and those for the 1 or 2 previous years (usually 1986 and 1985) are only semifinal. Aside from methodological revisions, quantitative information, on which macroeconomic estimates are based, is usually incomplete at the time of first compilation and is supplemented by "projections" of the recent past.

Finally, although most of the data come from national data bases to which the OECD Secretariat has had generous access, modifications have been required to improve cross-national comparability. Sometimes, the information supplied here differs from the customary national presentation of health trends. The cross-national presentation does not automatically entail a superiority of one set of data over the other. These data are published under the authority of the Secretary General of the OECD. Thus, national authorities are not formally committed to changes made to published national series in order to enhance cross-national comparability.

The first hurdle to overcome in developing these tables was a boundary problem. In most countries, health care is monitored by a ministry of health. However, ancillary activities, such as armed forces health services, school health services, industrial medicine, family planning centers, and old-age homes with varying degrees of medical services are treated in a number of ways by the agencies responsible for their administration. To date, recognition of the boundary problem has led to important convergences in individual countries' data reporting, thus increasing comparability across countries. However, significant differences among countries do not yet permit full homogeneity. Denmark, for example, does not classify "residential" beds provided under the auspices of its Social Affairs Ministry as inpatient medical care beds. Sweden, on the other hand, considers "nursing" beds to be part of inpatient medical care institutions. Dealing with ambulatory care (outpatient clinics, office-based medicine, etc.) results in similar problems. Chiropractors are licensed professionals in some countries and treated as quasi-healers in others.

In a number of cases, the statistical subsystems (for example, expenditure and manpower data) of different agencies have heterogeneous definitions, with detailed, underlying series inaccessible in the published sources. This factor alone suffices to explain important variations between successive versions of the data, such as that included in the 1985 version of *Measuring Health Care* and that included here. A still greater difficulty than accessing data is that of consistency, even in each country's own definitions. Moreover, in some cases, the definitions used in a country's most quoted reference vary slightly almost annually because the time series shown varies in response to the policy emphasis of each particular year. The most common pitfall consists in using parameters with identical names as if they were comparable. Although similar terms are used, the meanings may differ because they may not be based on formal prior agreement on concepts, definitions, estimating methodologies, etc.

In a comparative international data base, the problems encountered at the national level are magnified. The omission of data on pharmaceuticals distributed through mail-order houses would have no effect on French or Spanish health outlays, but it would create a sizable gap in the U.S. data. Over-the-counter pharmaceutical sales are not directly observed in many countries. Therefore, their estimation requires an apparent-consumption approach established on the basis of production data minus exports plus imports plus net changes in inventories (stocks). Such an approach obviously leads to misclassification of the containers of medicines that can be found in cabinets in many homes that have been purchased but not consumed.

The definitional problem is not confined to expenditure series, as students of the quality of medicine also experience. In his article in this issue, Enthoven cites the paucity of hospital records in some European countries that he visited. Simple breakdowns, such as the distinction made between admissions and readmissions, are not available in many countries. Yet, this is an important variable in considering whether the pressure to lower the length of hospital stays leads to the early discharge of frail patients who soon require new spells of inpatient care. The recording approaches of major hospital subsystems in some countries differ, so the lags in accessibility of complete data sets can be fairly long.

The medical evidence of death records also can rest on cultural differences. For instance, one OECD country may record little mortality from bronchitis, simply because this classification is not used in its medical schools; deaths from "other upper respiratory diseases" are correspondingly more frequent. International comparisons thus require the aggregation of two or more subcategories.

A single issue of the *Health Care Financing Review* cannot encompass a full description of each of 24 countries' statistical sources and methods and their possible reconciliation. Only brief discussions are provided in the following sections.

National accounting concept

The expenditure series (Tables 1-9) initially was conceived as a national accounting (income and product accounts) series meant to satisfy two criteria: quasi-comprehensiveness of the underlying identity and adherence to rigorous economic classification principles. The identity ensures that all costs incurred for a stated purpose or function are added up. The components are private consumption of medical care—hospital care, physician services, pharmaceuticals, therapeutic appliances, other insurable benefits (except those related to sickness benefits paid in cash, which belong to an income maintenance function)—and general government outlays on health care, including public health preventive services, administration and regulation, etc.

The qualification "quasi" is used for several reasons. For one, there is a grey area related to those services that contribute to the health status of the population but are classified differently in various countries: under agriculture, under health, or elsewhere. Because detailed information is not readily accessible, it has not been possible to reallocate these services systematically. Whenever detailed information was available and permitted it, the reallocation has been effected for armed forces health services, prison health services, school health services, and publicly funded medical research and development, which are treated as auxiliaries to defense, justice, education, or science support outlays in the national accounts. In the national accounts, expenditure for health on private business premises is treated as an "intermediate" outlay, although the same services rendered to civil servants are final expenditure. Eye tests for airline pilots and similar examinations are necessary for rendering services such as safely flying passengers, but mostly the primary purposes of these services are preventive screening, which implies that they should be added to the other "final" consumption outlays. This has been done to the extent possible.

Also, gross capital outlays have been added to the aggregate outlays. In some countries, such as France, a depreciation allowance is included in the pricing (for example, the price of hospital services) and has to be deducted to avoid double counting; this was not always possible. However, the range of errors and omissions has been amply reduced over time. The estimated size of the gap or the inclusion of unwanted categories of expenditure, errors, and omissions may be in the range of 96 to 102 percent of the desired amount, much less for many countries.

Another major problem is that certain national accounting systems still are rudimentary. In public debates in a few countries, such as Belgium, the OECD estimates have been criticized as being on the low side. Almost never is it suggested that OECD estimates are overstatements. However, in France, a 1987 benchmark reevaluation led to a substantial downward revision, which is still only partly documented. Underreporting in the basic national systems from which the data are extracted regularly leads to small reevaluations of the estimates. The publication of the tables in this issue of the *Health Care Financing Review* is likely to generate further changes in ongoing accounting methodologies. Countries, such as Switzerland, that had no health accounts have established a working party to create such a system. Tentative satellite accounts have been developed in Finland and Norway. The Health Care Financing Administration in the U.S. Department of Health and Human Services publishes detailed National Health Accounts data (which, with only a 1-percent difference, nearly correspond to the National Income and Product Account Health Outlays data, compiled by the Bureau of Economic Analysis in the U.S. Department of Commerce). Health and Welfare Canada publishes data according to the same accounting rules as those used in the United States. Details published in the Dutch accounts or made available by the Central Bureau of Statistics suggest that the boundaries and economic classification principles used in the Netherlands are close to those adopted in North America. In France, Germany, and the United Kingdom, the accounting system has gained in reliability over time. However, the international compilation for countries is still crude. It is hoped that greater cross-comparability will be reached in the 1990s through international harmonization of boundary concepts and classification principles.

The use of international classifications other than those proposed by the OECD should be mentioned.[2] An example is a classification based on institutional similarity, such as social security. Estimates from these other classification systems do not include purely private medical outlays, and a fair number of public health outlays included here are also omitted. The expenditure levels estimated by the OECD Secretariat are higher than those reported elsewhere.

The heterogeneity of sources for the segments of the expenditure series is another cause of gaps in the identity. Total expenditure equals institutional care plus ambulatory care plus pharmaceutical purchases plus therapeutic appliances plus collective services (such as armed forces medical care) plus public health programs plus biomedical research and development outlays plus administrative outlays. However, for most countries, the gaps are not large.

Prices and incomes

Detailed expenditure flows are only one prerequisite of the accounting substrata needed for health policy analyses. To obtain a measure of real resources devoted to health care across countries or over time requires controlling for price trends. Have the resources devoted to health care genuinely decreased in some countries? Have they merely been stabilized in most, as exhibited by the simple ratio of total health expenditure to gross domestic product (GDP) or gross national product (GNP)? The answers provided rest on the evidence collated or estimated by statisticians regarding prices. (Schieber and Poullier briefly address the relationship between economic growth and the rate of consumption of health services in their article in this issue.) The methods of elaboration of the implicit price indexes of GDP and GNP are well documented; those of the numerator (health care consumption) are less so.

In a dynamic economic process, individual prices vary as a reflection of new scarcities, gains in productivity, market power, and a host of other demand and supply factors. If an aggregate price index for medical consumption—GDP deflator or consumer price index (CPI)—is used, specific changes occurring in inpatient care, ambulatory care, pharmaceutical production, therapeutic appliances, and government-supplied services are not captured. The OECD Health Data File includes distinct price measures (shown as 1980 = 100 in the

[2] A quantitative expression of the differences among classification systems can be found in *Structural Problems of Social Security Today and Tomorrow*, Proceedings of the European Institute of Social Security, Leuven, Belgium, ACCO, 1988, Table A-1.

accompanying tables) for each consumption function. The indicators that are accessible are mostly details of private consumption price trends, and these often fail to reflect the impact of changes in real factor costs. Input price measures, however, also are gradually collated.

At a more aggregate level, a new "total" medical consumption price index is presented in Table 13. This replaces the measure of "private" consumption trends previously presented in *Measuring Health Care*. The old measure was a fair indicator for Belgium, Switzerland, and the United States, where private consumption constitutes from two-thirds to more than four-fifths of total consumption. However, it was deceptive for other countries. For instance, in Canada, it reflected barely more than pharmaceutical prices. For some countries (Australia, Austria, Denmark, Finland, Greece, Iceland, Italy, Japan, Norway, Sweden, and the United Kingdom), the new measure is a weighted index of private and general government consumption of medical care and health services. For other countries (Belgium, Germany, Ireland, Luxembourg, Spain, Switzerland, and the United States), the price index shown reflects only private consumption; this can be a source of serious bias. For Canada, France, and the Netherlands, total health consumption indexes are calculated by the national authorities, but the underlying methodology is not given along with the published figures.

The Canadian price index is a weighted sum of the following: physician services (i.e., fee-for-service increases in medical care insurance plans, not salaries), which are calculated for each province and tabulated by Health and Welfare Canada; dental care and optometrist services, which are measured by consumer prices; average wages and salaries in hospitals (80 percent) combined with hospital supplies (20 percent), which is information collected by Statistics Canada; and prescribed and nonprescribed drugs, which are two consumer price series collected by Statistics Canada. The hospital index is also applied to other institutions.

The French index appears to be equally divided between a weighted price measure of the consumer price components and a cost index for public institutional care. Information on both wage costs and supplies is obtained in an annual survey conducted since the early 1980s. Consumer prices were the only deflators available for public hospital costs in the earliest years.

The Netherlands annually publishes current and constant price data for a range of inpatient care institutions, several ambulatory services, medical goods, and health administration services. The estimates allow calculation of a measure of total costs since 1980; provisional figures were calculated for the period 1972-80 (the estimation for past years is not yet completed); and consumer price figures were derived from several national accounting versions prior to 1972.

The final Australian private consumption expenditure deflator is a weighted measure of doctors' and dentists' fees for a range of services paid for by consumers; hospital services (weighted the same as the general government index, described next); and hospital and medical fund administrative expenses (fixed wage for the salary component; CPI trends for meals, transportation, and telephone services; and producer prices for paper and printing). For the general government index, wages and salaries for hospital, medical, and ancillary staff are weighted by fixed-weight wage and salary rates, and supplies are weighted by the corresponding input prices.

Finland also uses separate deflators for intermediate consumption and each component of value added, summing up the costs. The consumption of fixed capital is based on a capital stock model. Private health services are mainly based on social security schedules for paying patient bills, the physician fees and laboratory billing serving as control measures for a range of services. Dental services are evaluated mainly by employment data and CPI-monitored fees.

Luxembourg uses consumer price data for dental care, inpatient bed days, laboratory tests, and pharmaceutical products when evaluating market goods and services. Government health consumption is not specifically deflated.

Spain deflates nonmarket services through a weighted index of wages and supplies, with detailed calculations based on previous year = 100. (This index is not published and is not included in the estimates shown here.) Private medical consumption is deflated by the relevant CPI components.

The United States deflates physician, dentist, and other professional services and care in for-profit hospitals by the relevant CPI components. The hospital room component is used for care in for-profit hospitals. Nonprofit hospital and nursing home prices are composite input prices established by the Health Care Financing Administration. Drug preparation and sundries are deflated by the relevant medical care commodities CPI components, and ophthalmic and orthopedic appliances are deflated by the relevant eye care CPI components. Medical and hospitalization insurance is deflated by the weighted average of physician and hospital services based on estimated benefits composition; it is not separated from income loss insurance and workers' compensation insurance in the published details, the latter two being deflated by the total CPI index. Government purchases are deflated by the appropriate wage and supplies indexes. (This information is not published and is not included in the estimates shown here.) Fixed investment is also deflated by a range of relevant measures for medical and surgical instruments, hospital furniture, hospital construction, etc., including separate measures for the relevant merchandise exports and imports.

Only a limited amount of input cost data is available, so the series shown does not, in principle, include adjustments for productivity. The headings used for Tables 10-13 reflect common acceptance of pricing trends in health economics, but strictly defined they are conventional deflators rather than input price indexes. The distinction relates to the level of observation. Similar services may have two prices. For example, physicians may be committed by law to apply one level of fees to insured patients but may have some freedom to

apply another price to private patients. Where two or more sets of prices and price trends exist for given commodities or services, the level of observation does not permit differentiation. The statistician is compelled to make decisions on the basis of partial knowledge, which is only gradually incremented. The data presented reflect a provisional state of the art that is believed to be superior to use of CPI, GDP, or GNP aggregate price trends. The widespread use of separate indexes for wage components and supply components suggests that, notwithstanding the extreme variety in the basic parameters observed (e.g., in inpatient care institutions), the underlying deflation approach is reasonably comparable across countries.

Social protection

The documentation of differences across countries in the level of social protection is essential to the understanding of variations in the private-public mix in the financing of health services. Typically, only descriptive documentation is accessible. The OECD Health Data File constitutes an attempt to translate such descriptive documentation into a series of indicators reflecting the extent to which social preferences have moved countries toward coverage of the population by a public scheme and toward substituting collective for individual financing of medical benefits.

The indicators of public coverage constitute an entitlement index. In countries with universal access to publicly funded health services, the measure is straightforward. For all others, an interpretation is required of institutions and regulations that, at times, are fairly detailed. An index of social security coverage only is insufficient. In the Netherlands and Spain, for example, specific schemes—run by entities that are legally private—exist for specific groups of public employees. Since the schemes are compulsory for the groups concerned, the outlays have been treated as public, and so should the potential beneficiaries. Various systems offer gradients of coverage. For instance, in the Netherlands, a universal tax-funded scheme for long-term hospitalization has been run since 1968, but one-quarter of the population has not been subject to compulsory insurance for shorter hospitalization and other medical benefits. Ireland has a three-tier system under which, in mid-1987 (but not in the first two decades monitored), public hospital accommodation was accessible to all. Category III of this system pays for physician care. The population with voluntary health insurance, or VHI (private coverage) is estimated to have increased from 17.3 percent in 1976 to 29.3 percent in 1987. The benefits of VHI are mainly in the ambulatory care and pharmaceutical functions (plus physician services in hospitals for category I). However, a measure of the covered population is not simply the difference between 100 and the percent of population with VHI, because a special entitlement program for pharmaceutical benefits exists, notably for chronic care.

The estimates shown in Tables 15-17 are, for most countries, best estimates from the OECD Secretariat.

These are likely to be revised as more knowledge is gained of the 24 health systems under study. Several of these systems, in turn, comprise distinct subsystems. The appropriate index for a country cannot be a simple weighted average for that country, as each subsystem exhibits a number of exemptions and special cases.

An estimate of the average level of public cost sharing is still more difficult to establish. The nomenclatures of services accessible without charge (full reimbursement), those for which there is nominal cost sharing (partial reimbursement), and those for which gratuitous supply or reimbursement is denied (such as some cosmetic surgery, services supplied by physicians working outside a social contract framework, and medicines listed as nonreimbursable) sometimes comprise several hundred entries, and no detailed spending data are available. In addition, personal status affects entitlement and cost sharing. Pensioners are exempt or pay lower rates in some countries, such as Belgium; children are entitled to free dental care in several countries of Northern Europe; war victims are entitled to zero cost sharing in France; the unemployed and/or other underprivileged groups have access to specific programs in some countries, such as the United Kingdom and the United States.

No OECD country publishes an index of cost sharing. The generosity index, as it is sometimes labeled, is not a simple ratio of public-to-total expenditure. In the nearly three decades spanned by the observations, notable changes have occurred. Most countries have liberalized access to or are partly subsidizing reproductive services (family planning, prenatal and postnatal care, abortion, etc.) Older social care services aimed at the killer diseases of the period before World War II (tuberculosis, poliomyelitis, etc.) have been displaced by programs aimed at a new killer—acquired immunodeficiency syndrome (AIDS)—and by a range of treatment options made possible by advancing medical technology (such as treatment of end stage renal disease and the prevention of congenital malformations). In the opposite direction, the development of thousands of new medicines has forced many governments to moderate or even slightly reduce the level of pharmaceutical benefits. In actuality, this range of trends is still ill-translated in Tables 18 and 19. However, data from these tables can be used to find signals about turning points (years during which public schemes increased or decreased benefit levels) and to generate awareness about the typically modest size of patient cost-sharing requirements in most OECD countries. In many public debates, the public effect of cost-sharing techniques is overstated. However imperfect, the indexes produced serve a didactic purpose.

Medical care use and personnel

Health planning has long been conducted in terms of ratios, such as hospital beds per 1,000 population, with better endowed neighboring countries serving as targets. Underutilized beds contribute little to raising the health status of populations, and the differences in countries' occupancy rates are startling. The OECD Health Data

File has thus been designed as a measure of usage in addition to a measure of actual inputs. Many previous international listings included licensed but retired or otherwise inactive physicians. Efforts to standardize definitions so as to include similar inpatient institutions or active medical personnel have yielded only partial results to date. Further progress is expected in subsequent versions of the Health Data File.

Time series are more reliable than cross-sections, although this is not always the case. For example, the data on inpatient care beds in Norway matches the expenditures reported in Tables 3 and 4 only from 1980; earlier data seriously underreport the input into the Norwegian health system.

Tables 20-30 also differ from other classic presentations in attempting to portray an annual average (obtained from a daily census or other recording system) or a midyear position. Retired medical and paramedical personnel and graduates who are not practicing are not counted.

Efforts to standardize concepts cannot always overcome cultural and institutional differences. For instance, in some countries, physicians are allowed to charge their patients for diagnostic and prescriptive advice given by phone; elsewhere, they are not. The frequency of doctor consultations may be correlated with payment methods (as discussed by Sandier in this issue). The trends shown in Table 23 are probably more reliable than cross-country comparisons.

Definitional differences contribute to the intercountry differences in pharmaceutical consumption observable in Table 24. Hospital outlays on pharmaceuticals are excluded. In some countries, medicines delivered in outpatient wards are also excluded. Physicians in rural areas of some countries are allowed to dispense medicine, a source of minor data distortion. In Japan, one of the largest medicine consumers of all OECD countries, physicians in urban areas can dispense medicine as well. The number of units of medicine reported in Table 24 reflects only residual sales in pharmacies. In most countries, prescriptions refer to the number of items listed by physicians on each prescription form. Typically, more than three items constitute one prescription form for French general practitioners. Records also vary across the spectrum of countries with respect to renewable items for chronic treatments: Should six boxes of beta-blockers prescribed for a hypertensive patient over one-half year be entered as one prescription or six? In compiling international data, one lacks the necessary details to ensure consistent treatment across countries.

Medical practice variations

The literature on the impact of cultural and other factors on medical consumption in adjacent catchment areas and on the appropriateness of care in similar socioeconomic conditions has become sizable. (In this issue, McPherson adds to the literature survey.) Smaller efforts have been devoted to highlighting similarities across countries, whether tied to cultural factors or to prevailing socioeconomic incentives. Some facets of these large area variations are illustrated in Tables 31-49.

In Tables 31-37, mean length-of-stay is shown by discharge category using the 18 classes of the *International Classification of Diseases* (ICD) adopted under the auspices of the World Health Organization and used by all OECD countries. However, several countries do not yet record all their hospital admissions exhaustively and systematically, as indicated in the Enthoven article in this issue. In principle, the surveys on which these tables are based cover the entire nation for which data are reported. However, data for Australia relates only to the most populous State (New South Wales), and data for the United Kingdom come from a one-tenth sample based on a British classification developed by the Office of Population and Census. (This classification is also used in Ireland.) By and large, the figures reported for the 1970s are based on the *Eighth Revision of the ICD*. Use of the *Ninth Revision* spread only slowly across the spectrum of countries, so the figures for the 1980s are partly *Eighth Revision* and partly *Ninth Revision*. This factor is even more important when considering the three-digit entries in Tables 38-44. In some countries, maternity data are not aggregated with general hospital data, introducing some distortion. The extent to which psychiatric care is provided in hospitals differs, too. The entries for mental disorders in Table 31 are the least comparable, and this affects the overall total. The occasional reallocation of services inside a nation's hospital structure influences total length-of-stay; this is the case with Sweden beginning in 1984. The data for Switzerland are for a hospital federation covering more than four-fifths of all beds. The data for Austria and Germany are only for patients belonging to the largest health insurance schemes. The average length-of-stay figures for New Zealand are weighted for private and public institutions.

These tables also reflect conceptual differences related to definitions of personnel per bed. Data on all staff employed by hospitals (Table 45) are not completely comparable because the extent of subcontracting differs among countries. The definitions of nurses also vary (Table 46). Although there are persistent conceptual differences, considerable efforts are brought to bear to reduce the comparability gap that occurs when national series are simply collated. By and large, the trends are consistent, and no amount of statistical massaging would crush the important intercountry variations observed.

Health status indicators

Although some progress has been achieved, OECD countries do not monitor the outputs of their health systems satisfactorily because appropriate indicators are few. International organizations have limited their collection of data to a small set of "standard" indicators. The data on life expectancy at birth and at various ages (Tables 50-57) and infant and perinatal mortality rates (Tables 58 and 59) originate from national yearbooks and are sometimes supplemented by demographic journals. Mortality rates (Table 60) are supplied from the annual OECD publication *Labour Force Statistics*.

Part of the progress in a longer life span in the 1950s and 1960s is attributable to a sharp drop in infant and perinatal mortality. New diagnostic techniques to cope with high-risk pregnancies and the advent of sophisticated gynecology-obstretrical centers to cope with difficult deliveries have been essential factors in accelerating the downward trend in perinatal mortality and, by limiting complications at birth, have contributed to the improved well-being of both mothers and babies. The death rates for infectious diseases have dropped in OECD countries by about nine-tenths in the past half-century. However, in macro-policy terms, these measures are usually held to be of limited value. They may reflect advances in medical knowledge and the diffusion of certain medical procedures, but they do not lend themselves to the measurement of the outcome of public health programs and policy.

Demographic and economic background

International comparisons require ratios or the use of a common numeraire to deal with differences in population sizes and currency units. In this data compendium, Tables 1-9 and selected other entries are supplied in their original national currency expression and without reduction for population sizes. The required denominators or multipliers are published, though not always at hand when needed for analytical purposes. General economic and demographic background data are provided in Tables 61-67. The principal source for these data is Volume 1 of *National Accounts 1960-1987*, published by OECD in 1989. This source was occasionally supplemented by the underlying corresponding national publications. The OECD National Accounts and accompanying demographic data reflect guidelines that have been gradually established by the statistics profession in a harmonization process started in the early 1950s.

Differences observed in, for example, hospital beds per 1,000 population or pharmaceutical outlays per person when using national sources or the OECD data are not necessarily attributable to the numerator but may be caused by the denominator. Although an effort has been made to "massage" the numerator entries, the harmonization process of working from details to publish the most comparable aggregates is still in its infancy, whereas the body of principles on which the denominators are based is considerable.

Population figures are mid-year estimates. International agencies have opted to publish gross domestic product (GDP) estimates, not gross national product (GNP) or gross national expenditure (GNE) estimates; the difference—net factor income from abroad—is typically not very large and is not the reason why OECD GDP and domestic GNP figures are often at great variance. Canada, the United Kingdom, and the United States, to mention three large countries, adopted estimation methods in the 1940s which have not been fully incorporated in the standardized national accounts of the United Nations, the OECD, and (with some specific developments) the Statistical Office of the European Community. The standardized approach is reported here, the data being calculated by the concerned national statistical offices and meeting with their official approval.

The implicit GDP price indices, shown as 1980 = 100, are originally established in each country's own base year prices, then rebased at a subaggregate level by the OECD Secretariat whenever the base was not 1980. Several countries have various bases for, say, 10-year periods. The subperiods are linked by a chain index.

Typically, past international comparisons converted national currencies at exchange rates (Table 66). The

estimates shown are an annual average of daily observations. The vagaries of foreign exchange markets lead to grievous underestimates or overestimates of the variables analyzed.

Purchasing power parities are presented in Table 67. Indices representing the average prices in each country relative to the average international prices to purchase the same market basket of goods and services were calculated for most OECD countries for 1980 and 1985. A regression method was used to determine 1975 data. Partial estimates also existed for 1950, 1955, and 1970. From these base years, and with national accounting details, the series has been retropolated and extended beyond 1985.

List of tables

Expenditure on health

Health care pricing trends

Social protection and public participation

Utilization of medical services and available personnel resources

Selected variations in common medical care practice

Selected health status indicators

Demographic and general economic background data

Total expenditure on health, by country: 1960-87

National currency in millions

Country	1960	1961	1962	1963	1964	1965	1966	1967	1969	1970	1971	1972	1973
Australia	681	824	843	909	1,006	1,034	1,126	1,321	1,668	1,711	1,992	2,310	2,619
Austria	7,500	8,400	9,050	10,000	10,800	12,250	13,500	15,300	18,300	20,473	22,797	25,814	30,159
Belgium	19,150	19,950	21,550	23,850	27,500	32,700	35,000	38,000	44,645	51,496	57,682	67,110	81,471
Canada	2,142	2,376	2,561	2,802	3,060	3,416	3,838	4,324	5,503	6,256	7,122	7,790	8,720
Denmark	1,500	1,930	2,280	2,530	2,840	3,410	4,164	4,930	6,681	7,197	8,416	9,506	11,166
Finland	636	720	808	911	1,087	1,308	1,469	1,753	2,374	2,608	2,948	3,508	4,177
France	12,742	14,750	16,974	19,771	22,976	25,568	28,906	32,065	41,349	46,184	53,361	60,951	70,215
Germany	14,230	16,002	17,964	18,640	20,542	23,510	26,840	28,020	34,540	37,260	44,510	50,830	60,100
Greece	3,326	3,607	4,044	4,563	5,305	6,415	7,122	7,841	10,457	12,071	13,337	14,799	18,176
Iceland	3	3	4	5	8	9	11	13	19	23	30	40	52
Ireland	25	26	30	33	37	42	49	58	75	90	122	149	184
Italy	894,999	988,000	1,084,000	1,318,000	1,569,000	1,810,000	2,053,000	2,329,000	2,928,000	3,481,000	4,027,000	4,746,000	5,720,000
Japan	480,000	665,000	797,000	980,000	1,046,000	1,465,000	1,739,000	2,091,000	2,892,000	3,339,000	3,768,000	4,416,000	5,235,000
Luxembourg	—	—	—	—	—	—	—	—	—	2,250	2,600	2,900	3,250
Netherlands	1,731	1,914	2,116	2,340	2,717	3,154	3,662	4,252	5,729	7,255	8,737	10,531	12,258
New Zealand	124	—	—	—	—	179	—	231	—	300	—	—	493
Norway	1,093	1,254	1,448	1,628	1,829	1,992	2,276	2,514	3,225	4,001	4,772	5,836	6,851
Portugal	—	—	—	—	—	—	—	—	—	—	—	—	—
Spain	15,750	18,000	21,300	25,300	29,000	38,000	49,000	61,000	88,000	105,999	134,000	161,000	187,000
Sweden	3,396	3,737	4,120	4,864	5,505	6,328	7,483	8,618	10,734	12,419	14,116	15,453	16,853
Switzerland	1,223	1,350	1,650	1,870	2,090	2,301	3,000	3,450	4,250	4,697	5,730	6,450	7,520
Turkey	—	—	—	—	—	—	—	—	—	—	—	—	—
United Kingdom	1,009	1,093	1,148	1,250	1,368	1,484	1,625	1,787	2,051	2,323	2,637	3,014	3,444
United States	26,895	28,783	31,295	33,530	37,461	41,929	46,267	51,456	65,633	74,995	83,484	93,968	103,382

Country	1974	1975	1976	1977	1978	1979	1980	1981	1982	1983	1984	1985	1986	1987
Australia	3,148	4,232	5,719	6,603	7,469	8,240	9,078	10,224	11,798	13,273	14,986	16,580	18,613	21,052
Austria	35,222	48,100	54,600	59,600	66,322	72,219	78,390	86,790	90,986	96,335	101,486	109,273	118,344	124,271
Belgium	96,973	133,999	158,000	181,382	202,850	215,790	231,019	255,972	279,818	304,289	325,200	348,300	366,750	386,000
Canada	10,248	12,314	14,091	15,470	17,214	19,378	22,658	26,600	31,127	34,653	37,342	40,406	44,276	47,807
Denmark	13,747	13,976	17,126	18,348	20,542	22,791	25,426	27,836	31,658	33,655	35,968	38,582	39,778	41,400
Finland	5,217	6,617	7,861	8,915	9,724	10,912	12,448	14,452	16,580	18,823	21,124	24,171	26,328	29,110
France	81,902	102,046	119,057	134,552	158,927	183,934	212,198	248,968	288,902	326,410	370,446	396,816	429,967	450,348
Germany	70,270	80,390	86,500	91,550	98,630	106,490	117,080	126,340	128,820	133,400	142,080	149,410	156,690	161,800
Greece	22,301	27,382	33,399	39,808	47,966	62,244	74,172	91,956	113,756	142,199	172,798	224,526	296,180	336,000
Iceland	82	126	170	247	407	626	995	1,632	2,646	5,012	6,151	8,712	12,218	16,273
Ireland	220	291	354	426	495	607	800	930	1,070	1,180	1,300	1,380	1,450	1,470
Italy	7,288,000	8,434,000	10,511,000	12,007,000	14,746,000	18,345,000	25,843,000	30,280,000	36,740,000	43,510,000	48,680,000	55,720,000	61,310,000	70,890,000
Japan	6,858,000	8,378,000	9,410,000	10,748,000	12,235,000	13,542,000	15,749,501	17,084,800	18,468,200	19,422,900	20,045,700	21,146,400	22,428,000	23,853,000
Luxembourg	3,900	4,900	5,705	6,373	7,370	8,075	9,082	10,056	10,977	11,832	12,861	13,918	14,945	16,680
Netherlands	14,433	16,969	19,252	21,342	23,445	25,411	27,585	29,582	31,641	32,811	33,354	34,365	35,730	36,550
New Zealand	605	744	846	991	1,200	1,386	1,560	1,932	2,090	2,267	2,408	2,956	3,670	4,100
Norway	7,987	9,959	11,693	13,595	16,364	16,480	18,335	21,543	24,492	27,437	29,481	32,231	36,308	41,527
Portugal	15,862	24,219	29,000	35,123	45,955	56,427	73,321	95,683	117,075	142,000	176,223	245,725	291,753	333,000
Spain	250,000	304,000	406,000	535,000	664,000	764,000	895,000	1,060,000	1,258,000	1,400,000	1,505,000	1,678,000	1,933,499	2,145,600
Sweden	19,558	24,007	28,228	33,967	38,158	42,076	50,057	55,194	61,128	67,922	74,679	80,764	84,972	92,211
Switzerland	8,760	9,810	10,240	10,570	10,909	11,408	12,373	13,482	14,619	15,908	16,635	17,474	18,613	19,700
Turkey	—	18,190	—	—	—	—	179,267	—	—	407,200	—	—	1,400,000	—
United Kingdom	4,398	5,784	6,851	7,776	8,923	10,409	13,333	15,384	16,436	18,607	19,696	21,135	22,677	24,798
United States	116,113	132,680	150,760	169,855	189,657	214,659	248,109	286,975	323,635	357,185	388,500	419,000	455,700	500,300

SOURCE: Organization for Economic Cooperation and Development: Health Data File, 1989.

Table 2

Public expenditure on health, by country: 1960-87

National currency in millions

Country	1960	1961	1962	1963	1964	1965	1966	1967	1968	1969	1970	1971	1972	1973
Australia	358	400	462	492	543	591	638	632	772	—	900	1,129	1,342	1,530
Austria	5,000	5,600	6,050	6,700	7,200	8,150	9,000	10,300	10,700	12,400	12,900	14,550	16,350	19,250
Belgium	11,800	12,750	13,800	15,900	18,350	24,629	27,010	28,364	32,759	38,861	44,777	49,622	57,953	68,015
Canada	915	1,045	1,173	1,339	1,527	1,779	2,129	2,551	3,074	3,650	4,392	5,218	5,786	6,455
Denmark	1,330	1,663	1,953	2,172	2,440	2,928	3,514	4,218	4,952	5,829	6,208	7,204	8,196	9,072
Finland	344	394	461	535	659	863	990	1,259	1,504	1,749	1,924	2,144	2,580	3,179
France	7,361	8,990	11,027	13,312	15,747	17,414	19,811	22,085	23,206	28,928	34,505	39,908	46,057	52,841
Germany	9,600	10,802	12,114	13,080	14,322	16,660	19,460	20,480	23,020	25,700	27,630	33,780	38,950	47,130
Greece	1,950	2,100	2,379	2,658	3,317	4,011	4,601	4,834	5,060	5,751	6,443	7,575	8,644	10,532
Iceland	2	3	4	4	6	7	9	11	13	16	19	25	33	43
Ireland	19	20	22	25	30	32	37	44	46	56	70	88	113	144
Italy	744,000	851,000	956,000	1,192,000	1,392,000	1,590,000	1,790,000	2,050,000	2,263,000	2,541,000	3,006,000	3,581,000	4,218,000	5,062,000
Japan	290,000	400,000	480,000	590,000	730,000	900,000	1,045,000	1,263,000	1,493,000	1,724,000	2,331,000	2,477,000	2,988,000	3,603,000
Luxembourg	—	—	—	—	—	—	—	—	—	—	—	—	—	—
Netherlands	576	782	1,061	1,440	1,766	2,166	2,656	3,257	3,944	4,941	6,113	6,688	7,658	9,029
New Zealand	100	107	116	123	135	150	164	170	181	202	241	296	352	410
Norway	850	980	1,132	1,292	1,469	1,612	1,950	2,194	2,435	2,855	3,664	4,285	5,562	6,477
Portugal	657	731	789	809	925	1,304	1,529	1,749	2,475	3,141	3,306	3,880	5,704	7,580
Spain	8,200	9,300	11,000	13,100	15,000	20,000	26,000	32,000	37,000	47,000	58,000	71,000	95,000	122,000
Sweden	2,467	2,745	3,051	3,734	4,314	5,032	6,047	7,025	8,201	9,016	10,682	12,249	13,383	14,509
Switzerland	750	880	1,010	1,140	1,270	1,400	1,900	2,150	2,400	2,650	3,000	3,660	4,270	4,980
Turkey	—	—	586	672	771	843	1,086	1,230	1,451	1,810	1,863	1,830	3,580	—
United Kingdom	861	930	971	1,035	1,130	1,274	1,407	1,558	1,693	1,770	2,020	2,295	2,646	3,017
United States	6,636	7,276	7,922	8,560	9,268	10,988	13,558	18,956	22,109	24,942	27,773	31,649	35,430	39,374

Country	1974	1975	1976	1977	1978	1979	1980	1981	1982	1983	1984	1985	1986	1987
Australia	1,909	2,703	4,166	4,415	4,624	5,149	5,597	6,426	7,364	8,086	9,704	11,921	13,312	14,835
Austria	22,950	33,500	38,000	41,600	46,300	49,350	53,950	60,330	61,634	64,212	67,406	72,937	79,880	83,340
Belgium	79,957	106,700	127,100	144,914	163,412	176,402	188,318	206,147	223,767	233,100	249,300	268,000	282,200	297,000
Canada	7,677	9,362	10,878	11,906	13,119	14,704	16,982	20,154	23,668	26,428	28,027	30,182	32,944	35,335
Denmark	11,165	12,841	14,629	15,543	17,416	19,425	21,666	23,659	27,026	28,555	30,396	32,588	34,109	35,400
Finland	4,038	5,203	6,155	7,021	7,577	8,540	9,837	11,514	13,265	14,883	16,583	19,014	20,710	22,894
France	62,208	78,787	90,348	103,570	123,242	143,768	167,163	197,881	228,352	254,400	286,681	305,255	326,990	336,750
Germany	55,920	64,460	69,140	73,010	78,400	84,530	92,950	100,200	101,410	103,850	110,710	116,550	122,040	126,930
Greece	13,416	16,485	22,526	29,341	36,480	45,543	60,957	77,578	103,858	125,080	151,340	181,880	222,809	253,000
Iceland	72	110	149	217	367	559	884	1,439	2,355	4,458	5,329	7,629	10,729	14,413
Ireland	178	240	286	344	422	539	736	867	997	1,086	1,146	1,226	1,278	1,279
Italy	6,412,000	7,260,000	9,114,000	10,487,000	13,193,000	16,183,000	21,620,000	24,710,000	29,610,000	35,010,000	38,710,000	43,930,000	47,400,000	56,110,000
Japan	5,084,000	6,035,000	7,069,000	7,824,000	9,305,000	10,064,000	11,154,800	12,074,000	12,987,500	14,065,300	14,521,100	15,284,000	16,274,000	17,402,000
Luxembourg	—	4,500	5,239	5,828	6,792	7,487	8,426	9,344	10,205	10,550	11,453	12,421	13,367	15,284
Netherlands	10,798	12,974	14,755	16,426	18,265	19,831	20,908	22,501	24,256	25,021	25,533	26,180	26,265	26,995
New Zealand	503	624	728	855	1,033	1,216	1,387	1,695	1,762	1,953	2,072	2,519	3,169	3,382
Norway	7,573	9,583	11,386	13,362	15,172	16,708	18,623	21,199	23,802	26,862	28,699	31,035	34,988	40,549
Portugal	9,953	14,270	19,136	24,572	30,828	39,083	53,438	68,146	74,652	88,550	112,789	139,653	172,000	202,000
Spain	159,000	214,000	270,000	362,000	469,000	527,000	658,000	758,000	911,000	1,012,536	1,076,077	1,199,533	1,382,000	1,533,600
Sweden	17,582	21,652	25,452	31,014	34,915	38,565	46,084	50,762	56,094	62,136	68,140	73,609	77,213	83,752
Switzerland	5,800	6,763	6,985	7,169	7,328	7,691	8,354	9,211	10,008	10,887	11,288	11,945	12,703	—
Turkey	—	8,796	—	8,175	10,170	21,330	47,600	45,610	56,740	71,220	—	—	525,000	831,449
United Kingdom	3,946	5,268	6,233	6,997	8,033	9,325	11,942	13,723	14,450	16,311	17,189	18,338	19,640	21,433
United States	47,030	56,324	62,790	69,738	79,567	90,477	105,172	121,193	135,278	147,500	159,600	175,000	188,900	207,300

Table 3
Total expenditure on inpatient care, by country: 1960-87

National currency in millions

Country	1960	1961	1962	1963	1964	1965	1966	1967	1968	1969	1970	1971	1972	1973
Australia	—	—	—	—	—	—	—	—	—	478	579	—	—	—
Austria	1,713	1,901	2,111	2,257	2,482	2,784	3,137	3,590	4,427	5,222	5,895	6,473	7,251	8,628
Belgium	7,361	7,604	7,644	8,371	8,776	9,706	10,596	11,770	12,052	12,537	13,225	15,067	18,627	23,303
Canada	934	1,084	1,199	1,331	1,486	1,668	1,908	2,189	2,530	2,856	3,263	3,669	4,067	4,604
Denmark	755	876	1,016	1,178	1,366	1,658	2,042	2,283	2,807	3,281	4,019	4,343	5,013	5,842
Finland	278	331	375	436	538	637	727	844	1,022	1,160	1,315	1,526	1,768	2,066
France	4,419	5,253	6,175	7,316	8,428	9,322	10,234	11,161	11,912	15,093	17,378	20,875	23,972	27,144
Germany	—	—	—	—	—	—	—	—	—	—	14,208	17,252	20,015	24,355
Greece	1,913	2,056	2,316	2,558	3,012	3,399	3,660	4,082	4,506	5,073	5,606	6,007	6,562	8,088
Iceland	—	—	—	—	—	—	—	—	—	—	—	—	—	—
Ireland	—	—	—	—	—	—	—	—	—	—	—	—	—	—
Italy	387,000	434,000	487,000	579,000	653,000	733,000	836,000	1,006,000	1,144,000	1,307,000	1,657,000	2,114,000	2,558,000	3,037,000
Japan	163,700	203,200	234,400	279,000	335,400	410,400	455,200	526,700	620,200	710,300	879,900	969,100	1,264,200	1,435,900
Luxembourg	—	—	—	—	—	—	—	—	—	—	—	—	—	—
Netherlands	—	—	—	—	—	—	—	—	—	—	—	—	5,601	6,656
New Zealand	—	—	—	—	—	—	—	—	—	—	—	—	—	—
Norway	416	—	—	—	654	740	837	946	1,066	1,193	2,727	3,354	4,126	4,884
Portugal	—	—	—	—	—	—	—	—	—	—	—	—	—	—
Spain	—	—	—	—	—	—	—	—	—	—	—	—	—	43,885
Sweden	545	—	—	—	—	—	—	—	—	—	—	—	—	—
Switzerland	—	—	—	—	—	1,010	—	—	—	—	1,960	—	—	3,250
Turkey	—	—	—	—	—	—	—	—	—	—	—	—	—	—
United Kingdom	—	—	—	—	—	—	—	—	—	—	—	—	—	—
United States	9,618	10,257	11,353	12,600	13,911	16,048	18,131	21,162	24,529	28,030	32,655	36,646	41,711	46,118

Country	1974	1975	1976	1977	1978	1979	1980	1981	1982	1983	1984	1985	1986	1987
Australia	1,747	2,100	2,795	3,284	3,846	4,198	4,678	5,412	6,276	7,010	7,711	8,365	9,203	10,490
Austria	10,509	12,139	14,275	15,575	17,712	19,602	22,209	23,861	26,558	28,751	30,163	32,076	34,152	36,353
Belgium	29,327	39,323	50,846	58,660	63,780	67,934	75,821	85,810	96,055	108,143	114,790	119,856	124,719	130,492
Canada	5,585	6,642	7,780	8,432	9,319	10,371	11,961	14,051	16,628	18,412	19,352	20,487	22,068	23,754
Denmark	7,350	8,742	11,466	11,839	13,269	14,912	16,560	18,128	20,821	21,930	23,348	24,925	25,783	—
Finland	2,542	3,211	3,843	4,324	4,692	5,363	6,122	6,915	7,846	8,700	9,627	11,125	12,010	12,903
France	32,609	42,537	52,811	61,604	73,250	87,121	101,560	118,328	139,341	153,801	179,177	186,672	198,679	207,020
Germany	28,478	31,654	33,873	35,703	38,523	40,406	44,712	47,985	50,709	52,041	54,462	58,129	61,249	63,795
Greece	10,328	12,228	15,695	19,063	22,569	31,132	36,290	44,695	58,633	71,046	88,557	118,328	145,807	—
Iceland	—	—	—	—	—	—	—	—	—	—	—	—	—	—
Ireland	—	—	—	—	—	—	—	—	—	—	—	—	—	—
Italy	3,859,000	4,330,000	5,059,000	5,903,000	7,428,000	9,597,000	13,190,000	15,790,000	18,360,000	21,860,000	24,270,000	27,050,000	29,400,000	33,200,000
Japan	2,092,700	2,542,700	3,042,600	3,370,300	4,032,100	4,404,100	4,834,100	5,321,600	5,816,300	6,129,700	6,514,400	7,083,300	7,483,800	7,810,900
Luxembourg	—	1,350	1,454	1,636	1,926	2,105	2,389	2,649	2,923	3,213	3,530	3,809	4,171	4,619
Netherlands	8,069	9,718	11,198	12,495	13,785	15,032	16,411	17,659	18,859	19,439	19,526	20,021	20,635	20,927
New Zealand	—	—	—	—	—	870	—	1,250	—	1,428	1,506	1,796	2,283	—
Norway	5,016	6,955	8,600	10,057	11,400	12,569	13,979	16,104	18,112	19,868	21,471	23,504	25,950	—
Portugal	—	—	—	—	—	—	—	—	—	—	—	—	—	—
Spain	68,322	101,695	130,917	191,620	247,460	300,368	356,537	428,123	514,563	609,916	673,626	734,533	—	—
Sweden	—	—	—	—	—	—	—	—	—	—	—	—	—	—
Switzerland	3,800	4,527	4,713	4,861	4,924	5,170	5,655	6,188	6,751	7,444	7,801	8,187	8,706	—
Turkey	—	—	—	—	—	—	—	—	—	—	—	—	—	—
United Kingdom	—	—	—	—	—	—	—	—	—	—	—	—	—	—
United States	53,547	62,472	72,177	81,179	91,329	104,381	122,005	142,953	161,903	176,187	187,500	201,400	215,800	235,300

SOURCE: Organization for Economic Cooperation and Development: Health Data File, 1989.

Table 4
Public expenditure on inpatient care, by country: 1960-87

National currency in millions

Country	1960	1961	1962	1963	1964	1965	1966	1967	1968	1969	1970	1971	1972	1973
Australia	–	–	–	–	–	–	–	236	268	314	388	–	–	1,093
Austria	743	851	981	1,047	1,172	1,284	1,487	1,730	2,017	2,342	2,595	2,833	3,261	3,858
Belgium	–	–	–	–	–	3,873	4,697	4,849	5,732	6,633	7,683	8,527	10,034	12,443
Canada	640	740	854	995	1,165	1,402	1,515	1,735	2,006	2,337	2,949	3,327	3,689	4,170
Denmark	755	876	1,016	1,178	1,366	1,658	2,042	2,383	2,807	3,281	4,019	4,343	5,013	5,842
Finland	208	258	230	355	446	537	624	738	880	1,027	1,168	1,353	1,569	1,872
France	3,902	4,631	5,440	6,417	7,395	8,221	9,062	9,846	10,532	13,279	15,863	19,150	22,000	24,930
Germany	1,568	1,777	2,036	2,295	2,572	2,947	3,397	3,851	4,385	4,954	11,543	14,235	16,618	20,562
Greece	511	554	679	791	929	1,100	1,200	1,322	1,365	1,447	1,700	1,847	2,112	2,468
Iceland	–	1	1	2	2	3	3	4	7	8	11	12	16	28
Ireland	–	–	–	–	–	–	–	–	–	–	–	–	73	94
Italy	372,000	418,000	470,000	556,000	624,000	700,000	794,000	953,000	1,083,000	1,236,000	1,555,000	1,977,000	2,400,000	2,852,000
Japan	–	–	–	–	–	–	–	–	–	–	723,000	–	–	–
Luxembourg	–	–	–	–	–	–	–	–	–	–	–	–	–	–
Netherlands	500	650	850	1,050	1,250	1,430	1,650	1,850	2,450	2,900	3,430	4,200	4,792	5,762
New Zealand	65	69	75	82	91	103	114	118	126	139	167	205	240	278
Norway	416	467	522	580	654	740	837	946	1,066	1,193	2,727	3,354	4,126	4,884
Portugal	–	–	–	–	–	–	–	–	–	–	1,539	1,911	2,373	3,189
Spain	–	–	–	–	–	–	–	–	–	–	–	–	–	–
Sweden	–	–	–	2,576	3,043	3,506	4,230	4,887	5,425	6,018	7,419	8,681	9,597	10,674
Switzerland	–	–	–	–	–	905	–	–	–	–	–	–	–	–
Turkey	–	–	–	–	–	222	275	340	421	523	646	828	1,061	1,359
United Kingdom	449	489	530	570	611	651	748	846	943	1,041	1,138	1,332	1,525	1,909
United States	3,861	4,257	4,627	4,955	5,264	6,291	7,862	11,344	13,248	15,118	16,940	19,294	21,627	24,199

Country	1974	1975	1976	1977	1978	1979	1980	1981	1982	1983	1984	1985	1986	1987
Australia	1,584	1,536	2,202	2,552	2,886	3,155	3,485	4,130	4,705	5,071	5,781	6,750	7,459	8,356
Austria	4,479	5,339	6,495	7,275	8,222	8,772	9,539	10,441	11,338	12,181	12,953	13,456	14,312	15,223
Belgium	16,202	22,626	27,624	30,359	31,695	34,577	39,063	42,701	45,048	52,009	57,975	55,198	63,430	68,539
Canada	5,049	5,849	6,872	7,432	8,136	8,963	10,306	12,187	14,426	15,934	16,879	18,867	19,325	20,786
Denmark	7,350	8,742	11,466	11,839	13,269	14,912	16,560	18,128	20,821	21,930	23,348	24,925	25,783	–
Finland	2,326	2,976	3,490	3,964	4,255	4,855	5,598	6,332	7,167	7,903	8,761	10,107	10,883	11,745
France	30,550	38,800	47,610	55,300	66,300	78,240	93,414	110,300	129,650	147,450	164,236	166,030	179,912	185,896
Germany	24,268	26,844	28,689	30,193	33,227	34,705	38,476	41,221	43,590	44,426	46,381	49,707	52,372	54,498
Greece	3,299	4,147	5,861	7,523	9,490	12,736	16,315	19,338	24,518	31,927	42,533	55,611	66,028	82,349
Iceland	47	69	93	137	224	355	665	1,078	1,723	3,160	3,786	5,287	7,362	10,020
Ireland	120	162	185	239	279	388	547	630	719	797	844	907	920	936
Italy	3,629,000	4,067,000	4,769,000	5,577,000	7,100,000	9,272,000	12,068,000	14,280,000	16,300,000	19,240,000	21,210,000	23,650,000	25,720,000	29,440,000
Japan	–	2,302,400	2,771,000	3,107,000	3,733,500	4,113,600	4,528,800	5,001,600	5,483,200	5,733,000	6,059,000	6,586,000	6,957,700	7,250,000
Luxembourg	–	1,217	1,327	1,534	1,844	2,012	2,322	2,565	2,831	3,038	3,336	3,603	3,968	4,414
Netherlands	7,033	8,756	9,812	10,939	12,185	13,233	13,862	14,981	16,154	16,606	16,812	17,122	17,052	17,454
New Zealand	337	414	481	569	697	851	918	1,224	1,226	1,396	1,465	1,745	2,215	2,233
Norway	5,016	6,955	8,600	10,057	11,400	12,569	13,979	16,104	18,112	19,868	21,471	23,504	25,950	–
Portugal	4,285	5,996	8,389	10,739	13,747	17,403	22,031	28,000	34,385	40,975	52,154	61,405	76,000	740,000
Spain	51,787	80,174	101,596	148,554	187,571	228,559	269,323	322,072	385,098	467,695	519,108	–	–	–
Sweden	12,724	15,598	18,458	22,800	25,581	28,502	34,111	37,447	40,792	45,237	49,335	53,091	54,920	63,212
Switzerland	–	3,671	3,948	–	–	–	4,390	–	5,711	–	6,554	–	7,143	–
Turkey	1,741	2,231	2,879	4,538	7,169	11,216	20,112	22,571	–	–	–	–	–	–
United Kingdom	2,292	2,928	3,564	4,417	5,058	5,814	7,483	8,613	9,036	10,052	10,531	11,085	11,823	12,149
United States	29,006	34,529	38,733	43,718	49,527	56,373	65,116	75,306	85,273	91,619	99,500	107,400	113,400	122,100

Total expenditure on ambulatory medical services, by country: 1960-87

National currency in millions

Country	1960	1961	1962	1963	1964	1965	1966	1967	1968	1969	1970	1971	1972	1973
Australia	—	—	—	—	—	—	—	—	—	—	—	—	—	—
Austria	1,782	1,973	2,159	2,413	2,611	2,858	3,260	3,640	4,071	4,494	4,893	5,436	6,247	6,924
Belgium	7,904	8,075	8,794	9,353	10,133	14,142	14,964	15,866	17,633	20,880	21,888	24,914	29,102	34,514
Canada	513	556	581	647	704	771	851	950	1,090	1,242	1,402	1,667	1,850	2,028
Denmark	—	—	—	—	—	—	1,582	1,821	2,075	2,363	2,767	3,181	3,456	3,906
Finland	146	161	180	199	236	270	310	373	441	498	560	645	799	980
France	3,513	3,725	4,220	5,030	6,021	6,656	7,767	9,048	9,337	10,996	12,306	13,848	15,230	18,683
Germany	—	—	—	—	—	—	—	—	—	—	11,477	13,695	15,932	17,208
Greece	—	—	—	—	—	—	—	—	—	—	4,669	5,235	5,865	7,349
Iceland	—	—	—	—	—	—	—	—	—	—	—	—	—	—
Ireland	—	—	—	—	—	—	—	—	—	—	—	—	—	—
Italy	320,000	350,000	375,000	482,000	615,000	716,000	803,000	878,000	956,000	1,101,000	1,260,000	1,338,000	1,525,000	1,865,000
Japan	—	—	302,200	386,600	499,800	597,800	718,600	832,700	993,000	1,160,600	1,371,400	1,493,000	1,821,100	2,165,400
Luxembourg	—	—	—	—	—	—	—	—	—	—	505	613	680	790
Netherlands	535	579	689	737	877	991	1,093	1,276	1,441	1,570	—	—	3,062	3,494
New Zealand	—	—	—	—	—	—	—	—	—	—	—	—	—	—
Norway	—	—	—	—	—	—	—	—	—	—	—	—	—	—
Portugal	—	—	—	—	—	—	—	—	—	—	—	—	—	—
Spain	—	—	—	—	—	—	—	—	—	—	—	—	—	—
Sweden	—	—	—	—	—	—	—	—	—	—	—	—	—	—
Switzerland	—	—	—	—	—	—	—	—	—	—	—	—	—	—
Turkey	—	—	—	—	—	—	—	—	—	—	—	—	—	—
United Kingdom	—	—	—	—	—	—	—	—	—	—	—	—	—	—
United States	8,523	8,844	9,634	10,089	11,653	12,314	13,299	14,760	16,200	18,316	20,684	22,614	24,589	27,578

Country	1974	1975	1976	1977	1978	1979	1980	1981	1982	1983	1984	1985	1986	1987
Australia	827	827	1,226	1,387	1,588	1,805	2,043	2,278	2,615	3,055	3,543	4,012	4,618	5,131
Austria	8,455	9,628	11,118	12,123	13,356	14,474	15,857	17,342	18,364	19,732	21,735	23,272	24,868	26,469
Belgium	41,023	50,727	59,164	67,850	77,709	84,032	88,604	97,302	108,364	118,161	129,774	141,196	151,099	158,092
Canada	2,278	2,658	3,019	3,389	3,834	4,351	4,999	5,762	6,690	7,593	8,282	9,078	9,978	10,932
Denmark	4,334	4,764	4,953	5,580	6,218	6,792	7,657	8,433	9,397	10,117	10,844	11,616	11,704	—
Finland	1,232	1,596	1,941	2,254	2,541	2,904	3,382	4,069	4,787	5,548	6,527	7,748	8,647	9,895
France	21,401	26,154	29,977	33,191	39,664	45,607	52,590	60,644	69,552	83,353	93,197	104,343	117,609	124,263
Germany	19,846	22,591	24,274	25,793	28,181	30,270	32,914	35,430	36,270	38,224	40,624	44,265	44,293	46,131
Greece	9,140	11,506	14,399	17,216	21,407	27,673	33,688	40,132	50,008	—	—	—	—	—
Iceland	—	—	—	—	—	—	—	—	—	—	—	—	—	—
Ireland	—	—	—	—	—	—	—	—	—	—	—	—	—	—
Italy	2,445,000	2,850,000	3,917,000	4,367,000	5,209,000	6,171,000	8,320,000	9,185,000	11,360,000	15,070,000	16,960,000	18,710,000	22,190,000	25,300,000
Japan	2,799,600	3,367,300	3,967,300	4,341,900	4,868,500	5,300,200	5,700,300	5,930,700	6,289,300	6,569,300	6,678,200	6,945,400	7,437,100	—
Luxembourg	948	1,201	2,736	3,079	3,625	3,961	4,496	4,985	5,500	6,047	6,643	7,169	7,849	8,692
Netherlands	4,001	4,617	5,177	5,737	6,320	6,918	7,480	7,903	8,300	8,604	8,677	8,905	9,207	9,497
New Zealand	—	—	—	—	—	—	—	—	—	—	—	—	617	—
Norway	—	—	—	—	—	—	—	—	—	—	—	—	—	—
Portugal	—	—	—	5,687	7,413	8,855	12,021	15,795	19,925	27,283	35,284	41,654	53,024	—
Spain	—	—	—	—	—	—	108,461	118,982	134,807	152,062	166,356	186,651	—	—
Sweden	—	—	—	—	—	—	—	—	—	—	—	—	—	—
Switzerland	—	4,390	4,578	4,745	4,999	5,245	5,629	6,114	6,594	7,117	7,462	7,836	8,379	—
Turkey	—	—	—	—	—	—	—	—	—	—	—	—	—	—
United Kingdom	—	—	—	—	—	—	—	—	—	—	—	—	—	—
United States	30,840	35,788	40,215	45,953	51,704	58,317	67,954	78,913	89,240	99,485	109,800	120,900	135,300	156,900

SOURCE: Organization for Economic Cooperation and Development: Health Data File, 1989.

133

Table 6
Public expenditure on ambulatory medical services, by country: 1960-87

National currency in millions

Country	1960	1961	1962	1963	1964	1965	1966	1967	1968	1969	1970	1971	1972	1973	1974	1975	1976	1977	1978	1979	1980	1981	1982	1983	1984	1985	1986	1987
Australia	68	74	80	86	103	122	145	158	173	188	206	224	245	261	276	276	763	598	432	610	718	799	902	1,084	1,619	2,520	2,871	3,139
Austria	1,062	1,193	1,299	1,493	1,631	1,778	2,010	2,270	2,521	2,774	2,993	3,326	3,707	4,144	5,085	6,018	7,018	7,733	8,526	9,094	10,027	10,892	11,444	12,132	12,905	13,882	14,858	15,629
Belgium	–	–	–	–	–	9,209	10,215	10,933	12,667	15,232	17,535	19,887	23,250	27,131	32,112	39,828	46,875	54,003	63,590	68,325	71,382	78,365	87,554	94,621	103,842	108,694	123,605	136,365
Canada	52	58	66	76	88	103	154	232	352	537	830	1,190	1,335	1,464	1,657	1,951	2,206	2,442	2,761	3,095	3,599	4,260	4,880	5,529	6,019	6,579	7,304	7,802
Denmark	330	387	454	533	626	734	862	1,012	1,187	1,392	1,634	1,914	2,140	2,269	2,563	2,862	3,044	3,585	4,016	4,366	4,944	5,347	5,995	6,407	6,816	7,379	8,018	–
Finland	64	65	73	82	99	123	146	215	253	287	321	360	470	617	808	1,056	1,354	1,573	1,796	2,075	2,430	3,005	3,582	4,094	4,785	5,704	6,440	7,372
France	2,465	2,623	2,971	3,532	4,246	4,467	5,429	6,103	6,499	7,657	9,084	10,220	11,750	13,780	15,790	19,835	22,720	25,160	30,060	34,570	36,113	45,760	52,440	62,850	69,782	69,114	75,850	78,291
Germany	2,342	2,603	2,926	3,143	3,531	4,148	5,110	5,399	5,843	6,369	8,358	10,206	11,394	13,039	15,172	17,471	18,702	19,840	21,320	22,783	24,652	26,462	26,875	27,949	29,760	30,800	32,401	33,728
Greece	–	–	445	517	611	722	790	868	864	1,004	1,115	1,165	1,273	1,528	1,945	2,299	3,256	3,779	4,861	6,576	7,914	9,550	12,729	–	–	–	–	–
Iceland	–	–	–	–	–	–	–	–	–	–	–	–	–	–	18	35	45	69	117	174	158	245	431	795	999	1,545	2,302	3,163
Ireland	–	–	–	–	–	–	–	–	–	–	–	–	–	–	–	–	–	42	47	61	82	95	115	158	166	182	–	–
Italy	251,000	299,000	328,000	427,000	529,000	602,000	668,000	720,000	772,000	857,000	969,000	1,063,000	1,184,000	1,400,000	1,863,000	2,197,000	3,128,000	3,396,000	4,298,000	5,051,000	6,934,000	7,299,000	8,994,000	11,930,000	13,330,000	14,449,000	17,660,000	19,420,000
Japan	–	–	–	–	–	–	–	–	–	–	1,096,800	–	–	–	–	2,845,200	3,352,400	3,750,300	4,196,400	4,560,200	4,932,300	5,129,500	5,458,000	5,687,400	5,717,300	5,906,300	6,312,000	–
Luxembourg	–	–	–	–	–	–	–	–	–	–	–	–	–	–	–	1,033	–	–	–	–	3,907	4,358	4,820	5,173	5,680	6,135	6,757	7,501
Netherlands	29	39	53	72	88	108	133	163	200	247	306	334	1,891	2,071	2,418	2,836	2,396	2,663	3,128	3,466	4,734	5,010	5,295	5,556	5,618	5,763	5,744	6,014
New Zealand	10	11	12	12	14	15	16	17	18	20	24	25	31	36	44	57	58	63	79	82	93	100	107	–	–	–	–	–
Norway	–	–	–	–	–	–	–	–	–	–	875	–	–	–	–	–	–	–	–	–	–	–	–	–	–	–	–	–
Portugal	–	–	–	–	–	–	–	–	–	–	–	–	1,280	–	2,139	–	4,152	–	6,761	–	11,787	–	14,927	18,347	26,446	48,111	–	–
Spain	–	–	–	–	–	–	–	–	–	–	–	–	16,000	21,000	28,000	39,000	52,000	66,000	82,000	92,000	110,000	–	–	–	–	–	–	–
Sweden	–	–	–	–	245	266	317	379	479	555	732	1,039	1,199	1,183	1,449	1,769	2,238	2,755	3,212	3,450	4,159	4,865	5,772	6,356	7,353	8,703	9,744	12,637
Switzerland	–	–	–	–	–	–	–	–	–	–	–	–	–	–	–	–	–	–	–	–	–	–	–	–	–	–	–	–
Turkey	–	–	–	–	–	–	–	–	–	–	–	–	–	–	–	–	–	–	–	–	12,867	27,435	–	–	–	–	–	–
United Kingdom	–	143	136	133	162	172	189	208	221	236	278	302	323	351	435	564	641	667	759	922	1,165	1,363	1,576	1,676	1,845	1,973	2,107	2,343
United States	385	430	495	531	575	670	992	2,323	2,916	3,225	3,432	3,943	4,477	5,059	6,124	7,599	8,265	9,408	10,750	12,470	14,666	17,417	19,718	22,756	25,000	28,400	32,800	37,900

Table 7
Total expenditure on pharmaceutical goods, by country: 1960-87

National currency in millions

Country	1960	1961	1962	1963	1964	1965	1966	1967	1968	1969	1970	1971	1972	1973
Australia	—	—	—	—	—	—	—	—	—	—	—	—	—	—
Austria	1,235	1,403	1,536	1,673	1,745	1,913	2,153	2,445	2,741	3,030	3,311	3,756	4,106	4,446
Belgium	4,653	5,170	6,029	6,406	6,596	8,797	9,322	10,874	11,912	12,113	14,477	16,310	18,542	22,443
Canada	276	284	298	328	356	411	445	504	558	622	657	727	764	892
Denmark	—	—	—	—	—	—	343	420	513	588	698	801	825	977
Finland	109	123	128	139	161	194	206	234	274	297	329	400	474	535
France	2,810	3,504	4,000	4,504	5,136	5,817	6,625	7,410	7,934	9,367	10,730	12,054	13,380	15,445
Germany	—	—	—	—	—	—	—	—	—	—	7,765	8,998	10,310	11,951
Greece	1,070	1,133	1,224	1,466	1,644	2,199	2,521	2,843	3,391	4,238	5,230	5,864	6,473	7,636
Iceland	—	—	—	—	—	—	—	—	—	—	—	—	—	—
Ireland	—	—	—	—	—	—	—	—	—	—	20	—	28	33
Italy	177,000	192,000	209,000	241,000	284,000	343,000	389,000	424,000	450,000	496,000	538,000	547,000	631,000	779,000
Japan	—	—	—	—	—	—	—	—	—	—	—	—	—	—
Luxembourg	165	170	172	196	224	276	328	390	451	507	545	580	626	682
Netherlands	—	—	—	—	—	—	—	—	—	—	—	—	1,350	1,500
New Zealand	—	—	—	—	—	—	—	—	—	—	—	—	—	—
Norway	—	—	140	162	173	178	197	223	245	277	313	348	380	439
Portugal	—	—	—	—	—	—	—	—	—	—	—	—	—	—
Spain	—	—	—	—	—	—	—	—	—	—	—	—	—	—
Sweden	—	—	—	—	—	—	—	—	—	—	—	—	—	1,436
Switzerland	—	—	—	—	—	—	—	—	—	—	897	1,020	1,113	1,205
Turkey	—	—	—	—	—	—	—	—	—	—	—	—	—	—
United Kingdom	—	—	—	—	—	—	—	—	—	—	—	—	—	—
United States	3,657	3,824	4,095	4,235	4,446	5,180	5,462	5,764	6,421	7,145	7,996	8,579	9,335	10,056

Country	1974	1975	1976	1977	1978	1979	1980	1981	1982	1983	1984	1985	1986	1987
Australia	—	517	560	596	631	693	694	810	950	1,056	1,221	1,320	1,439	1,775
Austria	5,434	6,211	6,928	7,582	7,766	8,555	9,392	10,007	10,657	11,311	11,786	12,748	13,599	14,326
Belgium	25,969	29,327	29,831	33,829	36,393	37,935	39,827	41,149	44,221	48,601	49,256	55,297	59,444	64,011
Canada	958	1,091	1,197	1,288	1,481	1,753	2,040	2,434	2,758	3,158	3,647	4,230	4,910	5,553
Denmark	1,167	1,253	1,355	1,534	1,799	2,020	2,308	2,524	2,849	3,136	3,343	3,676	3,977	—
Finland	648	789	940	1,061	1,162	1,243	1,328	1,490	1,622	1,880	2,105	2,346	2,539	2,801
France	17,076	20,256	21,357	21,857	26,187	28,990	33,687	40,688	46,587	51,385	57,037	64,200	70,520	73,764
Germany	13,758	15,502	17,109	17,778	19,482	21,062	23,225	25,196	25,642	27,206	29,377	31,257	33,042	35,212
Greece	8,812	11,338	12,925	15,019	18,578	21,625	25,820	30,209	32,263	41,813	51,346	64,851	84,955	—
Iceland	9	15	19	—	43	68	97	116	133	142	—	—	—	—
Ireland	33	41	49	57	67	78	—	—	—	—	—	—	—	—
Italy	935,000	1,192,000	1,461,000	1,633,000	1,973,000	2,411,000	3,704,000	4,475,000	5,972,000	7,182,000	7,990,000	10,190,000	11,410,000	13,560,000
Japan	—	—	—	—	—	—	3,480,600	3,719,200	3,572,500	3,892,100	3,550,000	3,555,300	3,917,300	3,917,000
Luxembourg	806	928	1,061	1,161	1,241	1,310	1,418	1,530	1,717	1,880	2,082	2,302	2,475	2,839
Netherlands	1,640	1,855	2,025	2,174	2,327	2,462	2,126	2,266	2,500	2,556	2,798	3,000	3,253	3,478
New Zealand	—	—	—	—	—	164	—	220	—	279	317	427	548	632
Norway	521	634	718	779	824	867	920	1,013	1,200	1,371	1,465	1,631	1,830	2,081
Portugal	—	—	—	6,943	10,539	13,357	16,543	19,255	23,418	29,238	37,602	44,670	53,124	—
Spain	—	—	—	—	—	—	180,288	204,627	247,599	269,883	273,931	307,625	—	—
Sweden	1,627	1,901	2,128	2,439	2,667	2,897	3,242	3,498	4,150	4,779	5,099	5,516	6,065	6,722
Switzerland	1,261	1,326	1,439	1,458	1,666	1,737	1,875	1,985	2,124	2,263	2,344	2,422	2,683	2,456
Turkey	—	—	—	—	—	—	—	—	—	—	—	—	—	—
United Kingdom	550	646	780	939	1,102	1,254	1,490	1,708	1,955	2,120	2,200	—	—	—
United States	10,999	11,940	13,022	14,074	15,420	17,129	18,752	20,704	22,129	24,474	26,537	28,500	31,300	34,000

SOURCE: Organization for Economic Cooperation and Development: Health Data File, 1989.

Table 8
Public expenditure on pharmaceutical goods, by country: 1960-87

National currency in millions

Country	1960	1961	1962	1963	1964	1965	1966	1967	1968	1969	1970	1971	1972	1973
Australia	–	–	–	–	–	–	–	–	–	–	–	–	–	–
Austria	645	723	816	883	925	1,013	1,173	1,375	1,511	1,740	1,971	2,226	2,486	2,616
Belgium	–	–	–	–	–	5,276	5,412	5,606	6,424	7,566	8,472	9,014	10,487	12,365
Canada	2	2	3	3	3	4	5	7	9	12	15	24	36	49
Denmark	48	60	76	92	109	126	150	182	219	260	288	334	386	447
Finland	–	–	–	–	9	43	49	63	83	94	111	142	182	221
France	2,078	2,561	2,921	3,285	3,735	4,217	4,790	5,314	5,680	6,674	7,632	8,570	9,520	10,980
Germany	1,574	1,753	1,953	2,185	2,410	2,794	3,367	3,790	4,390	5,364	4,812	5,729	6,717	8,079
Greece	102	142	174	196	232	284	307	306	319	386	404	471	559	709
Iceland	–	–	–	–	–	–	–	–	–	–	2	2	2	3
Ireland	–	–	–	–	–	–	–	–	–	–	–	2	3	7
Italy	121,000	134,000	158,000	209,000	239,000	288,000	328,000	377,000	408,000	448,000	482,000	541,000	634,000	810,000
Japan	–	–	–	–	–	–	–	–	–	–	–	–	–	–
Luxembourg	–	–	–	–	–	–	–	–	–	–	–	–	–	–
Netherlands	–	–	–	–	–	–	–	235	278	327	402	498	722	886
New Zealand	14	15	16	16	18	20	21	22	25	27	31	33	40	45
Norway	–	–	–	–	–	–	–	–	–	–	–	–	–	–
Portugal	–	–	–	–	–	–	–	–	–	–	515	–	1,119	–
Spain	–	–	–	–	–	–	–	–	–	–	–	–	35,000	48,000
Sweden	86	102	116	131	150	176	207	239	396	452	516	607	740	901
Switzerland	–	–	–	–	–	–	–	–	–	–	–	–	–	–
Turkey	–	–	–	–	–	–	–	–	–	–	–	–	–	–
United Kingdom	59	68	59	57	79	137	161	175	175	182	199	219	249	277
United States	–	74	93	109	126	196	239	280	334	416	484	590	668	745

Country	1974	1975	1976	1977	1978	1979	1980	1981	1982	1983	1984	1985	1986	1987
Australia	–	285	314	266	289	307	314	354	446	483	546	629	693	833
Austria	3,094	3,571	4,088	4,482	4,326	4,935	5,572	5,887	6,027	6,171	6,436	6,968	7,479	7,966
Belgium	14,612	16,577	18,124	19,843	20,263	21,597	22,834	22,833	23,508	26,224	26,662	28,204	32,428	35,934
Canada	81	150	206	254	313	372	447	546	659	787	933	1,110	1,308	1,420
Denmark	518	530	601	666	777	910	1,061	1,122	1,231	1,364	1,465	1,625	1,770	–
Finland	292	367	435	490	519	561	620	699	761	853	936	1,044	1,137	1,281
France	12,140	14,395	15,180	15,540	18,620	20,610	21,789	28,930	33,120	36,530	36,907	42,394	46,561	44,376
Germany	9,542	10,895	12,067	12,420	13,499	14,571	16,118	17,513	17,630	18,481	20,091	21,476	22,947	24,709
Greece	944	1,072	1,362	1,667	2,036	2,778	3,744	5,246	6,241	7,883	9,632	12,060	18,076	–
Iceland	5	10	11	19	31	45	71	116	201	503	544	797	1,065	–
Ireland	10	16	19	19	30	37	49	65	77	76	82	87	–	1,230
Italy	920,000	996,000	1,217,000	1,514,000	1,794,000	1,860,000	2,622,000	3,123,000	4,310,000	5,140,000	5,560,000	6,940,000	7,186,000	–
Japan	–	–	–	–	–	–	2,828,700	2,963,500	2,866,500	3,113,000	2,871,300	2,851,400	3,182,000	–
Luxembourg	–	693	812	846	970	1,051	1,139	1,256	1,384	1,406	1,572	1,766	1,958	2,195
Netherlands	981	1,139	1,261	1,379	1,488	1,566	1,417	1,519	1,683	1,594	1,754	1,899	1,988	2,121
New Zealand	56	70	85	98	113	133	147	176	196	222	255	346	444	513
Norway	597	729	861	994	1,137	1,258	1,418	1,554	–	–	1,025	1,148	1,348	–
Portugal	1,902	–	3,766	–	6,583	–	11,350	–	16,476	17,940	21,232	27,656	–	–
Spain	52,000	62,000	65,000	74,000	94,000	99,000	110,000	113,000	138,000	159,000	–	–	–	–
Sweden	1,042	1,276	1,416	1,694	1,870	2,038	2,326	2,403	2,919	3,362	3,490	3,830	4,199	4,763
Switzerland	–	–	–	–	–	–	–	–	–	–	–	–	–	–
Turkey	–	–	–	–	–	–	2,530	3,610	4,800	7,680	–	–	–	–
United Kingdom	377	446	558	686	818	916	1,078	1,247	1,427	1,592	1,736	1,855	1,994	2,164
United States	860	1,027	1,141	1,186	1,294	1,445	1,614	1,861	1,952	2,149	2,374	2,900	3,400	3,900

136

Public expenditure on capital goods for medical care, by country: 1960-87

National currency in millions

Country	1960	1961	1962	1963	1964	1965	1966	1967	1968	1969	1970	1971	1972	1973
Australia	–	–	–	–	63	71	75	71	81	91	–	104	118	122
Austria	278	351	434	444	550	717	742	827	973	1,093	1,134	1,314	1,514	2,088
Belgium	–	–	–	–	–	–	–	–	–	–	1,646	994	1,518	2,287
Canada	102	–	–	–	–	105	–	–	–	–	232	272	284	287
Denmark	–	–	–	–	–	–	–	–	–	–	–	978	991	999
Finland	62	60	78	86	78	116	124	187	212	257	228	175	216	282
France	–	–	–	–	–	–	–	–	–	–	–	–	–	–
Germany	–	–	–	–	–	–	–	–	–	–	2,484	2,839	3,130	3,890
Greece	57	43	71	53	50	115	207	170	166	199	203	245	296	554
Iceland	–	–	–	–	–	–	–	–	–	–	–	–	–	3
Ireland	–	–	–	–	–	–	–	–	–	–	5	5	6	7
Italy	29,000	34,000	39,000	38,000	45,000	55,000	67,000	113,000	125,000	142,000	173,000	188,000	289,000	342,000
Japan	–	–	–	–	–	–	–	–	–	–	130,000	152,000	174,000	195,000
Luxembourg	–	–	–	–	–	–	–	–	–	–	–	–	–	–
Netherlands	–	–	–	–	–	–	–	–	–	–	–	–	–	–
New Zealand	–	–	–	–	–	–	–	–	–	–	–	34	39	45
Norway	84	96	113	138	164	145	169	181	210	285	346	385	533	630
Portugal	–	–	–	–	146	53	89	104	191	251	330	176	417	543
Spain	–	–	–	–	–	–	–	–	–	–	–	–	–	–
Sweden	339	368	400	475	581	734	918	1,134	1,444	1,511	1,722	1,629	1,555	1,456
Switzerland	–	–	–	–	–	–	–	–	284	404	275	313	568	547
Turkey	–	–	–	–	–	–	–	–	–	–	–	–	406	504
United Kingdom	37	45	55	60	79	93	106	129	147	140	154	183	223	264
United States	512	518	541	545	564	705	728	821	843	938	1,086	1,351	1,240	1,272

Country	1974	1975	1976	1977	1978	1979	1980	1981	1982	1983	1984	1985	1986	1987
Australia	153	255	407	422	393	390	334	288	259	269	379	436	547	640
Austria	1,770	2,704	2,656	2,680	3,710	3,875	3,838	5,456	4,909	5,105	5,551	5,302	7,449	5,201
Belgium	2,175	2,300	3,073	3,888	4,893	5,115	4,800	8,596	6,157	4,342	–	–	–	–
Canada	330	377	368	386	451	610	699	830	978	1,191	1,145	1,223	1,324	1,386
Denmark	1,167	1,150	1,207	1,004	1,060	1,296	1,139	1,146	1,152	1,189	1,428	1,125	1,140	–
Finland	367	487	487	551	564	538	609	781	970	1,158	1,207	–	–	1,212
France	–	1,651	1,813	2,405	2,392	2,373	2,584	2,357	2,751	12,570	13,004	14,128	14,235	–
Germany	4,412	4,594	4,506	4,390	5,169	5,087	5,994	6,086	6,965	6,991	6,508	7,085	7,077	6,980
Greece	633	741	809	1,015	1,123	1,791	2,094	3,857	2,698	6,055	8,689	10,979	14,867	15,331
Iceland	6	10	12	28	21	24	43	86	136	208	178	334	457	618
Ireland	7	7	13	25	30	38	52	60	59	53	56	57	59	58
Italy	420,000	324,000	438,000	457,000	586,000	687,000	1,926,000	1,046,000	919,000	1,141,000	1,422,000	1,575,000	2,048,000	2,255,000
Japan	337,000	317,000	331,000	406,000	518,000	545,000	595,700	641,200	697,300	614,000	587,800	603,200	637,000	753,000
Luxembourg	–	–	–	412	486	466	623	804	873	919	992	1,172	1,027	1,270
Netherlands	–	–	372	1,287	1,510	1,424	1,734	1,783	–	–	–	–	–	–
New Zealand	55	76	95	99	110	119	123	115	108	101	105	–	–	–
Norway	787	1,033	1,251	1,337	1,505	1,497	1,717	1,689	1,685	1,567	1,431	1,426	1,873	2,499
Portugal	488	820	853	1,592	2,458	3,090	4,218	7,165	6,463	6,796	6,230	5,614	7,964	–
Spain	–	–	–	–	–	–	–	–	–	–	35,873	44,455	48,920	–
Sweden	1,470	1,798	2,015	2,294	2,629	2,825	3,357	3,862	4,374	4,901	5,435	5,320	5,570	5,197
Switzerland	625	572	489	522	520	448	412	491	470	442	395	382	396	–
Turkey	807	1,071	1,638	1,936	2,946	3,812	7,322	14,200	19,680	18,000	25,000	–	–	127,000
United Kingdom	277	359	410	420	459	555	616	700	817	854	945	1,005	1,078	998
United States	1,625	1,995	2,080	2,071	2,093	2,255	2,532	2,728	2,624	2,778	2,660	2,571	2,500	2,600

NOTE: Capital goods represent investment plus capital transfers.

SOURCE: Organization for Economic Cooperation and Development: Health Data File, 1989.

137

Table 10
Inpatient care price index, by country: 1960-87

Country	1960	1961	1962	1963	1964	1965	1966	1967	1968	1969	1970	1971	1972	1973
Australia	20.8	21.2	21.7	22.5	24.4	24.2	25.3	26.6	27.5	28.9	31.6	35.0	38.3	41.3
Austria	10.2	11.3	12.8	13.5	14.7	16.4	17.9	20.4	24.1	27.0	31.6	37.2	44.2	45.5
Belgium	17.4	19.1	20.9	22.8	25.0	27.3	29.9	32.7	35.8	39.1	42.8	43.8	46.0	48.9
Canada	19.1	20.4	20.9	21.3	22.2	23.4	25.3	27.1	29.1	32.5	35.4	37.9	40.9	44.8
Denmark	9.3	10.6	12.1	13.7	15.7	17.9	27.1	29.1	30.9	33.0	34.5	39.9	43.4	48.8
Finland	17.1	18.3	19.5	20.9	22.4	23.9	25.6	29.1	29.2	31.2	33.4	38.1	43.3	49.3
France	20.1	21.1	22.6	25.4	26.7	27.3	28.2	27.3	29.2	34.6	37.0	39.3	42.0	44.4
Germany	–	–	13.6	14.9	16.4	18.7	21.5	29.0	30.8	28.2	31.5	37.8	43.2	50.6
Greece	12.8	13.6	15.2	17.0	15.8	16.6	16.8	17.0	17.0	17.6	18.1	18.4	20.2	26.8
Iceland	–	–	–	–	–	–	–	–	–	–	–	–	–	–
Ireland	7.1	8.1	9.2	10.6	12.1	13.8	15.9	18.1	20.7	23.7	27.8	31.9	36.0	40.3
Italy	8.0	8.7	10.1	11.2	12.4	13.9	14.5	14.8	15.1	16.6	21.8	27.1	29.9	33.3
Japan	39.7	42.3	48.6	48.7	45.4	49.6	49.6	50.5	54.7	53.3	57.1	57.5	64.1	62.1
Luxembourg	–	–	–	–	–	–	–	–	–	–	–	–	–	–
Netherlands	12.9	14.6	16.6	18.8	21.4	24.3	–	–	–	–	–	–	–	–
New Zealand	13.4	13.7	14.5	15.3	16.0	16.7	17.1	18.2	19.3	20.8	24.7	28.9	35.5	40.9
Norway	19.5	21.3	23.2	25.4	27.0	30.2	30.2	34.7	37.1	39.7	42.6	46.9	51.7	57.0
Portugal	–	–	–	–	–	–	–	–	–	–	19.3	21.4	23.8	26.4
Spain	–	–	–	–	–	–	–	–	–	–	–	–	–	–
Sweden	13.8	15.1	16.5	18.0	19.7	21.5	23.2	24.9	26.7	28.8	30.9	34.9	39.5	44.6
Switzerland	–	–	–	–	–	–	–	–	–	–	–	–	–	–
Turkey	–	–	–	–	–	–	–	–	–	–	–	–	–	–
United Kingdom	11.5	12.1	12.7	13.3	13.9	14.6	15.5	16.5	17.5	18.5	19.7	21.9	24.3	27.1
United States	27.2	27.9	28.8	29.7	30.5	31.7	33.5	36.2	38.9	40.8	43.8	46.7	49.3	52.3

Country	1974	1975	1976	1977	1978	1979	1980	1981	1982	1983	1984	1985	1986	1987
Australia	47.7	61.3	71.1	80.2	86.8	91.9	100.0	112.1	124.9	138.7	147.4	156.1	165.6	180.4
Austria	51.4	57.7	62.8	73.3	89.3	94.7	100.0	109.1	123.0	131.9	142.5	151.1	162.0	175.8
Belgium	59.4	67.0	76.8	83.5	89.2	93.7	100.0	109.1	119.9	132.8	144.8	154.8	161.8	163.6
Canada	53.0	61.2	71.0	76.1	80.7	89.2	100.0	115.1	127.9	137.6	144.4	149.7	154.4	159.7
Denmark	57.6	66.7	73.0	79.0	84.5	90.2	100.0	110.3	126.9	137.9	151.6	157.5	161.8	173.4
Finland	56.2	63.1	71.6	77.6	81.5	89.1	100.0	112.9	123.9	136.4	148.7	161.6	169.2	177.3
France	50.9	60.4	70.8	72.3	80.0	88.5	100.0	112.8	128.3	141.4	151.4	159.7	165.8	168.6
Germany	60.5	71.2	78.0	82.2	86.5	93.0	100.0	109.1	117.1	124.4	129.2	133.9	139.3	146.3
Greece	32.7	41.5	55.9	62.0	78.7	85.9	100.0	119.3	155.0	184.1	224.9	292.5	355.4	–
Iceland	–	–	–	–	–	–	100.0	169.9	238.6	368.7	472.4	650.9	806.6	1,012.3
Ireland	43.1	52.9	61.6	63.9	72.5	88.2	100.0	110.8	129.6	146.2	160.3	201.9	212.4	237.0
Italy	40.2	46.7	54.8	66.6	74.4	85.3	100.0	127.4	145.8	167.6	185.8	201.9	212.4	120.7
Japan	66.0	74.5	82.0	85.4	96.8	99.0	100.0	101.5	104.0	103.9	106.0	115.2	118.1	120.7
Luxembourg	–	–	–	–	–	–	100.0	–	–	–	–	–	–	–
Netherlands	48.2	58.0	65.4	80.9	87.5	93.9	100.0	107.0	114.0	117.0	117.0	119.0	121.0	122.0
New Zealand	39.9	46.8	54.7	62.4	71.5	85.7	100.0	117.9	136.1	154.3	155.2	161.6	158.4	176.5
Norway	62.0	69.3	74.2	80.9	88.1	90.0	100.0	111.0	120.1	128.2	136.3	146.5	201.0	227.8
Portugal	29.3	32.6	35.8	44.6	53.4	76.9	100.0	119.9	136.8	176.2	213.0	255.0	303.0	–
Spain	–	–	–	–	–	–	100.0	117.0	134.4	154.8	180.1	194.4	212.0	–
Sweden	50.3	56.9	63.8	75.5	80.1	86.3	100.0	117.0	116.1	115.8	134.2	134.1	134.2	–
Switzerland	–	–	–	–	–	95.6	100.0	109.4	119.8	128.5	139.1	151.5	155.9	163.6
Turkey	–	–	–	–	–	–	100.0	–	–	–	–	–	–	–
United Kingdom	37.1	47.7	54.2	58.9	64.5	78.1	100.0	108.2	115.2	121.1	123.2	134.8	144.1	156.3
United States	57.6	63.7	69.3	74.9	81.2	89.4	100.0	112.1	123.4	131.8	139.6	147.3	151.0	160.3

NOTE: 1980 equals 100.

SOURCE: Organization for Economic Cooperation and Development: Health Data File, 1990.

Ambulatory medical care price index, by country: 1960-87

Country	1960	1961	1962	1963	1964	1965	1966	1967	1968	1969	1970	1971	1972	1973
Australia	21.5	22.5	24.9	25.8	27.0	27.8	29.3	30.5	32.2	31.6	35.1	36.7	41.1	43.6
Austria	18.1	19.4	20.7	23.1	24.6	25.8	28.5	29.5	32.9	34.7	36.5	39.3	42.7	50.2
Belgium	21.6	21.6	21.7	22.5	24.6	31.5	35.1	36.2	37.3	38.9	42.2	44.8	49.6	54.1
Canada	37.9	38.6	39.8	40.8	41.8	43.0	44.1	48.3	50.2	52.4	56.0	57.6	58.7	59.9
Denmark	—	—	—	—	—	—	25.1	26.6	27.5	29.2	41.8	46.2	50.2	54.2
Finland	25.7	—	—	—	—	24.5	25.5	26.6	27.7	28.9	30.1	33.6	37.4	41.8
France	—	24.9	26.8	28.9	31.2	32.4	34.2	35.6	37.9	41.5	43.3	46.0	48.8	53.3
Germany	—	—	23.4	24.9	26.3	29.6	33.0	35.5	40.2	42.3	46.5	52.1	57.2	62.5
Greece	—	—	—	11.9	12.1	13.5	14.4	15.4	14.9	15.1	15.8	16.2	16.3	20.6
Iceland	—	—	—	—	—	—	—	—	—	—	—	—	—	—
Ireland	—	—	—	—	—	—	—	—	—	—	—	—	—	—
Italy	10.9	11.5	12.1	14.6	18.4	20.0	20.8	22.9	23.4	24.2	27.1	30.8	34.2	38.1
Japan	39.7	42.3	48.6	48.7	45.4	49.6	49.6	50.5	54.7	53.3	57.1	57.5	64.1	62.1
Luxembourg	—	—	—	—	—	18.1	22.5	22.8	23.8	24.2	29.2	41.3	45.5	50.9
Netherlands	—	—	—	—	—	—	—	—	—	—	38.6	43.6	49.1	54.9
New Zealand	—	—	—	—	—	—	—	—	—	—	—	—	—	—
Norway	—	—	20.9	22.8	25.0	27.3	29.2	31.3	33.5	36.0	38.5	42.4	46.7	51.4
Portugal	—	—	—	—	—	—	—	—	—	—	19.6	21.8	24.2	26.8
Spain	—	—	—	—	—	—	—	—	—	—	—	—	—	—
Sweden	—	—	—	54.7	60.2	62.4	74.0	82.5	73.4	75.0	65.2	69.7	75.9	88.5
Switzerland	—	—	—	—	—	—	—	47.7	49.9	52.4	54.0	59.3	66.6	73.9
Turkey	—	—	—	—	—	—	—	—	—	—	—	—	—	—
United Kingdom	—	—	—	—	—	—	—	—	—	—	—	—	—	—
United States	30.1	30.5	31.2	32.4	33.0	35.0	37.1	39.7	41.8	44.6	47.5	50.6	52.4	54.1

Country	1974	1975	1976	1977	1978	1979	1980	1981	1982	1983	1984	1985	1986	1987
Australia	49.4	57.6	69.8	78.7	85.8	89.6	100.0	111.1	121.7	133.7	143.4	155.6	167.5	183.8
Austria	57.9	64.0	78.6	84.6	90.7	95.8	100.0	104.1	109.8	114.2	119.0	123.5	130.6	133.5
Belgium	60.2	70.6	76.7	83.1	89.6	94.4	100.0	103.9	111.0	115.7	120.6	126.0	132.6	138.7
Canada	63.1	68.0	73.0	79.6	85.4	91.2	100.0	111.5	125.5	137.3	145.2	151.2	158.5	166.9
Denmark	63.3	73.1	75.1	78.1	85.1	92.2	100.0	108.2	117.4	126.9	139.0	146.7	150.4	159.4
Finland	46.6	52.0	59.7	67.2	77.0	86.8	100.0	113.3	127.8	150.0	175.9	196.9	214.1	230.4
France	58.3	65.3	71.2	77.4	84.9	91.7	100.0	109.7	117.9	131.6	136.1	141.2	145.1	146.7
Germany	69.5	75.8	80.8	84.9	88.9	93.4	100.0	105.7	109.7	115.0	117.4	119.0	120.7	121.2
Greece	25.2	30.3	44.5	51.9	65.2	82.6	100.0	110.0	147.3	—	—	—	—	—
Iceland	—	—	—	—	—	—	100.0	—	—	—	—	—	—	—
Ireland	43.1	52.9	61.6	70.7	80.1	83.2	100.0	110.0	130.1	144.4	—	—	—	—
Italy	43.3	51.2	58.6	64.6	74.1	81.7	100.0	124.4	157.2	173.7	193.3	213.5	226.9	257.7
Japan	66.0	74.5	82.0	85.4	96.8	99.0	100.0	101.5	104.0	103.9	106.0	115.2	118.1	120.7
Luxembourg	59.3	71.9	79.5	84.4	87.0	94.2	100.0	106.5	111.4	111.6	119.6	117.5	124.0	—
Netherlands	62.2	72.4	78.8	88.6	92.7	96.3	100.0	103.0	106.0	107.0	107.0	108.0	108.0	—
New Zealand	—	—	—	—	—	—	100.0	—	—	—	—	—	—	108.0
Norway	56.7	62.4	66.5	73.1	79.5	81.3	100.0	109.7	118.9	126.5	134.8	145.2	156.1	162.3
Portugal	29.7	33.0	36.9	45.7	54.5	77.2	100.0	127.3	141.6	179.9	223.0	268.0	—	—
Spain	—	—	—	—	—	—	100.0	110.1	124.9	147.3	159.1	179.8	—	—
Sweden	48.2	60.3	71.3	72.0	78.7	83.7	100.0	108.5	123.6	137.5	157.5	171.1	—	—
Switzerland	80.8	89.8	91.4	92.5	93.7	96.9	100.0	105.2	113.2	117.9	120.0	123.3	125.8	128.4
Turkey	—	—	—	—	—	—	100.0	—	—	—	—	—	—	—
United Kingdom	39.6	50.8	56.4	61.3	69.2	81.8	100.0	110.8	119.9	126.0	134.7	141.8	149.3	160.0
United States	56.8	65.3	71.2	77.2	82.9	90.0	100.0	110.3	119.6	128.2	137.3	145.8	155.0	164.4

NOTE: 1980 equals 100.

SOURCE: Organization for Economic Cooperation and Development: Health Data File, 1989.

Table 12
Pharmaceutical price index, by country: 1960-87

Country	1960	1961	1962	1963	1964	1965	1966	1967	1968	1969	1970	1971	1972	1973
Australia	43.1	44.1	45.0	46.1	47.5	49.2	49.4	49.8	50.9	52.4	55.1	58.2	59.2	61.4
Austria	58.7	58.7	58.7	58.7	58.7	58.7	60.6	64.1	63.9	64.2	65.0	69.9	74.7	77.2
Belgium	66.3	67.8	69.2	66.3	66.3	75.4	76.8	77.8	78.9	78.9	79.6	80.0	82.2	85.5
Canada	67.1	67.1	67.2	65.5	65.3	64.7	65.7	65.9	63.5	64.0	64.2	62.9	63.5	64.2
Denmark	—	—	—	—	—	—	41.2	46.4	48.0	51.4	53.5	59.3	60.8	60.5
Finland	32.2	32.5	32.8	33.0	33.3	33.5	34.9	36.2	37.7	39.2	40.8	45.6	51.0	56.9
France	56.7	57.9	58.8	59.6	59.5	60.8	62.0	62.1	61.8	64.4	65.8	65.9	66.9	66.2
Germany	48.5	50.1	55.2	55.4	55.7	56.4	60.6	62.0	64.1	65.5	68.1	71.4	74.5	77.6
Greece	34.0	34.5	34.4	34.1	33.9	34.9	34.7	34.7	35.1	33.9	34.6	35.5	36.9	38.1
Iceland	—	—	—	—	—	—	—	—	—	—	—	—	—	—
Ireland	—	—	—	—	—	—	—	—	—	—	34.5	36.2	37.8	40.0
Italy	59.3	58.8	58.7	59.0	59.4	59.8	60.5	60.8	60.8	61.9	63.2	63.2	63.2	63.2
Japan	54.7	54.0	50.4	49.0	49.6	52.7	52.5	52.6	54.6	55.6	60.7	62.6	64.8	66.8
Luxembourg	—	—	—	—	—	81.1	81.1	81.1	81.1	81.1	81.1	80.6	82.2	83.5
Netherlands	—	—	—	—	—	—	—	—	—	—	67.7	70.0	74.0	76.1
New Zealand	—	—	—	—	—	—	—	—	—	—	—	—	—	—
Norway	—	—	32.7	33.7	34.8	35.8	37.8	39.9	42.1	44.4	46.8	50.8	55.1	59.7
Portugal	—	—	—	—	—	—	—	—	—	—	36.2	40.0	44.1	48.7
Spain	—	—	—	—	—	50.7	52.1	53.5	55.0	56.5	58.0	58.9	59.8	60.8
Sweden	—	—	—	37.0	37.0	37.8	38.8	40.3	40.3	40.4	43.3	47.3	53.8	54.5
Switzerland	—	—	—	—	—	—	—	65.4	67.2	68.9	70.0	73.6	77.0	79.9
Turkey	—	—	—	—	—	—	—	—	—	—	—	—	—	—
United Kingdom	33.1	33.0	32.8	32.7	32.5	32.3	32.2	32.0	31.9	31.8	31.7	32.9	34.6	35.7
United States	62.2	61.4	60.5	60.0	59.9	59.6	59.9	59.5	59.6	60.2	61.6	62.7	62.9	63.0

Country	1974	1975	1976	1977	1978	1979	1980	1981	1982	1983	1984	1985	1986	1987
Australia	61.4	65.5	74.0	80.1	87.1	93.4	100.0	110.3	121.8	131.7	136.9	143.2	151.7	163.3
Austria	82.6	91.5	93.1	95.8	95.2	98.5	100.0	103.5	105.0	108.6	112.8	116.9	119.2	121.4
Belgium	90.4	94.6	96.3	97.6	98.8	99.8	100.0	98.3	105.8	114.6	126.9	131.7	137.4	142.2
Canada	66.7	71.7	76.2	79.3	82.5	90.4	100.0	114.3	132.3	149.3	159.5	170.1	179.5	197.8
Denmark	68.6	78.8	84.3	87.1	94.4	95.3	100.0	116.1	131.7	140.4	150.6	165.1	168.0	173.8
Finland	63.6	71.1	78.4	84.5	90.2	93.9	100.0	107.5	115.0	130.5	152.3	160.5	167.7	172.2
France	70.2	74.6	75.8	78.3	86.6	91.4	100.0	110.4	117.0	120.9	125.1	128.2	130.4	132.4
Germany	81.6	85.7	87.5	90.1	92.1	95.6	100.0	102.3	117.4	132.9	135.1	137.7	139.1	140.2
Greece	43.6	50.4	55.7	63.2	69.8	83.9	100.0	118.8	126.8	147.3	176.1	202.4	249.7	—
Iceland	—	—	—	—	—	—	100.0	—	—	—	—	—	—	—
Ireland	41.6	48.8	59.2	70.1	79.3	82.7	100.0	125.4	144.9	159.6	143.0	162.1	162.4	167.6
Italy	66.2	67.6	70.8	69.7	72.8	76.3	100.0	106.7	121.0	135.0	122.0	123.7	125.5	128.0
Japan	70.7	80.1	84.8	91.0	93.6	96.9	100.0	105.4	109.6	113.0	—	—	—	—
Luxembourg	85.9	88.3	100.9	96.4	96.4	97.1	100.0	107.2	118.5	143.1	152.7	157.7	—	—
Netherlands	78.7	85.7	89.8	90.7	92.9	92.6	100.0	103.0	109.0	112.0	116.0	119.0	121.0	123.0
New Zealand	—	61.3	74.6	81.2	89.7	93.4	100.0	101.8	110.5	118.4	136.8	160.0	171.1	183.6
Norway	64.7	70.2	78.4	84.1	91.7	95.8	100.0	112.6	130.6	138.6	147.5	158.6	184.9	—
Portugal	53.6	59.2	69.8	80.7	82.2	90.3	100.0	110.8	121.6	142.2	190.0	225.0	196.5	—
Spain	61.7	62.7	67.2	70.2	88.0	94.9	100.0	116.7	141.4	161.4	182.1	192.8	—	—
Sweden	59.1	65.7	72.5	77.8	92.4	94.9	100.0	133.2	124.7	133.7	148.4	150.9	—	—
Switzerland	83.4	91.0	95.8	97.3	98.2	98.4	100.0	102.2	105.2	108.6	111.5	113.5	116.2	118.8
Turkey	—	—	—	—	—	—	100.0	—	—	—	—	—	—	—
United Kingdom	42.8	50.8	60.8	70.4	77.9	85.5	100.0	111.7	120.6	126.3	130.5	137.2	141.8	149.1
United States	65.2	70.7	75.0	79.8	85.4	91.6	100.0	111.0	122.4	132.9	142.7	152.9	162.8	173.8

NOTE: 1980 equals 100.

Table 13

Medical care and health services price index, by country: 1960-87

Country	1960	1961	1962	1963	1964	1965	1966	1967	1968	1969	1970	1971	1972	1973
Australia	17.5	17.8	18.4	19.6	20.7	21.7	22.5	23.8	24.6	29.6	34.2	34.7	37.9	40.9
Austria	20.6	22.0	24.5	26.2	28.0	29.8	32.0	35.0	38.2	41.8	41.2	45.7	50.4	55.4
Belgium	30.0	30.4	30.7	31.6	33.6	39.8	42.9	45.0	46.0	47.1	48.7	51.0	54.5	58.3
Canada	29.0	29.9	30.7	31.1	31.9	33.0	34.6	37.0	38.6	41.4	45.1	46.9	49.0	51.7
Denmark	21.7	22.6	24.1	25.5	26.7	28.7	30.6	33.3	35.2	37.7	42.7	47.4	51.2	54.0
Finland	25.4	26.4	26.0	26.3	28.8	30.0	31.2	32.1	35.7	36.6	35.5	36.8	39.4	45.8
France	27.7	28.3	29.9	32.2	33.7	34.6	35.9	37.0	38.6	42.1	43.6	47.0	50.8	54.8
Germany	34.3	34.9	36.0	36.9	38.0	40.7	44.6	46.1	51.5	53.2	56.9	61.5	65.7	70.1
Greece	20.8	21.7	23.5	25.0	24.0	25.1	25.3	25.5	25.6	25.8	26.4	26.9	28.7	33.0
Iceland	1.0	1.1	1.3	1.4	1.7	1.9	2.2	2.3	2.7	3.2	3.8	4.7	4.8	7.0
Ireland	17.5	17.9	18.7	19.2	20.8	21.7	22.6	23.3	25.9	26.3	27.3	33.8	36.5	39.2
Italy	15.1	15.4	15.9	17.8	20.6	21.9	22.6	23.4	23.6	24.5	26.0	28.1	29.9	33.5
Japan	26.2	27.4	29.5	31.3	32.6	35.0	37.2	38.5	40.3	42.2	50.3	51.1	56.2	57.1
Luxembourg	—	—	—	—	—	23.6	38.0	39.2	41.1	43.0	51.3	51.9	62.3	62.3
Netherlands	17.9	18.4	19.0	19.9	21.6	23.0	24.3	25.4	26.4	28.1	33.6	37.9	45.1	50.6
New Zealand	—	—	—	—	—	—	—	—	—	—	—	—	—	—
Norway	19.8	22.7	23.4	25.0	27.7	29.7	32.4	35.8	37.1	39.5	41.2	44.3	47.4	52.7
Portugal	—	—	—	—	—	—	—	—	—	—	—	—	—	—
Spain	11.6	11.8	12.5	13.6	14.4	15.5	17.0	18.9	18.9	20.7	24.1	27.1	30.8	34.5
Sweden	24.0	24.7	25.6	26.1	27.0	27.8	30.1	32.1	31.8	31.7	34.8	37.9	41.2	44.8
Switzerland	27.1	27.9	29.3	30.9	32.8	35.5	37.8	40.3	42.7	45.4	47.8	53.3	59.4	66.7
Turkey	—	—	—	—	—	—	—	—	—	—	—	—	—	—
United Kingdom	20.6	21.7	22.0	22.0	22.8	23.1	23.5	24.1	25.4	26.5	28.5	31.0	32.4	34.3
United States	33.8	34.8	35.5	35.9	36.6	37.7	39.3	41.5	44.4	46.6	49.2	51.7	53.4	55.4

Country	1974	1975	1976	1977	1978	1979	1980	1981	1982	1983	1984	1985	1986	1987
Australia	47.2	59.7	69.3	78.6	85.4	90.7	100.0	111.4	124.1	137.4	146.0	155.4	165.7	181.0
Austria	63.0	70.2	76.0	82.3	89.7	95.2	100.0	107.7	115.8	121.0	127.4	134.7	140.7	147.2
Belgium	66.0	74.1	80.4	85.9	91.0	95.1	100.0	104.7	113.0	121.7	130.1	136.5	142.9	147.5
Canada	57.7	64.6	72.3	77.5	82.1	90.1	100.0	113.8	127.4	138.2	145.5	151.6	165.0	175.0
Denmark	63.1	72.6	76.6	80.7	88.1	93.3	100.0	111.9	124.9	133.5	140.4	145.9	149.6	159.4
Finland	52.6	63.1	70.6	76.7	81.5	89.1	100.0	112.0	122.6	136.4	152.2	166.6	174.4	182.0
France	59.1	63.8	70.3	77.4	85.3	90.2	100.0	111.6	122.1	132.8	140.2	145.8	150.2	153.8
Germany	75.1	80.6	84.4	87.7	90.9	94.4	100.0	105.0	112.3	119.5	121.3	124.8	125.8	127.5
Greece	36.7	46.3	55.5	62.8	67.3	85.9	100.0	118.4	145.7	166.0	195.1	237.0	284.7	312.0
Iceland	11.9	16.0	20.8	29.3	37.0	65.0	100.0	165.9	232.7	372.0	457.0	664.7	823.3	1,019.1
Ireland	41.7	46.3	55.6	67.2	76.5	82.9	100.0	118.8	137.9	156.3	155.5	178.6	185.7	193.0
Italy	38.8	45.4	51.7	59.1	68.7	80.3	100.0	122.8	144.2	163.0	179.2	196.8	205.0	224.8
Japan	67.0	74.8	82.4	86.1	96.3	98.6	100.0	101.9	104.5	104.8	107.1	115.5	117.8	121.6
Luxembourg	68.9	77.1	85.6	88.4	90.2	94.7	100.0	107.2	113.9	121.0	126.7	135.2	142.8	—
Netherlands	57.6	68.3	76.2	82.3	88.5	94.4	100.0	105.0	111.0	113.0	114.0	116.0	118.0	118.0
New Zealand	—	40.0	48.0	58.0	69.9	80.9	100.0	122.0	147.5	152.5	166.3	192.9	237.5	302.8
Norway	55.9	65.4	70.5	77.0	83.4	86.2	100.0	110.9	120.3	128.4	136.7	146.8	158.6	174.4
Portugal	—	—	—	—	—	—	100.0	—	—	—	—	—	—	—
Spain	40.5	44.7	48.7	63.5	75.5	88.8	100.0	115.3	135.8	155.0	173.6	184.9	198.4	217.2
Sweden	48.6	57.1	64.6	75.5	80.4	86.6	100.0	107.7	116.7	127.4	136.1	143.2	168.8	178.0
Switzerland	74.1	83.4	89.3	91.1	93.5	96.8	100.0	105.9	113.8	119.4	124.0	129.3	134.8	140.3
Turkey	—	—	—	—	—	—	100.0	—	—	—	—	—	—	—
United Kingdom	38.8	48.9	56.4	62.9	69.9	78.8	100.0	110.7	119.2	131.5	137.0	144.5	152.2	164.7
United States	59.6	65.4	70.7	77.0	83.1	90.2	100.0	111.1	121.4	130.0	139.0	150.1	157.5	166.8

NOTE: 1980 equals 100.

SOURCE: Organization for Economic Cooperation and Development: Health Data File, 1989.

Table 14
Average income of physicians, by country: 1960-87

National currency units

Country	1960	1961	1962	1963	1964	1965	1966	1967	1968	1969	1970	1971	1972	1973
Australia	9,016	—	—	—	10,852	11,604	12,403	12,846	13,568	—	16,659	—	—	—
Austria	—	—	—	—	—	—	—	—	—	—	—	—	—	—
Belgium	—	—	—	—	—	—	—	—	—	—	—	—	—	—
Canada	15,735	—	16,970	18,688	20,484	22,064	23,262	26,093	28,615	30,861	34,360	39,203	39,977	41,220
Denmark	—	—	—	—	—	—	—	—	—	—	—	—	—	—
Finland	20,270	22,040	24,850	27,370	30,720	34,450	36,690	40,440	45,300	47,450	48,950	50,610	53,540	54,780
France	—	—	54,653	—	—	—	75,996	—	84,766	90,413	111,252	120,399	127,079	151,490
Germany	—	42,947	—	—	—	62,911	—	—	—	—	—	116,727	—	—
Greece	—	—	—	—	—	—	—	—	—	—	—	—	—	—
Iceland	—	—	—	—	—	—	—	—	—	—	—	—	—	—
Ireland	—	—	—	—	—	—	—	—	—	—	—	—	—	—
Italy	1,014	1,117	1,215	1,480	1,676	1,785	2,015	2,330	2,575	2,725	3,272	3,960	4,272	4,586
Japan	490,632	579,288	661,440	754,956	815,748	933,876	1,072,716	1,235,832	1,492,000	1,710,540	2,017,068	2,292,348	2,619,620	2,875,836
Luxembourg	—	—	—	—	—	—	—	—	—	—	—	—	—	—
Netherlands	—	—	—	—	—	—	—	—	—	—	—	—	—	—
New Zealand	6,865	—	7,746	7,814	8,207	8,366	8,612	9,366	9,665	10,682	12,630	14,523	16,530	18,810
Norway	—	—	—	—	—	—	—	—	—	—	—	—	—	—
Portugal	—	—	—	—	—	—	—	—	—	—	—	—	—	—
Spain	—	—	—	—	—	—	—	—	—	—	—	—	—	—
Sweden	—	—	—	—	—	—	60,270	68,037	73,703	81,383	109,564	118,434	116,845	124,609
Switzerland	—	—	—	—	—	—	—	—	—	—	92,222	104,663	—	129,273
Turkey	—	—	—	—	—	—	—	—	—	—	—	—	—	—
United Kingdom	—	—	—	—	—	—	—	—	—	—	—	—	—	—
United States	—	—	—	—	—	—	—	—	—	36,100	41,100	—	47,300	47,600

Country	1974	1975	1976	1977	1978	1979	1980	1981	1982	1983	1984	1985	1986	1987
Australia	—	33,812	33,812	35,697	34,934	37,158	35,941	38,018	39,051	42,726	44,595	46,463	51,286	52,829
Austria	—	—	—	—	—	—	—	—	—	—	—	—	—	—
Belgium	—	—	1,095,761	1,214,973	1,293,039	1,307,237	1,275,582	1,254,113	—	—	—	—	—	—
Canada	42,290	45,360	47,590	50,000	52,840	56,090	61,100	66,930	73,640	77,500	88,300	90,900	97,500	101,800
Denmark	—	—	—	—	—	—	285,000	—	—	281,900	298,800	210,800	316,000	346,000
Finland	57,260	65,700	70,360	75,000	75,640	88,790	104,840	111,870	135,040	148,460	151,610	166,680	180,280	188,950
France	154,576	188,741	204,975	205,176	233,682	239,713	—	—	—	—	—	—	—	—
Germany	143,769	150,300	153,600	159,275	166,300	172,400	180,858	189,500	187,200	179,592	194,900	195,900	198,000	—
Greece	—	—	—	—	—	—	—	—	—	—	—	—	—	—
Iceland	—	—	—	—	—	—	—	—	—	—	—	—	—	—
Ireland	—	—	—	—	—	—	—	—	—	—	—	—	—	—
Italy	5,245	5,625	6,240	5,795	6,471	7,194	7,823	9,096	11,165	11,695	12,075	12,810	13,194	13,727
Japan	3,615,672	4,205,448	4,806,144	5,424,308	5,760,480	6,202,740	6,785,784	7,275,552	7,661,280	7,833,456	8,207,292	—	9,510,696	—
Luxembourg	—	—	—	—	—	—	—	—	—	—	—	—	—	—
Netherlands	—	—	—	—	—	—	—	—	—	—	—	—	—	—
New Zealand	22,550	24,870	23,700	29,070	33,010	30,690	34,530	36,290	42,100	43,300	48,300	57,400	62,800	—
Norway	—	—	98,000	—	—	—	141,600	—	194,100	210,100	223,800	232,600	234,000	238,300
Portugal	—	—	—	—	—	—	—	—	—	—	—	—	—	—
Spain	—	—	—	—	—	—	—	—	—	—	—	—	—	—
Sweden	123,080	121,340	139,157	146,344	160,762	167,965	172,387	194,487	191,904	197,643	197,516	204,465	213,303	223,980
Switzerland	149,590	166,391	169,388	167,845	168,070	170,463	174,281	186,037	190,441	198,918	—	—	—	—
Turkey	—	—	—	—	—	—	—	—	—	—	—	—	—	—
United Kingdom	—	7,637	8,071	8,283	9,080	11,343	15,006	16,139	17,282	18,691	19,977	21,253	22,888	24,732
United States	50,900	55,300	—	60,400	64,600	77,400	—	89,900	97,700	104,100	—	112,200	119,500	132,300

NOTE: Italy is reported in millions of national currency units.

Public coverage against inpatient care costs, by country: 1960-87

Percent of total population

Country	1960	1961	1962	1963	1964	1965	1966	1967	1968	1969	1970	1971	1972	1973	1974	1975	1976	1977	1978	1979	1980	1981	1982	1983	1984	1985	1986	1987
Australia	77.0	77.0	77.0	77.0	77.0	77.0	77.0	79.0	77.0	77.0	79.0	100.0	100.0	100.0	100.0	100.0	100.0	100.0	100.0	100.0	100.0	100.0	100.0	100.0	100.0	100.0	100.0	100.0
Austria	78.0	78.0	78.0	79.0	79.0	92.0	92.0	91.0	91.0	91.0	91.0	92.0	93.0	95.0	96.0	96.0	96.0	98.0	98.0	99.0	99.0	99.0	99.0	99.0	99.0	99.0	99.0	99.0
Belgium	58.0	58.0	58.0	58.0	78.0	86.0	86.0	86.0	86.0	86.0	98.0	98.0	98.0	98.0	98.0	98.0	98.0	98.0	98.0	98.0	98.0	98.0	98.0	98.0	98.0	98.0	98.0	98.0
Canada	68.0	95.0	100.0	100.0	100.0	100.0	100.0	100.0	100.0	100.0	100.0	100.0	100.0	100.0	100.0	100.0	100.0	100.0	100.0	100.0	100.0	100.0	100.0	100.0	100.0	100.0	100.0	100.0
Denmark	95.0	95.0	95.0	95.0	95.0	95.0	100.0	100.0	100.0	100.0	100.0	100.0	100.0	100.0	100.0	100.0	100.0	100.0	100.0	100.0	100.0	100.0	100.0	100.0	100.0	100.0	100.0	100.0
Finland	100.0	100.0	100.0	100.0	100.0	100.0	100.0	100.0	100.0	100.0	100.0	100.0	100.0	100.0	100.0	100.0	100.0	100.0	100.0	100.0	100.0	100.0	100.0	100.0	100.0	100.0	100.0	100.0
France	80.0	80.0	80.0	80.0	85.0	88.0	88.0	88.0	88.0	90.0	96.0	98.0	98.0	98.0	98.0	98.0	98.0	98.0	99.0	99.0	99.0	99.0	99.0	99.0	99.0	99.0	99.0	99.0
Germany	84.0	84.0	84.0	84.0	84.0	85.8	88.0	88.0	88.0	88.0	88.2	90.0	90.0	90.0	90.0	90.3	91.0	91.0	91.0	91.0	91.0	91.0	91.0	91.0	91.0	92.2	92.2	92.2
Greece	30.0	30.0	30.0	40.0	40.0	40.0	40.0	40.0	91.0	91.0	91.0	91.0	95.0	98.0	98.0	98.0	98.0	98.0	98.0	98.0	98.0	98.0	98.0	98.0	100.0	100.0	100.0	100.0
Iceland	90.0	90.0	90.0	90.0	90.0	90.0	100.0	100.0	100.0	100.0	100.0	100.0	100.0	100.0	100.0	100.0	100.0	100.0	100.0	100.0	100.0	100.0	100.0	100.0	100.0	100.0	100.0	100.0
Ireland	85.0	85.0	85.0	85.0	85.0	85.0	85.0	85.0	85.0	85.0	85.0	85.0	85.0	85.0	85.0	85.0	85.0	85.0	85.0	100.0	100.0	100.0	100.0	100.0	100.0	100.0	100.0	100.0
Italy	87.0	87.0	88.0	88.0	90.0	91.0	91.0	91.0	92.0	92.0	93.0	94.0	94.0	94.0	95.0	100.0	100.0	100.0	100.0	100.0	100.0	100.0	100.0	100.0	100.0	100.0	100.0	100.0
Japan	88.0	99.0	100.0	100.0	100.0	100.0	100.0	100.0	100.0	100.0	100.0	100.0	100.0	100.0	100.0	100.0	100.0	100.0	100.0	100.0	100.0	100.0	100.0	100.0	100.0	100.0	100.0	100.0
Luxembourg	100.0	100.0	100.0	100.0	100.0	100.0	100.0	100.0	100.0	100.0	100.0	100.0	100.0	100.0	100.0	100.0	100.0	100.0	100.0	100.0	100.0	100.0	100.0	100.0	100.0	100.0	100.0	100.0
Netherlands	71.0	71.0	71.0	71.0	71.0	71.0	71.0	71.0	78.0	86.0	86.0	86.0	86.0	100.0	100.0	100.0	100.0	100.0	100.0	100.0	100.0	100.0	100.0	100.0	100.0	100.0	100.0	100.0
New Zealand	100.0	100.0	100.0	100.0	100.0	100.0	100.0	100.0	100.0	100.0	86.0	86.0	100.0	87.0	87.0	88.0	88.0	88.0	88.0	88.0	78.0	77.0	77.0	77.0	77.0	77.0	74.0	73.0
Norway	100.0	100.0	100.0	100.0	100.0	100.0	100.0	100.0	100.0	100.0	100.0	100.0	100.0	100.0	100.0	100.0	100.0	100.0	100.0	100.0	100.0	100.0	100.0	100.0	100.0	100.0	100.0	100.0
Portugal	18.0	20.0	24.0	27.0	29.0	32.0	32.0	35.0	44.0	48.0	52.0	62.0	69.0	78.0	87.0	90.0	98.0	98.0	100.0	100.0	100.0	100.0	100.0	100.0	100.0	100.0	100.0	100.0
Spain	50.0	50.0	50.0	50.0	50.0	55.0	55.0	55.0	55.0	58.0	61.0	67.0	72.0	77.0	87.0	90.0	98.0	98.0	100.0	100.0	100.0	100.0	100.0	100.0	100.0	100.0	100.0	100.0
Sweden	100.0	100.0	100.0	100.0	100.0	100.0	100.0	100.0	100.0	100.0	100.0	100.0	100.0	100.0	78.0	81.0	84.0	84.0	84.0	82.0	83.0	84.0	85.5	90.0	92.0	95.0	96.0	97.1
Switzerland	72.0	74.0	75.0	77.0	79.0	82.0	84.0	86.0	87.0	88.0	89.0	90.0	91.0	93.0	94.0	94.0	94.4	94.8	95.3	96.0	95.5	97.0	97.4	97.7	97.8	98.0	98.3	98.7
Turkey	–	–	–	–	–	–	–	–	–	–	–	–	–	–	–	–	–	–	–	–	–	–	–	–	–	–	–	–
United Kingdom	100.0	100.0	100.0	100.0	100.0	100.0	100.0	100.0	100.0	100.0	100.0	100.0	100.0	100.0	100.0	100.0	100.0	100.0	100.0	100.0	100.0	100.0	100.0	100.0	100.0	100.0	100.0	100.0
United States	20.0	22.0	22.0	22.0	22.0	22.0	38.0	38.0	38.0	38.0	40.0	40.0	40.0	40.0	40.0	40.0	40.0	40.0	40.0	40.0	42.0	42.0	42.0	42.0	42.6	43.0	43.0	43.0

SOURCE: Organization for Economic Cooperation and Development: Health Data File, 1989.

Table 16

Public coverage against costs of ambulatory care, by country: 1960-87

Percent of total population

Country	1960	1961	1962	1963	1964	1965	1966	1967	1968	1969	1970	1971	1972	1973
Australia	78.0	78.0	78.0	78.0	78.0	78.0	78.0	78.0	78.0	78.0	76.0	78.0	79.0	80.0
Austria	78.0	78.0	78.0	79.0	79.0	92.0	92.0	91.0	91.0	91.0	91.0	92.0	93.0	95.0
Belgium	58.0	58.0	58.0	58.0	78.0	86.0	86.0	86.0	86.0	86.0	93.0	93.0	93.0	93.0
Canada	2.0	2.0	6.0	6.0	6.0	7.0	14.0	16.0	24.0	66.0	95.0	99.0	100.0	100.0
Denmark	95.0	95.0	95.0	95.0	95.0	95.0	100.0	100.0	100.0	100.0	100.0	100.0	100.0	100.0
Finland	100.0	100.0	100.0	100.0	100.0	100.0	100.0	100.0	100.0	100.0	100.0	100.0	100.0	100.0
France	76.0	76.0	76.0	76.0	85.0	85.0	88.0	88.0	88.0	88.0	96.0	98.0	98.0	98.0
Germany	84.0	84.0	84.0	84.0	84.0	85.8	88.0	86.0	86.0	86.0	88.2	89.0	90.0	90.0
Greece	75.0	75.0	75.0	88.0	88.0	88.0	88.0	88.0	88.0	88.0	90.0	90.0	97.0	97.0
Iceland	75.0	75.0	75.0	75.0	75.0	100.0	100.0	100.0	100.0	100.0	100.0	100.0	100.0	100.0
Ireland	30.0	30.0	30.0	30.0	30.0	30.0	30.0	30.0	30.0	30.0	30.0	30.0	30.0	33.0
Italy	87.0	87.0	88.0	88.0	90.0	91.0	91.0	91.0	92.0	92.0	93.0	94.0	94.0	94.0
Japan	88.0	99.0	100.0	100.0	100.0	100.0	100.0	100.0	100.0	100.0	100.0	100.0	100.0	100.0
Luxembourg	100.0	100.0	100.0	100.0	100.0	100.0	100.0	100.0	100.0	100.0	100.0	100.0	100.0	100.0
Netherlands	71.0	71.0	71.0	71.0	71.0	71.0	71.0	71.0	71.0	72.0	72.0	72.0	72.0	73.0
New Zealand	100.0	100.0	100.0	100.0	100.0	100.0	100.0	100.0	100.0	100.0	100.0	100.0	100.0	100.0
Norway	100.0	100.0	100.0	100.0	100.0	100.0	100.0	100.0	100.0	100.0	100.0	100.0	100.0	100.0
Portugal	18.0	20.0	24.0	27.0	29.0	32.0	32.0	35.0	44.0	48.0	52.0	62.0	69.0	78.0
Spain	50.0	50.0	50.0	50.0	50.0	55.0	55.0	55.0	55.0	58.0	61.0	67.0	72.0	77.0
Sweden	100.0	100.0	100.0	100.0	100.0	100.0	100.0	100.0	100.0	100.0	100.0	100.0	100.0	100.0
Switzerland	72.0	74.0	75.0	77.0	79.0	82.0	84.0	86.0	87.0	88.0	89.0	90.0	91.0	93.0
Turkey	–	–	–	–	–	–	–	–	–	–	–	–	–	–
United Kingdom	100.0	100.0	100.0	100.0	100.0	100.0	100.0	100.0	100.0	100.0	100.0	100.0	100.0	100.0
United States	20.0	22.0	22.0	22.0	22.0	25.0	38.0	38.0	38.0	38.0	40.0	40.0	40.0	40.0

Country	1974	1975	1976	1977	1978	1979	1980	1981	1982	1983	1984	1985	1986	1987
Australia	78.0	100.0	45.0	43.0	100.0	100.0	100.0	84.0	84.0	84.0	97.0	100.0	100.0	100.0
Austria	96.0	96.0	96.0	98.0	98.0	99.0	99.0	99.0	99.0	99.0	99.0	99.0	99.0	99.0
Belgium	93.0	93.0	93.0	93.0	93.0	93.0	93.0	93.0	93.0	93.0	93.0	93.0	93.0	93.0
Canada	100.0	100.0	100.0	100.0	100.0	100.0	100.0	100.0	100.0	100.0	100.0	100.0	100.0	100.0
Denmark	100.0	100.0	100.0	100.0	100.0	100.0	100.0	100.0	100.0	100.0	100.0	100.0	100.0	100.0
Finland	100.0	100.0	100.0	100.0	100.0	100.0	100.0	100.0	100.0	100.0	100.0	100.0	100.0	100.0
France	98.0	98.0	98.0	98.0	98.0	99.0	99.0	99.0	99.0	99.0	99.0	99.0	99.0	98.0
Germany	90.0	90.3	91.0	91.0	90.0	90.0	90.3	91.0	91.0	91.0	92.0	92.2	92.2	92.2
Greece	97.0	97.0	97.0	97.0	97.0	97.0	97.0	97.0	98.0	98.0	99.0	100.0	100.0	100.0
Iceland	100.0	100.0	100.0	100.0	100.0	100.0	100.0	100.0	100.0	100.0	100.0	100.0	100.0	100.0
Ireland	35.0	37.0	37.0	38.0	37.0	36.0	35.0	36.0	37.0	38.0	37.0	37.0	37.0	37.0
Italy	95.0	96.0	96.0	96.0	96.0	97.0	100.0	100.0	100.0	100.0	100.0	100.0	100.0	100.0
Japan	100.0	100.0	100.0	100.0	100.0	100.0	100.0	100.0	100.0	100.0	100.0	100.0	100.0	100.0
Luxembourg	100.0	100.0	100.0	100.0	100.0	100.0	100.0	100.0	100.0	100.0	100.0	100.0	100.0	100.0
Netherlands	74.0	74.0	75.0	75.0	76.0	76.0	72.0	72.0	72.0	71.0	71.0	71.0	68.0	67.0
New Zealand	100.0	100.0	100.0	100.0	100.0	100.0	100.0	100.0	100.0	100.0	100.0	100.0	100.0	100.0
Norway	100.0	100.0	100.0	100.0	100.0	100.0	100.0	100.0	100.0	100.0	100.0	100.0	100.0	100.0
Portugal	87.0	90.0	98.0	98.0	100.0	100.0	100.0	100.0	100.0	100.0	100.0	100.0	100.0	100.0
Spain	78.0	81.0	84.0	84.0	84.0	82.0	83.0	84.0	85.5	90.0	92.0	92.0	96.0	97.1
Sweden	100.0	100.0	100.0	100.0	100.0	100.0	100.0	100.0	100.0	100.0	100.0	100.0	100.0	100.0
Switzerland	94.0	94.0	94.4	94.8	95.3	96.0	96.5	97.0	97.4	97.7	97.8	98.0	98.3	98.7
Turkey							52.0							
United Kingdom	100.0	100.0	100.0	100.0	100.0	100.0	100.0	100.0	100.0	100.0	100.0	100.0	100.0	100.0
United States	40.0	40.0	40.0	40.0	40.0	40.0	42.0	42.0	42.0	42.0	42.6	43.0	43.0	43.0

Table 17
Public coverage against costs of medical goods, by country: 1960-87

Percent of population

Country	1960	1961	1962	1963	1964	1965	1966	1967	1968	1969	1970	1971	1972	1973
Australia	100.0	100.0	100.0	100.0	100.0	100.0	100.0	100.0	100.0	100.0	100.0	100.0	100.0	100.0
Austria	78.0	78.0	78.0	79.0	79.0	92.0	92.0	91.0	91.0	91.0	91.0	92.0	93.0	95.0
Belgium	58.0	58.0	58.0	58.0	78.0	86.0	86.0	86.0	86.0	86.0	93.0	93.0	93.0	85.0
Canada	5.0	5.0	5.0	5.0	5.0	5.0	5.0	5.0	6.0	6.0	6.0	7.0	16.0	17.0
Denmark	95.0	95.0	95.0	95.0	95.0	95.0	100.0	100.0	100.0	100.0	100.0	100.0	100.0	100.0
Finland	0.0	0.0	0.0	0.0	100.0	100.0	100.0	100.0	100.0	100.0	100.0	100.0	100.0	100.0
France	76.0	76.0	76.0	76.0	76.0	85.0	88.0	88.0	88.0	88.0	96.0	98.0	98.0	98.0
Germany	84.0	84.0	84.0	84.0	84.0	85.8	88.0	88.0	88.0	88.0	88.2	89.0	90.0	90.0
Greece	25.0	25.0	25.0	40.0	40.0	40.0	40.0	40.0	44.0	44.0	46.0	46.0	48.0	49.0
Iceland	50.0	50.0	50.0	50.0	50.0	50.0	100.0	100.0	100.0	100.0	100.0	100.0	100.0	100.0
Ireland	30.0	30.0	30.0	30.0	30.0	30.0	30.0	30.0	30.0	30.0	30.0	30.0	30.0	37.0
Italy	87.0	87.0	88.0	88.0	90.0	91.0	91.0	91.0	92.0	92.0	93.0	94.0	94.0	94.0
Japan	88.0	99.0	100.0	100.0	100.0	100.0	100.0	100.0	100.0	100.0	100.0	100.0	100.0	100.0
Luxembourg	100.0	100.0	100.0	100.0	100.0	100.0	100.0	100.0	100.0	100.0	100.0	100.0	100.0	100.0
Netherlands	71.0	71.0	71.0	71.0	71.0	71.0	71.0	71.0	71.0	71.0	72.0	72.0	72.0	73.0
New Zealand	100.0	100.0	100.0	100.0	100.0	100.0	100.0	100.0	100.0	100.0	100.0	100.0	100.0	100.0
Norway	100.0	100.0	100.0	100.0	100.0	100.0	100.0	100.0	100.0	100.0	100.0	100.0	100.0	100.0
Portugal	18.0	20.0	24.0	27.0	29.0	32.0	32.0	35.0	44.0	48.0	52.0	62.0	69.0	78.0
Spain	50.0	50.0	50.0	50.0	50.0	55.0	55.0	55.0	55.0	58.0	61.0	67.0	72.0	77.0
Sweden	100.0	100.0	100.0	100.0	100.0	100.0	100.0	100.0	100.0	100.0	100.0	100.0	100.0	100.0
Switzerland	72.0	74.0	75.0	77.0	79.0	82.0	84.0	86.0	87.0	88.0	89.0	90.0	91.0	93.0
Turkey	—	—	—	—	—	—	—	—	—	—	—	—	—	—
United Kingdom	100.0	100.0	100.0	100.0	100.0	100.0	100.0	100.0	100.0	100.0	100.0	100.0	100.0	100.0
United States	3.0	3.0	3.0	4.0	4.0	5.0	5.0	6.0	7.0	8.0	9.0	10.0	10.0	10.0

Country	1974	1975	1976	1977	1978	1979	1980	1981	1982	1983	1984	1985	1986	1987
Australia	100.0	100.0	100.0	100.0	100.0	100.0	100.0	100.0	100.0	100.0	100.0	100.0	100.0	100.0
Austria	96.0	96.0	96.0	98.0	98.0	99.0	99.0	99.0	99.0	99.0	99.0	99.0	99.0	99.0
Belgium	85.0	85.0	85.0	85.0	93.0	93.0	93.0	93.0	93.0	93.0	93.0	93.0	93.0	93.0
Canada	18.0	19.0	22.0	25.0	28.0	31.0	33.0	33.0	33.0	33.0	33.0	34.0	34.0	34.0
Denmark	100.0	100.0	100.0	100.0	100.0	100.0	100.0	100.0	100.0	100.0	100.0	100.0	100.0	100.0
Finland	100.0	100.0	100.0	100.0	100.0	100.0	100.0	100.0	100.0	100.0	100.0	100.0	100.0	100.0
France	98.0	98.0	98.0	98.0	98.0	99.0	99.0	99.0	99.0	99.0	99.0	99.0	99.0	99.0
Germany	90.0	90.3	91.0	91.0	91.0	91.0	90.3	91.0	91.0	92.0	92.0	92.2	92.2	92.2
Greece	50.0	52.0	52.0	52.0	60.0	60.0	60.0	60.0	60.0	98.0	98.0	100.0	100.0	100.0
Iceland	100.0	100.0	100.0	100.0	100.0	100.0	100.0	100.0	100.0	100.0	100.0	100.0	100.0	100.0
Ireland	37.0	37.0	37.0	37.0	37.0	37.0	37.0	37.0	40.0	40.0	40.0	40.0	40.0	40.0
Italy	95.0	96.0	96.0	96.0	96.0	97.0	100.0	100.0	100.0	100.0	100.0	100.0	100.0	100.0
Japan	100.0	100.0	100.0	100.0	100.0	100.0	100.0	100.0	100.0	100.0	100.0	100.0	100.0	100.0
Luxembourg	100.0	100.0	100.0	100.0	100.0	100.0	100.0	100.0	100.0	100.0	100.0	100.0	100.0	100.0
Netherlands	74.0	74.0	75.0	75.0	76.0	76.0	68.0	68.0	67.0	67.0	67.0	66.0	62.0	61.0
New Zealand	100.0	100.0	100.0	100.0	100.0	100.0	100.0	100.0	100.0	100.0	100.0	100.0	100.0	100.0
Norway	100.0	100.0	100.0	100.0	100.0	100.0	100.0	100.0	100.0	100.0	100.0	100.0	100.0	100.0
Portugal	87.0	90.0	98.0	98.0	100.0	100.0	100.0	100.0	100.0	100.0	100.0	100.0	100.0	100.0
Spain	78.0	81.0	84.0	84.0	84.0	82.0	33.0	84.0	85.5	90.0	92.0	95.0	96.0	97.1
Sweden	100.0	100.0	100.0	100.0	100.0	100.0	100.0	100.0	100.0	100.0	100.0	100.0	100.0	100.0
Switzerland	94.0	94.0	94.4	94.8	95.3	96.0	96.5	97.0	97.4	97.7	97.8	98.0	98.3	98.7
Turkey	—	—	—	—	—	—	52.0	—	—	—	—	—	—	—
United Kingdom	100.0	100.0	100.0	100.0	100.0	100.0	100.0	100.0	100.0	100.0	100.0	100.0	100.0	100.0
United States	10.0	10.0	10.0	10.0	10.0	10.0	10.0	10.0	10.0	10.0	10.0	10.0	10.0	10.0

SOURCE: Organization for Economic Cooperation and Development: Health Data File, 1989.

Table 18
Public share of inpatient care billing, by country: 1960-87

Percent of billing

Country	1960	1961	1962	1963	1964	1965	1966	1967	1968	1969	1970	1971	1972	1973
Australia	50.0	50.0	50.0	50.0	50.0	50.0	50.0	50.0	50.0	50.0	75.0	75.0	75.0	75.0
Austria	90.0	90.0	90.0	90.0	90.0	90.0	90.0	90.0	90.0	90.0	90.0	90.0	90.0	90.0
Belgium	75.0	75.0	75.0	78.0	78.0	78.0	80.0	80.0	80.0	80.0	85.0	85.0	85.0	70.0
Canada	72.4	78.0	80.0	83.0	86.0	89.1	90.0	91.0	92.0	93.0	93.9	94.3	94.6	94.4
Denmark	80.0	80.0	80.0	80.0	86.0	100.0	100.0	100.0	100.0	100.0	100.0	100.0	100.0	100.0
Finland	79.0	82.0	81.0	84.0	85.0	87.0	88.0	89.0	89.0	89.0	91.0	89.0	90.0	90.0
France	85.0	85.0	85.0	85.0	85.0	85.0	85.0	85.0	85.0	85.0	91.0	90.0	90.0	90.0
Germany	99.0	99.0	99.0	99.0	99.0	99.0	99.0	99.0	99.0	99.0	99.0	99.0	99.0	99.0
Greece	75.0	75.0	75.0	75.0	75.0	88.0	88.0	88.0	88.0	88.0	90.0	90.0	90.0	90.0
Iceland	—	—	—	—	—	—	—	—	—	—	—	—	—	—
Ireland	—	—	—	—	—	—	—	80.0	80.0	80.0	80.0	82.0	82.0	82.0
Italy	96.0	96.0	96.0	96.0	95.0	95.0	95.0	94.0	94.0	94.0	93.0	93.0	93.0	93.0
Japan	79.0	79.0	79.0	79.0	79.0	79.0	80.0	80.0	80.0	81.0	82.0	82.0	82.0	82.0
Luxembourg	75.0	75.0	75.0	75.0	75.0	75.0	75.0	75.0	75.0	75.0	75.0	75.0	75.0	75.0
Netherlands	64.0	64.0	64.0	64.0	64.0	64.0	64.0	64.0	86.0	86.0	86.0	86.0	86.0	87.0
New Zealand	93.0	93.0	93.0	93.0	93.0	93.0	93.0	93.0	93.0	93.0	93.0	93.0	93.0	93.0
Norway	100.0	100.0	100.0	100.0	100.0	100.0	100.0	100.0	100.0	100.0	100.0	100.0	100.0	100.0
Portugal	—	—	—	—	—	—	—	—	—	—	—	—	—	—
Spain	—	—	—	—	—	—	—	—	—	—	—	—	—	—
Sweden	100.0	100.0	100.0	100.0	100.0	100.0	100.0	100.0	100.0	100.0	100.0	100.0	100.0	80.6
Switzerland	100.0	100.0	100.0	100.0	100.0	100.0	100.0	100.0	100.0	100.0	100.0	100.0	100.0	100.0
Turkey	—	—	—	—	—	—	—	—	—	—	—	—	51.0	—
United Kingdom	98.0	99.0	99.0	99.0	99.0	99.0	99.0	99.0	99.0	99.0	99.0	99.0	99.0	99.0
United States	41.0	40.0	40.0	40.0	40.0	39.0	44.0	55.0	55.0	54.0	53.0	53.0	53.0	53.0

Country	1974	1975	1976	1977	1978	1979	1980	1981	1982	1983	1984	1985	1986	1987
Australia	75.0	82.0	78.8	77.7	75.0	75.2	74.5	76.3	75.0	72.3	75.0	80.7	81.0	79.7
Austria	90.0	90.0	90.0	90.0	90.0	90.0	90.0	90.0	90.0	90.0	90.0	90.0	90.0	90.0
Belgium	70.0	70.0	70.0	70.0	72.0	72.0	72.0	72.0	70.0	68.0	68.0	68.0	68.0	68.0
Canada	94.3	94.2	94.1	93.9	93.0	92.3	92.0	91.8	91.7	91.4	90.1	90.6	90.7	90.6
Denmark	100.0	100.0	100.0	100.0	100.0	100.0	100.0	100.0	100.0	100.0	100.0	100.0	100.0	100.0
Finland	92.0	93.0	92.0	92.0	90.0	89.0	90.0	89.0	89.0	89.0	92.0	90.0	90.0	90.0
France	90.0	90.1	91.0	91.0	91.0	91.0	92.0	92.0	92.0	92.0	92.0	92.0	92.4	92.2
Germany	99.0	99.0	99.0	99.0	99.0	99.0	99.0	98.0	98.0	98.0	98.0	98.0	98.0	98.0
Greece	90.0	90.0	90.0	90.0	90.0	90.0	90.0	90.0	90.0	90.0	90.0	90.0	90.0	90.0
Iceland	100.0	100.0	100.0	100.0	100.0	100.0	100.0	100.0	100.0	100.0	100.0	100.0	100.0	100.0
Ireland	88.0	88.0	88.0	88.0	90.0	90.0	94.6	95.0	95.0	95.0	95.4	95.0	95.0	95.0
Italy	93.0	93.0	94.0	94.0	95.0	96.0	91.4	90.6	88.8	93.5	93.0	87.4	87.5	88.7
Japan	82.0	80.5	81.1	82.2	82.6	83.4	83.7	84.0	84.3	95.0	95.0	93.0	93.0	93.0
Luxembourg	100.0	100.0	100.0	100.0	100.0	100.0	100.0	100.0	100.0	95.0	95.0	95.0	95.0	95.0
Netherlands	87.0	88.0	88.0	88.0	88.0	88.0	85.0	85.0	85.0	85.0	85.0	84.0	81.0	82.0
New Zealand	93.0	93.0	93.0	93.0	93.0	93.0	93.0	93.0	93.0	93.0	92.0	92.0	92.0	92.0
Norway	100.0	100.0	100.0	100.0	100.0	100.0	100.0	100.0	100.0	100.0	100.0	100.0	100.0	100.0
Portugal	—	100.0	100.0	100.0	100.0	100.0	100.0	100.0	100.0	100.0	100.0	100.0	100.0	100.0
Spain	82.5	85.6	84.4	84.3	82.6	82.9	82.4	82.0	81.6	83.4	84.0	84.0	84.0	84.0
Sweden	100.0	100.0	100.0	100.0	100.0	100.0	100.0	100.0	100.0	100.0	100.0	100.0	100.0	100.0
Switzerland	100.0	100.0	100.0	100.0	100.0	100.0	100.0	100.0	100.0	100.0	100.0	100.0	100.0	100.0
Turkey	48.0	—	33.0	—	—	25.0	—	—	—	—	—	—	—	—
United Kingdom	99.0	99.0	99.0	99.0	99.0	99.0	99.0	99.0	99.0	99.0	99.0	99.0	99.0	99.0
United States	55.0	55.0	55.0	54.0	54.0	54.0	54.0	54.0	54.0	54.0	55.0	55.0	55.0	55.0

Table 13

Public share of ambulatory care billing, by country: 1960-87

Percent of billing

Country	1960	1961	1962	1963	1964	1965	1966	1967	1968	1969	1970	1971	1972	1973
Australia	-	-	-	-	-	-	-	-	-	-	-	-	-	-
Austria	80.0	80.0	80.0	80.0	80.0	80.0	80.0	80.0	80.0	80.0	80.0	80.0	80.0	80.0
Belgium	69.0	69.0	69.0	69.0	55.0	66.0	66.0	66.0	66.0	66.0	68.0	68.0	68.0	52.0
Canada	32.0	-	-	-	-	28.8	-	-	-	-	62.9	74.7	74.3	73.9
Denmark	-	-	-	37.0	-	-	58.0	59.0	62.0	64.0	64.0	64.0	65.0	62.0
Finland	41.0	38.0	37.0	37.0	39.0	42.0	42.0	54.0	56.0	56.0	56.0	56.0	57.0	60.0
France	60.0	60.0	60.0	60.0	60.0	60.0	62.0	64.0	66.0	68.0	68.0	68.0	68.0	68.0
Germany	93.0	93.0	93.0	93.0	93.0	93.0	93.0	93.0	93.0	93.0	93.0	93.0	93.0	93.0
Greece	85.0	85.0	85.0	85.0	85.0	85.0	85.0	85.0	85.0	85.0	85.0	85.0	85.0	85.0
Iceland	-	-	-	-	-	-	-	-	-	-	-	-	-	-
Ireland	100.0	100.0	100.0	100.0	100.0	100.0	100.0	100.0	40.0	40.0	40.0	40.0	44.0	44.0
Italy	71.0	81.0	83.0	84.0	81.0	78.0	76.0	76.0	74.0	70.0	70.0	73.0	70.0	67.0
Japan	79.0	79.0	79.0	79.0	79.0	79.0	80.0	80.0	80.0	81.0	80.0	82.0	84.0	84.0
Luxembourg	-	-	-	-	-	-	-	-	-	-	-	-	-	-
Netherlands	53.0	53.0	53.0	53.0	53.0	53.0	53.0	53.0	53.0	53.0	53.0	53.0	62.0	59.0
New Zealand	56.0	55.0	48.0	48.0	48.0	48.0	48.0	48.0	48.0	44.0	44.0	44.0	44.0	44.0
Norway	-	-	-	-	-	-	-	-	-	-	-	-	-	-
Portugal	-	-	-	-	-	-	-	-	-	-	-	-	-	-
Spain	-	-	-	-	-	-	-	-	-	-	-	-	-	-
Sweden	47.0	47.0	47.0	47.0	47.0	47.0	47.0	47.0	78.0	78.0	78.0	78.0	78.0	78.0
Switzerland	-	-	-	-	-	-	-	-	-	-	-	-	-	-
Turkey	-	-	-	-	-	-	-	-	-	-	-	-	-	-
United Kingdom	88.0	88.0	88.0	88.0	89.0	89.0	90.0	90.0	90.0	90.0	90.0	89.0	88.0	87.0
United States	18.0	20.0	20.0	20.0	20.0	20.0	25.0	39.0	44.0	43.0	42.0	44.0	45.0	46.0

Country	1974	1975	1976	1977	1978	1979	1980	1981	1982	1983	1984	1985	1986	1987
Australia	33.0	62.0	62.2	43.1	27.2	33.8	35.1	35.1	34.5	35.5	45.7	62.8	62.2	61.2
Austria	80.0	80.0	80.0	80.0	80.0	80.0	80.0	80.0	80.0	80.0	80.0	80.0	80.0	80.0
Belgium	54.0	54.0	58.0	52.0	52.0	53.0	54.0	53.0	52.0	50.0	50.0	50.0	50.0	50.0
Canada	74.3	74.1	73.8	72.7	72.5	71.6	72.6	74.7	73.8	73.6	73.5	73.1	73.9	72.1
Denmark	65.0	66.0	68.0	72.0	73.0	72.0	73.0	72.0	73.0	72.0	71.0	73.0	76.0	76.0
Finland	63.0	66.0	71.0	71.0	70.0	71.0	73.0	75.0	76.0	75.0	71.0	70.0	70.0	70.0
France	68.0	67.6	67.0	67.0	67.0	67.0	66.3	66.0	66.0	66.0	65.0	64.9	63.2	62.1
Germany	93.0	93.0	93.0	93.0	93.0	93.0	93.0	93.0	93.0	93.0	92.0	92.0	92.0	92.0
Greece	85.0	85.0	85.0	85.0	85.0	85.0	85.0	85.0	85.0	85.0	85.0	85.0	85.0	85.0
Iceland	-	-	-	-	-	-	80.0	80.0	80.0	80.0	80.0	80.0	80.0	80.0
Ireland	45.0	45.0	47.5	48.0	48.5	49.0	49.6	50.0	50.0	50.0	50.0	48.0	47.0	47.0
Italy	67.0	70.0	71.0	69.0	76.0	76.0	83.3	79.6	79.2	80.1	79.2	78.6	77.4	79.6
Japan	84.0	84.5	84.5	86.4	86.2	86.0	86.5	86.8	86.8	86.6	85.6	85.0	84.9	85.0
Luxembourg	-	100.0	100.0	100.0	100.0	100.0	100.0	100.0	100.0	98.0	98.0	98.0	98.0	98.0
Netherlands	60.0	61.0	62.0	64.0	64.0	63.0	48.0	47.0	47.0	48.0	47.0	46.0	44.0	44.0
New Zealand	47.0	47.0	47.0	47.0	47.0	47.0	47.0	47.0	47.0	47.0	47.0	47.0	47.0	47.0
Norway	-	-	-	-	-	-	-	-	-	-	-	-	-	-
Portugal	-	100.0	100.0	100.0	100.0	100.0	100.0	100.0	100.0	100.0	100.0	100.0	100.0	100.0
Spain	-	-	-	-	-	-	-	-	-	-	-	-	-	-
Sweden	78.0	78.0	-	-	-	-	-	-	-	-	-	-	-	-
Switzerland	-	-	89.0	90.0	90.0	91.0	91.0	91.0	91.0	91.0	90.0	90.0	90.0	90.0
Turkey	-	-	-	-	-	-	-	-	-	-	-	-	-	-
United Kingdom	88.0	91.0	90.0	90.0	90.0	90.0	89.0	89.0	88.0	88.0	88.0	88.0	88.0	88.0
United States	50.0	53.0	52.0	52.0	53.0	54.0	55.0	56.0	56.0	56.0	56.0	56.0	56.0	56.0

SOURCE: Organization for Economic Cooperation and Development: Health Data File, 1989.

147

Table 20
Use of inpatient care, by country: 1960-87

Bed days per person

Country	1960	1961	1962	1963	1964	1965	1966	1967	1968	1969	1970	1971	1972	1973
Australia	–	–	–	2.4	2.5	2.5	2.6	2.6	2.7	2.7	3.5	–	–	–
Austria	3.5	3.5	3.6	3.5	3.5	3.5	3.4	3.4	3.4	3.5	3.4	3.4	3.4	3.4
Belgium	–	–	–	–	–	1.6	1.7	1.7	1.8	1.9	2.3	2.4	2.5	2.5
Canada	1.8	1.8	1.9	2.0	2.0	2.0	2.0	2.0	2.0	2.0	2.0	2.1	2.0	2.0
Denmark	2.6	2.6	2.6	2.8	2.6	2.6	2.6	2.6	2.6	2.6	2.6	2.6	2.6	2.6
Finland	4.2	4.3	4.3	4.4	4.5	4.6	4.7	4.7	4.8	4.9	5.0	5.0	5.1	5.1
France	2.6	3.0	3.2	3.3	3.5	3.1	2.9	3.0	3.2	3.3	3.4	3.4	3.6	3.5
Germany	3.6	3.6	3.6	3.6	3.6	3.6	3.6	3.6	3.6	3.6	3.6	3.6	3.6	3.6
Greece	1.3	1.3	1.4	1.5	1.5	1.5	1.5	1.5	1.5	1.5	1.6	1.6	1.6	1.6
Iceland	3.4	3.5	3.5	3.1	3.0	3.0	2.9	2.9	3.3	3.4	3.6	3.6	3.6	3.7
Ireland	–	–	–	–	–	–	–	–	–	–	–	1.8	2.1	1.7
Italy	2.2	2.2	2.3	2.3	2.4	2.4	2.4	2.5	2.5	2.5	2.6	2.6	2.6	2.6
Japan	2.1	2.2	2.3	2.5	2.6	2.6	2.7	2.8	2.9	3.0	3.0	3.0	3.0	3.0
Luxembourg	3.4	3.5	3.5	3.5	3.3	3.6	3.5	3.6	3.6	3.6	3.6	3.6	3.5	3.4
Netherlands	–	–	–	–	–	–	–	–	3.8	3.8	3.8	3.8	3.8	4.0
New Zealand	3.3	3.2	3.2	3.2	3.2	3.2	3.1	3.1	3.2	3.0	3.0	2.9	2.9	2.7
Norway	3.1	3.1	3.1	3.1	3.1	3.1	3.1	3.1	3.1	3.1	2.8	2.9	2.6	2.7
Portugal	0.8	0.8	0.9	0.9	0.9	0.9	0.8	0.9	0.9	0.9	1.1	1.1	1.1	1.1
Spain	–	–	–	–	–	–	0.8	0.8	–	–	1.3	1.3	1.3	1.3
Sweden	4.3	4.3	4.3	4.2	4.2	4.3	4.3	4.3	4.4	4.5	4.5	4.5	4.6	4.7
Switzerland	3.9	–	–	–	–	3.7	–	–	–	–	3.4	–	2.6	2.7
Turkey	–	–	–	–	–	0.4	–	–	–	–	0.4	0.1	0.1	0.1
United Kingdom	3.4	3.3	3.2	3.2	3.2	3.1	3.1	3.1	3.0	3.0	2.9	2.7	2.8	2.7
United States	2.8	2.8	2.8	2.8	2.7	2.6	2.6	2.5	2.5	2.4	2.3	2.2	2.1	2.0

Country	1974	1975	1976	1977	1978	1979	1980	1981	1982	1983	1984	1985	1986	1987
Australia	–	3.5	–	3.5	–	–	3.5	3.5	3.4	–	–	3.2	3.2	–
Austria	3.5	3.5	3.5	3.5	3.5	3.5	3.5	3.5	3.4	3.4	3.4	3.3	3.3	3.3
Belgium	2.6	2.6	2.6	2.7	2.6	2.7	2.7	2.8	2.9	2.8	2.8	2.8	2.8	–
Canada	2.0	2.0	2.0	2.1	2.1	2.1	2.1	2.1	2.1	2.1	2.1	2.0	–	–
Denmark	2.6	2.6	–	2.5	2.5	2.4	2.3	2.3	2.2	2.2	2.1	2.1	2.1	1.9
Finland	5.0	4.9	4.8	4.8	4.8	4.8	4.9	4.8	4.8	4.8	4.4	4.4	4.2	4.2
France	3.5	3.5	3.5	3.5	3.5	3.5	3.5	3.5	3.4	3.4	3.4	3.4	3.3	–
Germany	3.6	3.6	3.6	3.6	3.6	3.6	3.6	3.5	3.4	3.4	3.4	3.5	3.5	3.5
Greece	1.6	1.6	1.6	1.5	1.6	1.5	1.6	1.6	1.6	1.5	1.4	1.4	1.4	1.4
Iceland	3.8	3.9	4.0	4.0	4.0	3.9	3.4	4.0	3.8	3.9	–	3.5	4.0	–
Ireland	1.7	1.8	1.7	1.8	1.7	1.7	1.7	2.0	1.6	1.8	1.5	1.7	1.6	1.3
Italy	2.6	2.6	2.5	2.4	2.3	2.2	2.1	2.0	1.9	1.8	1.8	1.7	1.6	1.6
Japan	3.0	3.0	3.1	3.1	3.2	3.3	3.4	3.5	3.6	3.7	3.8	3.8	3.9	–
Luxembourg	3.4	3.4	3.4	3.4	3.6	3.7	3.9	4.0	3.8	3.7	3.7	3.8	–	3.8
Netherlands	4.0	4.0	4.1	4.1	4.1	4.1	4.1	4.0	4.0	4.0	4.0	3.9	3.8	3.8
New Zealand	2.9	2.6	2.6	2.6	2.6	2.7	2.7	2.6	2.7	2.7	–	–	2.1	–
Norway	2.4	2.4	2.4	2.3	5.3	5.3	5.3	5.2	5.2	5.2	5.2	5.2	5.2	4.9
Portugal	1.1	1.1	1.2	1.1	1.2	1.4	1.3	1.4	0.6	0.7	0.8	1.1	1.2	1.1
Spain	1.3	1.3	1.3	1.1	1.3	1.4	1.4	1.3	1.3	1.3	1.3	1.2	1.2	1.1
Sweden	4.6	4.7	4.6	4.5	4.6	4.6	4.7	4.8	4.8	4.8	4.8	4.5	4.4	4.2
Switzerland	2.8	2.8	2.9	3.0	3.0	3.0	3.0	3.0	3.1	3.0	3.1	3.1	3.0	3.0
Turkey	0.1	0.1	0.1	0.1	0.1	0.1	0.1	0.1	0.1	–	–	0.7	–	–
United Kingdom	2.7	2.6	2.6	2.5	2.5	2.4	2.4	2.4	2.3	2.3	2.2	2.2	2.1	–
United States	2.0	1.9	1.8	1.8	1.7	1.7	1.7	1.7	–	–	–	–	–	–

Table 21
Inpatient care admission rates, by country: 1960-87

Percent of population

Country	1960	1961	1962	1963	1964	1965	1966	1967	1968	1969	1970	1971	1972	1973
Australia	–	12.5	–	–	12.8	–	–	–	16.4	16.8	19.8	20.5	22.0	–
Austria	14.1	14.4	14.3	14.4	14.6	14.5	14.5	14.7	14.8	15.4	15.5	15.8	15.7	15.9
Belgium	–	–	–	–	–	8.0	8.1	8.2	8.6	9.1	9.3	9.7	10.2	10.5
Canada	15.0	15.2	15.5	15.9	16.0	15.9	15.8	15.7	15.9	16.0	16.5	16.8	16.8	16.8
Denmark	–	–	–	12.7	12.3	12.7	12.8	13.1	13.6	13.9	14.4	14.9	15.9	16.4
Finland	13.1	13.2	13.5	13.8	14.3	15.0	15.4	15.7	16.0	17.4	18.2	19.2	19.5	19.5
France	–	–	–	–	–	–	6.7	6.9	7.1	7.1	7.4	7.9	14.9	15.3
Germany	13.3	13.3	13.2	13.4	13.6	13.8	14.0	14.3	14.7	15.0	15.4	15.7	15.9	16.1
Greece	–	7.0	7.8	8.0	8.5	8.9	9.2	9.7	10.2	10.4	10.5	10.8	10.9	10.9
Iceland	–	–	–	11.8	12.9	12.7	12.3	12.3	13.3	14.2	16.2	16.9	17.4	17.7
Ireland	–	–	–	–	–	–	–	–	–	–	12.4	13.2	14.8	13.7
Italy	7.8	8.2	8.7	9.4	9.9	10.5	11.0	11.5	12.2	13.1	13.8	13.7	13.9	14.7
Japan	3.7	3.9	4.1	4.3	4.5	4.6	4.7	5.0	5.2	5.3	5.4	5.5	5.6	5.6
Luxembourg	11.6	11.9	12.0	12.1	12.6	12.8	12.4	12.8	12.8	13.0	13.4	13.9	13.6	13.5
Netherlands	–	–	–	8.6	8.8	9.0	9.2	9.4	9.6	9.9	10.0	10.1	10.5	10.7
New Zealand	7.9	7.9	8.1	8.3	8.5	8.7	8.7	8.8	9.1	9.0	9.3	9.2	9.6	9.9
Norway	–	–	–	11.7	12.0	12.1	12.2	12.6	13.0	13.2	13.2	13.5	13.6	13.6
Portugal	4.2	4.4	4.6	4.7	5.0	4.9	5.0	5.1	5.4	5.6	5.9	6.3	6.5	6.8
Spain	–	–	–	–	–	–	–	–	–	–	–	–	7.1	7.3
Sweden	13.4	13.4	13.6	14.0	14.3	14.5	14.8	15.2	16.3	16.3	16.6	16.8	17.0	17.2
Switzerland	12.4	–	–	–	–	13.5	–	–	–	–	13.1	–	10.4	10.8
Turkey	3.4	–	–	–	–	3.8	–	–	–	–	4.4	–	4.6	4.8
United Kingdom	9.1	9.3	9.4	9.7	10.0	10.1	10.2	10.4	10.6	10.8	10.9	11.1	12.0	11.9
United States	13.9	13.9	14.2	14.5	14.7	14.8	14.8	14.8	14.8	15.2	15.5	15.7	15.8	16.2

Country	1974	1975	1976	1977	1978	1979	1980	1981	1982	1983	1984	1985	1986	1987
Australia	–	–	26.7	19.7	20.0	20.3	20.1	20.2	20.4	20.5	20.7	20.6	21.1	21.6
Austria	16.6	17.0	17.4	17.8	18.4	18.9	19.5	19.6	20.2	20.7	21.1	21.6	22.2	22.6
Belgium	10.8	11.8	11.7	12.0	12.5	12.7	13.8	13.8	14.0	14.4	14.6	14.5	14.6	–
Canada	16.8	16.5	16.7	15.7	15.4	15.1	14.9	14.8	14.7	14.6	14.5	14.5	14.5	14.5
Denmark	16.4	17.7	18.2	18.2	18.5	18.2	18.3	18.2	18.7	19.2	19.5	19.9	20.3	20.5
Finland	19.2	18.9	19.4	20.1	20.4	20.7	21.0	21.4	21.7	20.9	21.6	22.6	22.3	22.6
France	15.8	16.5	17.2	17.9	18.8	19.3	20.0	20.8	19.6	18.3	19.7	20.6	21.1	21.2
Germany	16.6	16.9	17.3	17.8	18.3	18.5	18.8	18.7	18.7	18.8	19.4	19.9	20.6	21.1
Greece	10.7	10.8	11.3	11.1	11.3	11.5	11.8	11.8	11.9	11.9	12.0	11.9	12.0	12.1
Iceland	18.2	19.5	19.4	19.7	20.4	20.9	20.9	20.9	20.2	20.9	–	–	–	–
Ireland	14.3	15.6	15.9	16.2	16.7	16.7	17.2	17.6	17.6	17.3	17.1	–	17.0	16.9
Italy	14.9	15.4	15.9	16.0	15.9	15.9	16.0	15.8	15.6	15.2	15.2	15.2	15.2	15.0
Japan	5.6	5.5	5.6	5.7	5.7	5.3	6.0	6.2	6.4	6.7	7.0	7.0	7.2	7.5
Luxembourg	13.8	13.7	14.3	14.9	15.9	16.1	16.6	17.0	17.8	18.1	18.5	18.8	19.0	–
Netherlands	10.8	11.0	11.3	11.3	11.5	11.6	11.7	11.8	11.9	11.8	11.5	11.4	11.2	11.0
New Zealand	12.2	12.5	12.8	13.0	13.1	13.1	13.3	14.3	15.6	15.7	–	–	13.0	13.0
Norway	14.0	14.7	14.1	15.0	14.3	15.6	15.5	15.4	15.6	15.8	16.3	16.6	16.6	16.3
Portugal	7.0	7.2	7.3	7.5	7.6	9.2	9.2	9.5	9.6	9.4	9.5	8.5	8.7	9.3
Spain	7.7	8.1	8.5	8.9	9.0	9.2	9.3	9.2	9.1	9.1	9.3	9.1	9.0	–
Sweden	18.1	18.1	18.4	18.2	18.1	18.4	18.3	18.6	18.9	19.2	19.1	20.0	19.7	20.0
Switzerland	11.3	11.4	11.8	12.0	12.1	12.2	12.6	12.6	12.8	12.8	12.9	13.1	13.3	13.2
Turkey	4.8	4.3	4.4	4.5	4.4	4.1	3.9	4.1	4.1	4.5	4.8	4.8	5.2	5.5
United Kingdom	12.0	11.6	12.3	12.6	12.7	12.8	13.6	13.8	13.7	14.6	15.1	15.5	15.7	15.8
United States	16.6	16.7	16.9	16.8	16.7	16.8	17.1	17.0	16.5	16.2	15.7	14.8	14.8	14.7

SOURCE: Organization for Economic Cooperation and Development: Health Data File, 1989.

149

Table 22
Average length-of-stay in inpatient care institutions, by country: 1960-87

Patient days per admission

Country	1960	1961	1962	1963	1964	1965	1966	1967	1968	1969	1970	1971	1972	1973	1974	1975	1976	1977	1978	1979	1980	1981	1982	1983	1984	1985	1986	1987
Australia	-	-	-	-	-	-	-	9.8	9.6	9.3	9.3	9.1	9.0	8.8	8.7	8.5	8.3	8.3	8.0	7.8	7.7	7.6	7.4	7.3	7.1	6.9	6.7	6.1
Austria	24.8	24.4	24.8	24.0	24.2	24.0	23.8	23.3	24.3	22.5	22.2	21.5	21.6	21.1	21.0	20.4	20.1	19.8	19.0	18.6	17.9	17.6	15.2	14.8	14.6	14.1	13.7	13.4
Belgium	-	-	-	-	-	-	-	-	-	-	-	-	-	-	-	-	21.1	20.7	20.0	19.6	19.5	18.5	18.5	17.8	17.2	16.9	16.3	-
Canada	11.1	11.1	11.3	11.5	11.5	11.6	11.7	11.5	11.7	11.7	11.5	11.3	11.1	10.8	11.0	11.2	12.2	13.0	12.6	12.8	12.9	13.1	13.3	13.6	13.6	13.4	13.3	13.2
Denmark	-	-	-	22.2	20.6	20.1	20.0	19.4	19.0	18.5	18.1	17.3	16.9	15.8	15.9	14.6	13.8	13.8	13.5	13.1	12.7	12.4	11.9	11.5	11.0	10.7	10.2	9.1
Finland	31.7	32.5	32.1	32.2	31.8	30.1	30.7	30.0	29.9	28.1	27.3	26.2	26.3	26.1	25.9	26.0	24.7	23.7	23.3	23.2	23.2	22.5	22.2	20.5	20.3	19.3	18.9	18.4
France	-	22.8	22.6	22.0	21.7	21.1	20.7	20.1	19.6	18.9	18.3	17.3	16.2	16.0	15.6	15.0	14.4	14.0	13.8	13.8	13.9	13.6	13.7	14.2	13.7	13.2	12.7	12.5
Germany	28.7	28.6	28.7	28.2	27.7	27.4	26.8	26.4	25.9	25.3	24.9	24.3	23.9	23.4	22.7	22.2	21.5	20.8	20.3	20.1	19.7	19.2	18.7	18.6	18.4	18.0	17.5	17.1
Greece	-	18.8	18.5	18.9	17.6	17.0	15.9	15.2	15.2	14.4	15.0	15.2	14.6	14.4	14.5	14.5	14.5	13.4	13.7	13.3	13.3	13.2	13.0	12.2	12.1	12.0	12.0	11.0
Iceland	-	-	-	30.0	30.5	30.5	30.9	31.7	32.7	31.4	28.8	27.5	27.4	27.2	27.1	26.3	20.5	20.1	19.5	18.8	19.1	19.1	19.0	19.0	-	-	16.1	16.0
Ireland	-	-	-	-	-	-	-	-	-	-	13.3	14.0	13.9	12.4	11.3	11.4	10.8	10.9	10.3	10.4	9.7	9.4	9.0	8.6	9.0	11.5	8.0	11.0
Italy	27.9	26.9	25.9	24.9	23.9	22.9	22.2	21.4	20.4	19.4	18.8	18.9	18.6	17.9	17.3	16.3	15.5	15.1	14.4	13.7	13.1	12.7	12.4	12.1	11.7	11.5	11.2	11.0
Japan	57.3	56.9	57.7	57.9	57.3	56.7	58.1	56.5	56.7	56.3	55.3	54.1	53.9	54.0	54.4	54.8	55.0	55.3	55.8	55.9	55.9	56.4	56.1	55.1	54.6	54.2	54.0	52.9
Luxembourg	29.0	29.0	29.0	29.0	26.0	28.0	28.0	28.0	28.0	28.0	27.0	26.0	26.0	25.0	24.0	25.0	24.0	23.1	22.7	23.1	23.2	23.0	21.0	21.0	20.0	20.0	19.8	-
Netherlands	-	-	-	-	-	-	-	-	39.4	38.5	38.2	37.8	37.7	37.4	37.1	36.8	35.9	35.9	35.3	35.2	34.7	34.4	34.1	33.9	34.3	34.3	34.1	34.8
New Zealand	18.9	18.8	18.3	17.4	17.4	17.0	16.7	16.4	16.5	16.1	-	15.4	14.7	13.9	14.5	13.2	12.9	13.2	13.3	14.1	13.8	12.6	12.3	12.4	12.0	12.7	12.9	-
Norway	-	-	-	26.3	26.0	25.7	25.3	24.8	24.0	23.6	21.0	19.4	19.0	18.3	17.4	16.9	16.7	16.3	15.7	15.0	14.3	14.4	13.6	12.2	12.0	11.6	11.3	11.0
Portugal	19.5	19.6	19.1	18.2	17.3	18.9	18.1	17.9	16.4	15.8	18.4	17.4	16.2	15.5	15.4	15.5	16.0	14.4	15.4	14.9	14.4	14.6	13.6	14.1	13.6	13.9	13.5	12.4
Spain	-	-	-	-	-	-	-	-	-	-	-	-	-	-	17.0	16.8	16.0	15.5	15.2	15.0	14.8	14.6	14.6	14.6	13.6	14.0	13.0	-
Sweden	31.8	31.7	31.4	30.4	29.9	29.2	28.7	28.3	26.9	27.4	27.2	27.2	27.4	27.1	25.9	25.8	25.0	24.6	24.9	24.6	24.4	23.0	22.9	22.7	22.7	21.3	20.8	19.7
Switzerland	31.7	-	31.4	-	-	27.5	-	-	-	-	26.0	-	26.4	26.2	25.7	25.8	25.8	25.8	25.4	25.2	24.7	25.3	25.4	24.6	24.4	24.4	23.7	25.2
Turkey	-	-	-	-	-	11.0	-	-	-	-	9.0	-	9.1	8.7	8.4	9.0	9.0	9.0	8.0	8.5	9.0	8.8	-	-	-	7.6	-	-
United Kingdom	35.9	34.4	33.4	32.1	30.9	30.1	29.7	28.5	28.0	26.6	25.7	24.5	23.9	23.6	23.0	22.9	22.1	21.3	20.8	20.3	19.1	18.6	18.3	17.4	16.5	15.8	15.2	15.0
United States	20.5	20.0	19.4	19.0	18.4	17.8	17.5	17.2	16.9	16.0	14.9	13.8	13.3	12.6	12.0	11.4	10.8	10.5	10.2	10.1	10.0	9.9	9.8	9.6	-	-	-	-

Table 23
Patient contact, by country: 1960-87

Consultations and visits per capita

Country	1960	1961	1962	1963	1964	1965	1966	1967	1968	1969	1970	1971	1972	1973	1974	1975	1976	1977	1978	1979	1980	1981	1982	1983	1984	1985	1986	1987
Australia	–	–	–	–	–	–	–	–	–	–	4.4	4.6	5.0	4.8	5.4	5.9	5.6	5.8	5.8	6.5	6.3	6.5	6.8	6.7	7.5	7.5	7.8	8.2
Austria	4.3	4.5	4.4	4.7	4.8	4.9	4.9	5.0	5.0	5.2	5.2	5.2	5.2	5.1	5.2	5.3	5.4	5.3	5.3	5.3	5.4	5.4	5.3	5.4	5.4	5.5	5.5	5.6
Belgium	–	–	–	–	–	–	5.4	–	–	5.8	–	–	6.2	–	6.4	6.4	6.5	6.4	6.7	6.7	7.1	7.1	–	–	–	7.3	7.3	7.4
Canada	–	–	4.0	–	–	–	–	–	–	–	–	–	–	4.4	4.6	4.9	4.9	5.0	5.1	5.3	5.4	5.5	5.1	5.9	6.0	6.2	6.4	6.6
Denmark	–	–	–	–	–	–	–	–	–	–	–	–	–	–	3.0	3.0	3.0	3.0	3.0	3.1	3.2	3.3	3.3	3.4	3.4	3.6	3.6	3.7
Finland	–	–	–	–	1.6	1.7	1.7	1.8	2.0	2.2	2.4	2.7	2.8	2.8	3.5	3.8	3.8	3.8	4.0	4.0	4.1	4.4	4.5	4.7	4.7	4.9	5.2	–
France	–	–	–	2.9	–	–	–	–	3.1	3.1	3.2	3.2	3.3	3.4	5.6	5.4	5.1	5.1	4.9	5.0	5.0	5.0	5.3	4.7	4.7	4.9	5.2	–
Germany	–	–	–	–	–	–	–	–	–	–	–	–	–	–	–	10.9	–	–	–	–	11.5	11.6	11.6	–	–	–	11.5	–
Greece	–	–	–	4.0	4.3	4.8	4.8	5.1	5.1	4.9	5.2	5.5	5.5	5.6	–	–	–	–	–	–	–	–	–	–	–	–	–	–
Iceland	–	–	–	–	–	–	–	–	–	–	–	–	–	–	–	–	–	–	–	–	–	–	–	–	–	–	–	–
Ireland	–	–	–	–	–	–	–	–	–	–	–	–	–	5.3	5.5	5.5	5.4	5.3	5.6	5.6	5.8	6.0	6.0	5.9	6.1	6.4	6.4	6.5
Italy	3.9	4.0	4.0	4.1	4.5	4.9	5.8	5.4	5.7	6.0	6.3	6.3	6.4	6.6	6.8	7.0	7.2	7.2	7.6	7.9	8.0	8.3	8.5	9.0	9.5	10.1	10.9	10.9
Japan	–	–	–	–	–	–	–	–	–	–	–	13.6	14.3	15.0	15.0	14.9	14.9	14.8	14.5	14.5	14.4	14.6	14.1	13.3	13.1	12.7	12.8	–
Luxembourg	–	–	–	–	–	–	–	–	–	–	–	–	–	–	–	–	–	–	–	–	–	–	–	–	–	–	–	–
Netherlands	–	–	–	–	–	–	4.2	4.2	4.2	–	–	–	–	–	–	–	–	3.7	3.2	–	3.2	3.6	3.4	3.4	3.5	3.6	3.5	3.7
New Zealand	–	–	–	–	–	–	–	–	–	–	–	–	–	–	–	–	–	3.7	3.7	3.8	3.7	3.8	–	–	–	–	–	–
Norway	–	–	–	–	–	–	–	–	–	–	–	–	–	–	2.9	4.5	–	–	–	–	–	–	–	–	–	5.7	–	–
Portugal	1.0	1.1	1.1	1.2	1.4	1.4	1.5	1.6	1.7	1.6	1.5	2.6	2.5	2.9	3.4	3.1	3.3	3.3	3.5	3.5	3.7	3.6	3.3	3.0	3.0	2.8	2.4	2.4
Spain	–	–	1.3	1.4	1.4	1.5	1.7	1.8	2.0	2.2	2.6	2.6	3.0	3.2	2.5	3.7	4.1	4.4	4.7	4.6	4.7	4.7	4.7	4.7	4.4	4.0	4.0	–
Sweden	–	–	–	–	–	–	–	–	–	–	–	1.9	1.9	1.9	2.5	2.6	2.5	2.5	2.5	2.6	2.6	2.7	2.7	2.7	2.7	2.7	2.7	2.7
Switzerland	–	–	–	5.3	5.4	5.4	4.3	4.4	5.1	5.9	6.3	4.5	4.0	4.0	4.9	5.1	5.4	5.3	5.4	5.6	5.6	5.7	5.6	5.8	5.8	6.0	6.1	–
Turkey	–	–	–	–	–	–	–	–	–	–	–	–	1.2	1.2	1.2	1.2	1.2	1.2	1.2	1.2	1.2	1.2	–	–	–	–	–	–
United Kingdom	–	–	–	–	–	–	–	–	–	–	–	–	3.8	3.5	3.5	3.5	3.3	3.7	4.0	4.0	4.2	3.8	4.3	4.2	4.0	4.0	4.5	–
United States	–	–	–	4.5	4.5	4.5	4.3	4.3	4.2	4.3	4.6	4.9	5.0	5.0	4.9	5.1	4.9	4.8	4.8	4.7	4.8	4.6	5.2	5.1	–	–	5.3	6.0

SOURCE: Organization for Economic Cooperation and Development: Health Data File, 1989.

Table 24
Pharmaceutical consumption, by country: 1960-87

Country	1960	1961	1962	1963	1964	1965	1966	1967	1968	1969	1970	1971	1972	1973
	Average number of medicines per person													
Australia	2.7	3.3	3.9	4.3	4.4	4.7	4.7	5.1	5.1	5.4	5.7	6.0	6.0	6.1
Austria	14.4	14.9	15.0	15.8	15.9	16.3	16.5	16.8	16.1	16.6	16.6	16.3	16.2	15.9
Belgium	—	—	—	—	—	—	9.0	—	—	—	—	—	—	—
Canada	—	—	—	—	—	—	—	—	—	—	—	—	—	—
Denmark	4.8	4.8	4.8	4.9	5.1	5.2	5.3	5.5	5.7	5.9	5.9	6.0	6.1	6.0
Finland	2.2	2.4	2.5	2.5	2.7	3.1	3.1	3.3	3.5	3.8	4.0	4.4	4.5	4.6
France	—	—	—	—	—	—	—	—	—	—	17.4	—	19.0	—
Germany	—	—	—	—	—	—	—	—	—	—	—	—	—	11.0
Greece	—	—	—	3.3	3.6	4.4	4.5	4.8	4.9	5.2	5.8	6.6	7.1	7.6
Iceland	—	—	—	—	—	—	—	—	—	—	—	—	—	—
Ireland	—	—	—	—	—	—	9.0	—	—	—	—	—	—	9.2
Italy	6.3	7.0	8.3	9.3	10.4	11.4	11.7	13.0	14.4	15.5	15.7	16.7	17.3	18.2
Japan	8.9	—	—	—	—	—	—	—	—	—	—	—	—	—
Luxembourg	—	—	—	—	—	11.7	—	—	—	—	11.3	—	11.1	—
Netherlands	—	—	—	6.8	7.2	7.5	7.7	7.7	8.4	8.8	9.1	—	—	—
New Zealand	6.2	6.2	6.1	6.4	6.1	6.4	6.4	6.3	6.3	6.6	6.8	6.7	7.0	7.0
Norway	—	—	—	—	—	—	—	—	—	—	—	—	—	—
Portugal	5.9	—	—	—	—	10.0	—	—	—	—	—	14.8	—	13.5
Spain	—	—	—	4.7	5.0	5.6	6.4	7.8	8.5	9.0	9.2	9.9	10.6	11.7
Sweden	—	—	—	—	—	—	—	—	—	—	—	—	—	—
Switzerland	—	—	—	—	—	—	—	—	—	—	—	—	—	—
Turkey	—	—	—	—	—	—	—	—	—	—	—	—	—	—
United Kingdom	4.7	4.4	4.2	4.3	4.4	5.1	5.5	5.6	5.5	5.5	5.5	5.4	5.6	5.8
United States	—	—	—	—	4.7	—	—	—	—	—	—	—	—	5.8

Country	1974	1975	1976	1977	1978	1979	1980	1981	1982	1983	1984	1985	1986	1987
Australia	6.9	7.5	7.8	6.9	7.1	7.0	6.7	7.0	7.5	7.5	7.7	8.4	8.3	7.1
Austria	16.6	17.4	17.8	17.9	14.4	14.5	14.9	14.9	14.2	14.2	13.8	14.3	14.7	14.8
Belgium	—	9.0	—	—	—	10.1	10.3	9.9	—	—	—	8.2	8.3	8.4
Canada	—	—	—	—	—	—	—	—	—	—	—	—	—	—
Denmark	6.2	6.2	6.2	6.3	6.4	6.4	6.5	6.4	6.5	6.3	5.9	5.9	6.1	5.6
Finland	4.8	4.8	4.8	4.8	4.8	4.8	4.9	4.9	4.9	5.1	5.1	5.5	5.5	5.6
France	21.3	—	23.8	24.1	26.2	26.1	27.6	28.9	—	—	—	—	—	—
Germany	—	—	—	—	—	—	—	—	13.5	12.3	12.0	12.1	12.5	12.2
Greece	7.5	8.2	7.4	7.1	7.1	6.9	6.9	7.2	7.4	—	—	—	—	—
Iceland	7.4	6.4	5.9	—	4.9	4.8	4.8	—	—	—	5.0	5.4	5.3	5.3
Ireland	9.8	10.1	10.2	10.2	10.6	10.8	11.4	11.9	9.5	7.9	8.5	9.1	9.4	9.9
Italy	18.2	20.2	21.0	19.8	20.7	20.7	19.9	20.1	20.1	19.6	18.6	19.6	19.2	19.3
Japan	0.1	0.1	0.2	0.2	0.3	0.4	0.5	0.6	0.7	0.8	0.9	0.9	0.9	—
Luxembourg	11.6	—	12.3	—	12.4	—	—	—	—	—	—	—	—	—
Netherlands	4.5	—	—	—	—	—	—	—	—	—	—	—	—	—
New Zealand	7.1	7.3	8.6	8.1	7.6	7.7	7.7	9.6	8.8	8.5	8.9	8.8	9.1	9.0
Norway	5.4	5.3	5.7	5.6	—	—	—	—	—	—	6.0	6.3	6.3	6.6
Portugal	—	14.5	13.7	19.6	—	14.7	15.4	15.5	14.7	14.2	13.3	14.2	14.2	17.2
Spain	12.0	12.2	14.4	14.4	15.6	14.7	14.4	14.5	12.1	11.9	11.3	—	—	—
Sweden	4.7	4.9	4.8	4.8	4.7	4.7	4.4	4.5	4.5	4.6	4.7	4.8	4.7	4.8
Switzerland	—	—	—	—	—	—	—	—	—	—	—	—	—	—
Turkey	—	—	—	—	—	—	—	—	—	—	—	—	—	—
United Kingdom	6.0	6.2	6.4	6.5	6.7	6.7	6.6	6.6	6.8	6.9	7.0	6.9	7.0	7.3
United States	—	6.9	6.7	6.4	5.9	6.1	6.1	6.2	6.4	6.4	6.5	—	—	—

SOURCE:

Table 25

Inpatient medical care beds, by country: 1960-87

Average daily census

Country	1960	1961	1962	1963	1964	1965	1966	1967	1968	1969	1970	1971	1972	1973
Australia	—	—	98,923	103,001	106,479	102,583	105,410	115,506	118,290	121,544	123,991	129,971	129,971	137,610
Austria	76,170	76,398	77,067	77,693	78,239	78,520	78,422	78,703	79,293	80,269	80,549	81,348	81,391	83,136
Belgium	55,214	—	—	—	—	60,528	—	—	—	—	80,392	80,400	83,448	—
Canada	—	—	—	—	—	—	—	—	—	—	—	—	—	—
Denmark	—	37,200	37,400	39,700	37,600	37,800	38,700	38,700	39,300	39,800	40,100	40,600	41,700	41,900
Finland	50,956	57,506	58,297	59,329	59,940	61,723	63,187	64,567	65,544	67,725	69,376	69,467	69,653	70,269
France	—	451,571	—	—	—	—	—	487,292	—	—	—	—	477,259	—
Germany	583,513	594,642	613,641	615,685	619,388	631,447	640,372	649,590	665,546	677,695	683,254	690,236	701,263	707,460
Greece	48,239	48,779	49,247	49,786	48,363	50,323	51,638	52,173	53,260	53,733	54,633	56,232	55,958	56,118
Iceland	1,727	1,740	1,800	1,902	2,089	2,133	2,143	2,153	2,564	2,543	2,575	2,645	2,752	2,823
Ireland	60,608	—	—	—	—	—	59,091	—	—	53,428	37,200	35,500	34,500	33,500
Italy	445,216	455,245	466,132	478,825	489,450	498,337	509,359	521,942	535,555	551,585	566,320	570,382	571,811	575,953
Japan	852,025	890,254	932,715	984,313	1,030,457	1,077,971	1,130,930	1,188,997	1,239,685	1,276,825	1,312,628	1,338,339	1,364,001	—
Luxembourg	3,729	3,812	3,890	3,925	4,058	4,126	4,114	4,254	4,297	4,306	4,289	4,246	4,616	4,661
Netherlands	125,900	127,600	129,300	131,000	133,500	136,000	138,500	141,000	143,400	145,400	148,550	151,300	156,306	162,216
New Zealand	27,789	27,774	27,756	27,905	28,038	28,247	28,932	29,309	29,212	29,554	30,337	30,513	30,916	31,959
Norway	—	—	—	34,110	35,074	34,534	34,437	34,796	35,039	35,450	32,031	32,123	32,130	32,097
Portugal	48,249	48,821	48,619	52,493	53,709	53,669	54,816	55,528	55,927	55,395	54,514	54,427	53,524	54,478
Spain	—	—	135,293	156,819	—	—	—	—	—	—	157,598	159,254	177,385	180,547
Sweden	102,394	104,736	105,882	106,953	109,071	110,142	110,984	112,739	114,569	117,790	119,679	117,349	117,996	117,934
Switzerland	67,722	—	—	—	—	71,742	—	—	—	—	69,932	—	—	—
Turkey	45,807	—	—	—	55,126	55,316	57,833	59,173	64,966	69,263	71,210	74,556	77,108	81,175
United Kingdom	—	543,457	532,922	533,404	537,151	537,210	534,009	532,898	533,001	528,917	524,682	516,097	509,926	505,620
United States	1,658,000	1,670,000	1,689,000	1,702,000	1,696,000	1,703,500	1,679,000	1,671,000	1,663,000	1,650,000	1,615,800	1,555,600	1,549,700	1,534,700

Country	1974	1975	1976	1977	1978	1979	1980	1981	1982	1983	1984	1985	1986	1987
Australia	142,051	143,674	146,089	148,324	151,187	155,530	159,047	162,012	164,711	166,668	168,601	169,006	168,536	165,453
Austria	86,746	85,461	84,856	84,790	84,959	85,204	84,382	84,310	82,957	83,141	83,572	82,388	82,443	81,721
Belgium	87,164	87,457	87,983	89,596	90,291	91,899	92,436	92,686	92,093	91,638	90,790	89,589	88,554	83,090
Canada	—	—	—	—	—	—	—	—	—	—	—	—	—	—
Denmark	42,900	42,900	43,400	42,500	43,497	42,955	42,504	40,182	39,273	37,900	36,405	35,976	35,606	32,325
Finland	70,301	71,115	72,418	72,547	73,667	74,513	74,381	74,441	75,026	74,796	68,938	68,704	68,220	67,246
France	538,551	550,639	557,531	562,421	575,935	585,399	587,150	601,051	589,728	594,238	—	580,325	592,525	—
Germany	716,530	729,791	726,846	722,953	714,879	712,055	707,710	695,603	683,624	682,747	678,708	674,742	674,384	673,687
Greece	56,885	58,501	58,574	58,994	59,100	60,073	60,067	59,914	58,938	57,496	57,081	54,438	52,864	51,575
Iceland	2,899	3,049	3,077	3,144	3,198	3,195	3,197	3,185	3,332	3,423	3,506	3,508	3,521	3,564
Ireland	34,000	33,800	33,300	33,600	33,600	—	33,028	—	—	—	—	—	—	36,670
Italy	580,195	585,875	585,053	577,963	568,126	558,462	548,428	535,741	522,314	508,742	495,054	479,638	457,210	441,682
Japan	—	1,428,482	1,451,972	1,477,199	1,510,702	1,552,812	1,607,482	1,647,818	1,688,152	1,726,496	1,750,768	1,778,979	1,816,194	1,860,315
Luxembourg	4,225	4,170	4,225	4,391	4,603	4,539	4,667	4,778	4,816	4,740	4,688	4,587	4,616	4,661
Netherlands	165,793	166,731	168,674	169,856	171,146	172,494	173,462	174,393	171,686	172,122	172,420	172,393	172,614	172,650
New Zealand	31,577	32,485	32,397	32,636	32,552	32,537	32,035	31,637	31,586	31,653	31,344	30,999	30,397	30,433
Norway	31,915	31,834	31,550	31,760	31,289	30,646	67,328	—	—	—	—	66,321	66,536	65,886
Portugal	53,454	52,268	52,047	51,449	52,327	51,701	51,254	51,246	51,173	51,274	50,210	45,818	46,066	46,448
Spain	185,218	190,444	194,097	200,134	202,043	203,819	201,035	202,969	206,567	196,959	193,042	181,985	186,051	—
Sweden	118,967	118,324	118,972	118,836	119,246	117,235	117,657	116,739	116,528	116,688	115,859	114,202	111,091	106,885
Switzerland	—	72,438	72,300	72,300	72,000	72,000	71,900	72,900	74,600	71,500	72,800	72,400	73,000	72,100
Turkey	83,693	81,264	82,945	83,027	86,526	96,752	99,117	97,765	96,138	99,396	100,496	103,918	107,152	111,135
United Kingdom	496,482	488,006	479,359	469,849	470,900	463,400	458,000	454,923	452,600	446,400	430,815	421,195	409,962	388,711
United States	1,512,700	1,465,800	1,433,500	1,407,100	1,380,600	1,371,800	1,364,500	1,361,500	1,359,800	1,350,400	1,338,700	1,318,000	1,288,000	—

SOURCE: Organization for Economic Cooperation and Development: Health Data File, 1989.

153

Table 26
Total health employment, by country: 1960-87

Number of persons or man-years in thousands

Country	1960	1961	1962	1963	1964	1965	1966	1967	1968	1969	1970	1971	1972	1973
Australia	–	128	–	–	–	155	–	–	–	–	–	259	279	293
Austria	–	–	–	–	–	–	–	–	–	–	–	–	–	–
Belgium	–	–	–	–	–	–	55	–	–	–	91	–	–	–
Canada	–	198	–	–	–	–	–	–	–	–	–	326	–	–
Denmark	58	–	–	–	–	–	–	–	–	–	86	–	96	–
Finland	46	48	52	54	56	60	65	68	73	76	80	84	87	93
France	–	–	–	–	–	–	–	–	–	–	–	438	–	–
Germany	–	–	–	–	664	679	681	707	748	827	774	799	875	921
Greece	–	–	–	–	–	–	–	40	40	41	44	45	46	49
Iceland	–	–	–	–	–	–	–	2	3	3	4	4	4	4
Ireland	–	–	–	–	–	–	–	–	–	–	–	35	–	–
Italy	148	156	165	176	185	194	202	212	225	243	271	301	328	357
Japan	637	–	–	754	–	–	900	–	–	1,032	–	–	1,162	–
Luxembourg	–	–	–	–	–	–	–	–	–	–	–	–	–	–
Netherlands	–	–	–	–	–	–	–	–	–	–	205	–	–	–
New Zealand	–	–	–	–	–	–	–	–	–	–	–	–	–	–
Norway	44	45	50	52	54	58	59	61	63	66	69	72	80	83
Portugal	27	30	31	34	35	35	36	36	37	48	58	59	59	63
Spain	–	–	–	–	–	–	–	–	–	–	–	–	–	–
Sweden	117	121	123	128	129	134	141	145	151	160	168	175	192	202
Switzerland	66	–	–	–	–	87	–	–	–	–	107	–	–	–
Turkey	–	–	–	–	–	–	–	–	–	–	–	–	–	–
United Kingdom	–	575	598	612	627	650	676	690	710	716	741	785	821	848
United States	1,763	1,788	1,838	1,909	1,991	2,101	2,262	2,426	2,585	2,768	2,878	3,074	3,393	3,618

Country	1974	1975	1976	1977	1978	1979	1980	1981	1982	1983	1984	1985	1986	1987
Australia	321	341	360	380	380	399	411	406	421	439	454	459	487	512
Austria	–	118	–	–	–	–	–	–	175	–	–	–	–	–
Belgium	112	120	128	136	145	153	159	167	–	–	–	–	–	–
Canada	–	–	–	–	–	–	–	519	–	–	–	–	599	–
Denmark	103	–	109	–	113	–	118	–	–	–	–	–	–	–
Finland	96	103	109	115	119	124	126	131	135	139	143	154	162	159
France	–	–	573	–	–	–	–	727	760	1,203	1,325	–	–	–
Germany	986	979	1,054	1,065	1,110	1,176	1,210	1,232	1,274	1,309	1,330	1,412	1,419	1,471
Greece	51	54	56	59	60	65	67	69	84	88	90	97	103	109
Iceland	5	5	6	6	6	6	7	7	7	8	8	8	9	10
Ireland	42	44	48	51	51	54	56	66	–	–	63	–	62	58
Italy	387	414	437	452	468	485	499	511	519	515	508	506	506	505
Japan	1,335	–	–	–	1,524	–	–	1,724	–	–	1,824	–	–	–
Luxembourg	–	–	–	–	–	–	–	6	–	–	–	–	–	–
Netherlands	–	266	–	284	290	297	306	313	318	321	323	327	335	341
New Zealand	–	–	68	–	–	–	73	76	–	–	–	–	81	–
Norway	87	94	102	110	115	121	126	130	131	135	138	140	142	150
Portugal	70	76	80	83	91	94	86	103	106	101	99	102	103	101
Spain	–	–	270	292	293	322	304	294	329	365	320	350	–	–
Sweden	215	222	240	252	273	287	304	315	323	329	–	–	–	–
Switzerland	–	140	143	146	150	155	161	167	173	174	175	176	178	–
Turkey	–	–	–	–	–	–	–	–	–	–	–	–	–	–
United Kingdom	911	1,042	1,096	1,099	1,120	1,152	1,174	1,207	1,227	1,227	1,223	1,223	1,215	1,212
United States	3,827	4,046	4,219	4,432	4,662	4,878	5,119	5,374	5,667	5,821	5,971	6,142	–	–

Table 27
Practicing physicians, by country: 1960-87

Number of active physicians

Country	1960	1961	1962	1963	1964	1965	1966	1967	1968	1969	1970	1971	1972	1973
Australia	10,881	—	—	—	10,086	13,085	13,873	—	—	—	—	16,105	10,154	10,416
Austria	9,573	9,851	9,995	10,063	10,119	10,169	10,222	10,062	10,079	10,137	10,137	10,153	15,888	16,478
Belgium	11,380	11,703	12,394	12,888	13,236	13,473	13,793	14,176	14,517	14,922	14,991	32,942	34,508	35,923
Canada	—	21,290	23,248	24,082	24,847	25,481	26,528	27,544	28,209	29,659	31,166	—	—	—
Denmark	—	—	5,900	6,200	6,300	6,450	6,650	6,800	7,000	7,100	7,200	7,500	8,100	8,500
Finland	2,827	2,961	3,104	3,261	3,384	3,553	3,797	3,956	4,185	4,486	4,798	5,112	5,475	5,826
France	44,600	46,492	48,465	58,522	52,665	54,900	56,819	59,065	60,861	62,989	65,191	68,778	70,711	73,552
Germany	79,350	80,825	82,097	83,025	84,203	85,801	86,700	88,559	90,882	93,934	99,654	103,910	107,403	110,980
Greece	10,424	10,423	10,723	11,265	11,980	12,072	12,383	12,839	13,159	13,712	14,263	14,883	15,351	16,984
Iceland	205	212	224	228	232	238	239	241	254	263	291	305	333	343
Ireland	—	2,952	—	—	—	—	3,011	—	—	—	—	3,565	—	—
Italy	22,655	23,685	24,951	26,044	27,077	28,131	29,274	30,430	31,557	33,143	35,605	38,028	40,847	44,228
Japan	96,038	97,329	98,562	99,471	101,021	102,015	103,956	104,990	107,028	109,595	113,214	116,746	119,084	120,107
Luxembourg	318	322	326	329	331	338	346	349	359	365	384	397	403	410
Netherlands	12,809	13,027	13,238	13,642	13,904	14,362	14,550	14,774	15,128	15,644	16,292	17,381	18,142	19,330
New Zealand	2,573	2,573	—	—	—	—	2,838	—	—	—	—	3,080	—	3,444
Norway	4,260	—	4,215	4,215	4,556	4,681	4,847	5,020	5,175	5,412	5,361	5,690	6,005	6,367
Portugal	7,075	7,368	7,673	7,541	7,561	7,320	7,619	7,838	8,482	8,019	8,156	8,410	8,972	9,111
Spain	35,685	36,562	37,374	37,743	39,064	39,709	40,840	41,932	42,460	44,102	45,335	47,419	49,256	51,594
Sweden	7,130	7,376	7,630	7,970	8,220	8,520	8,840	9,240	9,840	10,380	10,560	11,250	11,920	12,610
Switzerland	4,908	—	—	—	—	5,174	—	—	—	—	5,508	—	—	—
Turkey	8,214	—	—	—	—	10,895	11,335	11,875	12,389	13,331	15,856	16,514	17,365	18,511
United Kingdom	—	—	—	—	—	—	—	—	—	—	—	55,150	57,135	58,909
United States	259,400	264,659	271,700	289,189	297,089	305,115	313,559	322,045	330,111	338,379	326,500	337,400	348,300	355,700

Country	1974	1975	1976	1977	1978	1979	1980	1981	1982	1983	1984	1985	1986	1987
Australia	—	—	20,480	—	—	—	—	27,127	—	—	—	—	32,789	—
Austria	10,575	—	11,012	—	—	—	—	12,374	12,747	13,066	13,400	13,898	14,215	14,512
Belgium	17,272	18,506	19,872	20,725	22,143	23,415	24,536	25,629	26,593	27,726	28,826	29,776	30,942	31,718
Canada	37,297	39,104	40,130	41,398	42,238	43,192	44,275	45,542	47,384	48,860	49,916	51,948	53,207	55,275
Denmark	9,000	9,397	9,900	10,250	10,548	10,845	11,143	12,120	12,463	10,579	12,806	12,975	13,047	13,144
Finland	6,234	6,701	7,068	7,603	8,134	8,543	9,016	9,538	10,057	10,579	10,822	8,747	9,047	9,340
France	77,143	80,954	86,306	91,442	97,168	104,073	108,054	113,026	114,951	118,000	125,000	128,000	132,138	138,835
Germany	114,661	118,726	122,075	125,274	130,033	135,711	139,431	142,934	146,221	147,467	153,895	160,902	165,015	171,487
Greece	17,942	18,421	19,340	20,484	21,320	22,337	23,469	24,724	25,909	27,607	28,212	29,103	30,481	33,290
Iceland	372	400	408	424	439	459	488	509	532	545	574	626	632	665
Ireland	—	3,758	3,925	—	—	4,174	4,440	5,119	—	—	5,160	—	—	5,000
Italy	47,568	49,552	50,242	52,596	56,246	59,758	60,140	63,765	64,732	63,216	62,366	62,930	63,906	63,900
Japan	122,096	125,970	128,448	131,628	136,164	143,125	148,815	155,422	160,379	163,216	173,452	173,452	183,128	191,346
Luxembourg	425	452	456	455	530	575	621	563	605	627	637	663	686	666
Netherlands	20,200	21,892	22,913	23,769	24,878	25,947	26,887	28,037	28,807	29,951	31,185	32,193	33,330	34,573
New Zealand	—	—	4,048	4,257	4,377	4,557	4,881	5,037	—	5,403	5,437	5,556	5,747	—
Norway	6,602	6,899	7,140	7,485	7,648	7,813	8,332	8,311	8,630	8,691	8,822	9,176	9,443	9,443
Portugal	10,312	11,101	11,863	13,816	15,958	18,088	16,332	20,997	22,009	22,917	24,095	24,629	25,696	26,381
Spain	52,599	54,533	64,597	69,080	75,081	81,658	86,253	96,569	104,759	115,251	119,103	126,677	131,080	—
Sweden	13,260	14,050	14,650	15,410	16,340	16,840	18,300	19,000	19,500	20,100	21,596	21,596	22,485	22,485
Switzerland	—	6,248	6,399	6,634	6,925	7,209	7,473	7,799	8,330	8,602	9,009	9,298	9,646	9,947
Turkey	20,868	21,714	23,388	23,920	25,230	26,298	27,241	28,411	30,956	32,263	34,195	36,435	37,143	38,829
United Kingdom	60,182	62,344	63,675	65,034	66,473	68,268	71,081	72,781	73,370	75,334	76,080	77,124	77,192	78,128
United States	370,000	384,500	399,500	405,900	424,000	440,400	457,500	466,600	483,700	501,200	506,400	534,800	545,000	570,000

SOURCE: Organization for Economic Cooperation and Development: Health Data File, 1989.

Table 28
Practicing dentists, by country: 1960-87

Number of active dentists

Country	1960	1961	1962	1963	1964	1965	1966	1967	1968	1969	1970	1971	1972	1973
Australia	4,001	–	–	–	–	–	–	–	–	–	–	3,477	4,653	4,517
Austria	–	3,952	3,896	3,846	3,788	3,715	3,652	3,578	3,476	3,416	3,322	3,217	3,170	3,110
Belgium	–	–	–	–	–	1,969	–	–	2,135	2,303	2,718	2,261	–	2,369
Canada	5,708	5,906	5,999	6,103	6,218	6,396	6,532	6,713	6,738	6,933	7,115	7,453	7,611	7,825
Denmark	1,571	1,619	–	–	–	–	–	–	–	–	–	–	–	–
Finland	1,806	1,853	1,909	2,006	2,092	2,195	2,281	2,379	2,448	2,562	2,655	2,803	2,916	3,050
France	–	–	–	–	–	–	–	–	–	–	–	20,571	–	–
Germany	32,509	32,979	32,649	32,364	32,047	31,660	31,599	31,370	31,413	31,300	31,262	31,405	31,149	31,182
Greece	2,998	3,269	3,261	3,479	3,282	3,485	3,589	3,606	4,307	4,169	4,395	4,109	4,428	4,991
Iceland	50	51	54	58	67	69	73	82	87	89	101	106	117	122
Ireland	–	567	–	–	–	–	–	–	–	–	–	659	–	1,123
Italy	–	–	–	–	–	–	–	–	–	–	–	–	–	–
Japan	31,797	32,249	32,825	33,148	33,756	34,127	34,547	35,115	35,485	35,977	36,468	37,627	38,765	38,993
Luxembourg	117	112	103	100	95	88	80	74	73	67	106	–	–	–
Netherlands	2,492	2,592	2,383	2,502	2,837	2,955	3,034	3,133	3,243	3,205	3,364	3,444	3,648	3,889
New Zealand	–	–	–	–	–	–	–	959	–	1,008	–	1,000	1,002	1,057
Norway	–	–	–	–	–	–	–	–	–	–	–	–	–	–
Portugal	–	–	–	–	–	–	–	–	–	–	669	666	669	–
Spain	–	–	–	–	2,924	3,005	3,126	3,195	3,226	3,376	3,361	3,534	3,537	3,613
Sweden	5,090	5,280	5,410	5,600	5,860	6,080	5,880	6,130	6,300	6,630	6,720	6,680	6,990	7,000
Switzerland	1,367	–	–	–	1,769	1,932	2,140	2,246	2,381	–	1,982	2,440	2,544	2,553
Turkey	–	–	–	–	–	–	–	–	–	3,025	3,245	3,517	3,789	4,279
United Kingdom	–	–	–	–	–	–	–	–	–	–	–	–	–	–
United States	90,120	–	–	–	–	95,990	–	–	–	–	102,220	–	105,400	–

Country	1974	1975	1976	1977	1978	1979	1980	1981	1982	1983	1984	1985	1986	1987
Australia	4,601	4,861	4,630	5,208	5,209	5,206	5,547	5,586	5,277	5,635	5,643	5,739	6,311	–
Austria	3,051	3,065	3,050	3,091	3,087	3,061	3,059	3,095	3,158	3,139	3,162	3,002	3,078	3,062
Belgium	2,547	2,685	2,986	3,283	3,396	3,878	4,291	4,604	5,126	5,561	5,911	6,214	–	–
Canada	8,487	8,738	9,401	10,058	10,451	10,763	11,095	11,484	11,880	12,271	12,624	13,027	13,164	13,503
Denmark	–	2,315	2,072	2,153	2,193	–	2,321	2,321	2,351	–	–	3,492	3,586	3,644
Finland	3,151	3,254	3,366	3,536	3,658	3,827	3,938	4,068	4,234	4,337	4,430	4,519	4,736	4,795
France	–	–	–	–	–	–	–	–	–	–	–	–	–	–
Germany	31,538	31,774	31,858	32,121	32,482	32,958	33,240	33,501	33,679	33,713	34,082	34,578	38,055	38,826
Greece	5,283	5,930	6,160	6,386	6,825	7,177	7,677	7,777	8,007	8,222	8,379	8,337	9,131	9,104
Iceland	126	138	151	155	154	167	168	176	180	191	193	197	205	213
Ireland	1,144	1,270	1,296	1,302	1,313	1,303	1,319	1,375	1,418	1,440	1,463	–	–	1,201
Italy	–	–	–	–	–	–	–	–	–	–	–	–	–	–
Japan	40,088	41,951	42,704	43,906	46,902	48,899	51,597	54,954	56,327	–	61,283	–	64,804	66,797
Luxembourg	–	110	–	–	118	117	131	121	141	147	158	168	181	–
Netherlands	4,110	4,462	4,608	4,817	5,052	5,346	5,688	5,970	6,271	6,586	6,865	7,118	7,405	7,585
New Zealand	1,061	1,046	1,073	–	–	–	1,145	1,204	–	1,160	–	–	1,204	–
Norway	–	3,842	3,930	4,010	–	3,236	–	3,484	3,562	3,581	–	3,702	–	–
Portugal	712	1,191	759	836	857	904	958	958	820	818	738	745	732	797
Spain	3,664	3,446	3,703	3,785	3,820	3,532	3,946	4,032	4,065	4,458	4,682	5,137	5,722	–
Sweden	7,180	7,060	7,380	7,540	7,813	8,030	8,263	8,533	8,803	8,863	9,338	–	9,293	–
Switzerland	2,582	2,582	2,737	2,728	2,745	2,717	2,841	2,854	2,927	3,038	3,070	3,117	3,110	–
Turkey	4,269	5,046	5,379	5,954	6,826	7,021	7,077	6,790	6,802	–	8,183	8,305	8,410	8,589
United Kingdom	15,449	15,856	16,211	16,583	16,841	17,135	17,457	18,005	18,550	18,996	19,408	19,776	19,909	20,103
United States	112,020	115,000	117,890	120,620	123,500	126,240	129,180	132,010	135,120	137,950	140,770	143,230	–	–

SOURCE: Organization for Economic Cooperation and Development: Health Data File, 1989.

Table 29
First- and second-level nurses, by country: 1960-87

Number of active nurses

Country	1960	1961	1962	1963	1964	1965	1966	1967	1968	1969	1970	1971	1972	1973
Australia	—	—	—	—	—	—	—	—	—	—	—	89,502	—	—
Austria	17,058	17,742	18,730	19,990	19,760	20,829	21,774	22,299	22,543	23,257	24,384	25,062	26,223	27,916
Belgium	—	—	—	—	—	—	—	—	—	—	—	—	—	—
Canada	—	—	—	—	—	—	108,318	115,512	124,049	132,064	135,047	145,683	152,005	159,274
Denmark	—	—	—	—	—	—	—	—	—	—	—	—	—	—
Finland	10,283	12,489	13,499	13,858	14,582	15,884	17,150	17,803	18,472	19,200	19,950	20,875	21,870	22,280
France	—	—	—	—	—	—	—	—	—	—	—	151,441	—	—
Germany	93,332	94,654	96,641	98,231	99,784	103,884	114,526	119,901	125,895	132,290	143,598	156,552	168,619	180,705
Greece	—	—	—	—	—	—	—	14,525	14,649	15,000	16,082	16,622	17,184	18,012
Iceland	424	455	461	476	512	457	490	568	599	626	713	732	766	852
Ireland	—	15,230	—	—	—	—	—	—	—	—	—	19,284	—	—
Italy	48,608	51,735	54,776	58,508	62,165	65,578	69,325	73,874	79,952	88,065	99,839	117,078	125,377	138,123
Japan	171,961	—	191,584	202,314	212,537	226,609	245,478	255,958	271,062	287,752	309,744	325,179	339,456	—
Luxembourg	—	—	—	—	—	—	—	—	—	—	—	—	—	—
Netherlands	—	—	—	—	—	—	—	—	—	—	—	—	—	—
New Zealand	—	—	—	—	—	—	—	—	—	—	—	—	—	—
Norway	—	—	—	—	—	—	—	—	—	—	—	—	—	—
Portugal	6,225	6,582	7,344	7,285	7,647	7,905	8,445	8,887	9,070	9,551	12,989	15,148	14,639	16,428
Spain	—	—	—	—	26,234	26,185	26,304	26,304	26,268	26,415	26,757	27,499	28,543	29,811
Sweden	23,110	23,600	22,030	22,943	23,620	24,950	25,570	27,110	29,630	32,760	34,860	37,160	42,891	46,230
Switzerland	—	—	18,202	—	—	—	22,097	—	—	—	26,235	—	—	30,279
Turkey	8,427	—	—	—	—	13,587	—	—	—	27,822	30,071	31,897	34,840	38,002
United Kingdom	—	—	—	—	—	—	—	—	—	—	—	—	—	—
United States	527,000	—	—	—	—	621,000	—	—	—	—	750,000	—	—	—

Country	1974	1975	1976	1977	1978	1979	1980	1981	1982	1983	1984	1985	1986	1987
Australia	—	—	—	—	—	—	—	139,433	—	—	—	—	173,441	—
Austria	29,629	31,510	34,051	35,505	36,931	37,921	39,221	40,481	41,542	43,342	44,013	45,888	47,387	48,638
Belgium	—	—	—	45,143	—	49,289	—	55,448	—	54,896	—	57,516	—	60,689
Canada	168,530	177,182	179,567	187,062	202,039	192,919	203,849	206,184	214,989	218,344	222,960	229,650	237,181	241,955
Denmark	—	—	22,905	23,615	24,494	25,155	26,002	27,011	28,457	28,918	28,656	29,892	—	30,749
Finland	22,653	23,881	24,918	26,204	26,853	27,833	28,432	29,283	30,113	30,791	31,479	32,823	33,509	34,708
France	—	180,480	188,820	220,348	229,748	238,564	249,450	257,929	271,253	280,745	286,162	294,260	292,015	300,457
Germany	198,182	207,287	213,180	213,180	—	—	248,564	252,058	258,671	267,376	274,677	284,894	—	—
Greece	17,788	19,043	19,737	20,677	21,251	22,694	23,593	18,793	21,164	21,907	22,805	24,499	26,108	26,461
Iceland	915	997	987	1,083	1,215	1,301	1,329	1,427	1,542	1,640	1,708	1,754	1,846	1,890
Ireland	—	19,475	—	—	—	—	—	—	—	—	25,261	—	—	25,000
Italy	151,976	167,296	180,092	187,466	194,366	203,656	211,128	216,335	219,793	219,429	218,193	219,912	221,838	221,820
Japan	—	400,678	—	—	467,355	—	—	551,492	—	—	627,389	—	—	699,698
Luxembourg	—	—	—	—	—	—	—	—	—	—	—	—	—	—
Netherlands	—	—	—	—	—	—	—	—	—	—	—	—	—	—
New Zealand	—	—	17,981	—	—	—	19,195	—	—	23,200	—	—	27,750	—
Norway	30,136	32,106	34,863	40,550	43,948	45,183	—	69,103	—	66,126	—	72,448	—	—
Portugal	18,393	18,593	19,715	20,654	22,273	22,060	22,144	23,751	24,846	25,194	25,349	24,677	25,217	25,777
Spain	32,202	35,548	36,051	81,743	97,110	111,107	125,313	130,373	136,992	130,846	136,690	140,901	147,462	—
Sweden	48,240	49,010	53,590	56,200	55,640	57,560	58,334	59,860	63,972	66,570	71,300	72,386	—	—
Switzerland	34,014	35,952	38,121	38,981	40,597	42,577	45,270	47,755	51,101	50,345	52,107	52,782	53,992	56,691
Turkey	33,348	38,802	41,596	47,917	48,326	51,307	54,424	55,551	—	—	—	30,854	32,392	34,855
United Kingdom	—	—	—	188,000	188,260	192,010	197,900	212,100	219,300	223,620	227,730	234,130	236,770	239,360
United States	—	961,000	981,000	1,028,000	1,075,000	1,119,000	1,272,900	1,316,000	1,357,000	1,404,200	1,485,725	1,531,200	1,592,600	1,627,000

SOURCE: Organization for Economic Cooperation and Development: Health Data File, 1989.

Table 30
Practicing pharmacists, by country: 1960-87

Number of active pharmacists

Country	1960	1961	1962	1963	1964	1965	1966	1967	1968	1969	1970	1971	1972	1973
Australia	–	–	–	–	–	–	–	–	–	–	–	9,466	–	–
Austria	1,720	1,723	1,716	1,714	1,705	1,688	1,689	1,681	1,659	1,658	1,668	1,662	1,657	1,665
Belgium	5,383	5,622	5,714	5,844	5,968	6,078	6,171	6,249	6,533	6,735	–	–	–	–
Canada	–	9,022	9,136	9,310	9,432	9,604	9,863	10,147	10,390	10,587	11,084	11,330	11,629	11,779
Denmark	–	–	–	–	–	–	–	–	–	–	–	–	–	–
Finland	2,758	2,915	2,922	2,937	3,101	3,260	3,340	3,420	3,497	3,592	3,704	3,796	3,814	3,846
France	–	–	–	–	–	–	–	–	–	–	–	25,460	–	27,835
Germany	15,803	16,148	16,468	16,879	17,201	17,725	18,268	18,794	19,669	20,151	20,866	22,551	23,152	24,052
Greece	1,600	1,620	1,660	1,690	1,690	1,760	1,715	1,780	2,000	2,090	2,120	2,250	2,290	2,680
Iceland	–	–	–	46	75	80	85	90	86	95	93	96	98	100
Ireland	–	–	–	–	–	–	–	–	–	–	–	–	–	1,176
Italy	32,923	33,238	33,393	33,945	34,433	35,492	36,636	37,591	39,296	40,380	42,308	44,005	45,702	46,690
Japan	–	–	–	–	–	–	–	–	–	–	–	–	–	–
Luxembourg	171	–	165	174	176	173	170	172	176	172	181	179	183	183
Netherlands	856	856	856	845	947	974	999	1,008	1,008	1,019	1,057	1,084	1,114	1,138
New Zealand	–	–	–	–	–	–	–	–	–	–	–	–	–	–
Norway	–	–	1,246	1,246	1,271	1,273	1,287	1,290	1,299	1,305	1,311	1,339	1,339	1,379
Portugal	2,178	2,266	2,273	2,308	2,334	2,338	2,403	2,458	2,512	6,291	6,571	7,959	7,022	7,494
Spain	11,965	12,174	12,548	12,496	13,139	13,494	13,805	13,858	14,552	15,519	15,963	16,550	16,925	17,498
Sweden	2,210	2,320	2,360	2,470	2,470	2,540	2,640	2,700	2,720	3,000	3,230	3,220	3,400	3,420
Switzerland	1,114	1,118	1,109	1,120	1,122	1,129	1,130	1,127	1,137	1,161	1,140	1,148	1,144	1,150
Turkey	1,390	–	–	–	1,650	1,771	1,933	2,203	2,307	2,546	3,011	3,477	3,981	4,781
United Kingdom	–	–	–	–	–	–	–	–	–	–	–	–	–	–
United States	101,000	–	–	–	–	104,100	–	–	–	–	113,700	–	126,000	–

Country	1974	1975	1976	1977	1978	1979	1980	1981	1982	1983	1984	1985	1986	1987
Australia	–	–	9,876	–	–	–	–	10,189	–	–	–	–	10,637	–
Austria	1,671	1,687	1,704	1,727	1,754	1,744	1,760	1,791	1,815	1,873	1,896	1,912	1,969	2,003
Belgium	6,610	7,688	8,688	8,850	9,187	9,389	9,682	9,942	10,177	10,363	10,608	10,792	11,027	–
Canada	13,267	13,872	14,687	15,322	15,709	16,052	16,588	17,039	17,569	18,460	19,028	18,813	19,410	20,001
Denmark	–	–	1,338	–	1,364	–	1,381	1,344	1,091	–	1,470	–	–	1,476
Finland	3,817	3,884	3,856	3,893	3,894	3,946	3,961	4,052	4,054	4,020	4,006	4,027	4,086	4,160
France	30,059	30,616	30,616	33,510	–	–	–	37,820	39,533	41,113	42,694	43,965	45,521	47,531
Germany	24,787	25,597	25,885	26,811	27,480	27,889	28,674	29,454	29,831	29,536	30,865	32,234	33,025	33,903
Greece	2,710	2,040	3,420	3,600	4,250	4,600	5,170	5,850	5,082	5,384	5,732	5,994	6,261	6,611
Iceland	96	100	119	134	150	144	151	157	160	168	166	178	180	183
Ireland	1,199	1,145	1,146	1,106	1,117	1,110	1,106	1,116	1,115	1,114	1,110	–	–	1,085
Italy	48,362	49,838	51,770	53,985	56,531	60,228	63,765	67,274	69,971	–	74,676	–	78,548	–
Japan	–	–	–	–	–	–	–	–	–	–	–	–	–	–
Luxembourg	174	173	182	192	205	212	223	239	236	246	251	254	262	274
Netherlands	1,116	1,197	1,257	1,309	1,382	1,463	1,529	1,601	1,672	1,728	1,800	1,900	1,991	2,103
New Zealand	–	2,374	–	–	–	2,242	2,277	2,290	–	2,300	–	–	2,499	–
Norway	1,413	1,435	–	1,924	2,308	2,464	2,663	2,820	2,902	3,041	–	–	–	–
Portugal	7,511	7,920	8,527	8,204	8,568	8,888	9,605	10,030	9,519	9,678	10,071	10,023	9,484	10,253
Spain	17,926	18,952	19,253	19,871	20,855	21,986	23,299	24,832	26,274	27,646	28,748	29,969	31,118	–
Sweden	3,630	3,840	3,850	3,900	3,840	3,944	3,972	3,875	3,850	3,900	3,945	4,107	4,234	–
Switzerland	1,145	1,160	1,172	1,197	1,201	1,200	1,217	1,237	1,251	1,302	1,323	1,366	1,389	–
Turkey	4,715	7,002	7,828	10,572	11,280	11,305	11,578	11,610	11,428	–	11,586	11,602	12,866	13,668
United Kingdom	–	–	–	–	–	–	–	–	–	–	–	–	–	–
United States	–	122,480	127,280	132,080	136,670	140,360	144,260	–	–	–	–	–	–	–

Table 31
Mean length-of-stay in days for disease categories, by country: 1980

International Classification of Disease categories	Australia	Austria	Belgium	Canada	Denmark	Finland	France	Germany	Greece	Iceland	Ireland	Italy
Infectious and parasitic diseases (001-139)	5.8	18.2	—	10.5	9.2	12.9	—	17.7	18.0	—	12.4	—
Neoplasms (140-239)	10.7	15.6	—	16.2	11.0	13.5	—	18.9	15.0	—	15.9	—
Endocrine and metabolic diseases (240-279)	12.8	16.1	—	16.9	12.6	14.2	—	22.4	13.0	—	11.7	—
Diseases of the blood (280-289)	8.1	12.5	—	11.1	10.1	11.5	—	17.9	5.0	—	9.2	—
Mental disorders (290-319)	65.3	24.1	—	24.7	13.7	35.7	—	38.1	112.0	—	—	—
Diseases of the nervous system (320-389)	10.7	16.5	—	18.3	9.0	14.5	—	18.5	16.0	—	10.5	—
Diseases of the circulatory system (390-459)	20.4	18.2	—	24.5	15.9	24.6	—	23.5	13.0	—	17.1	—
Diseases of the respiratory system (460-519)	6.9	11.5	—	7.9	8.3	14.6	—	13.7	9.0	—	11.4	—
Diseases of the digestive system (520-579)	6.7	13.2	—	8.4	8.8	9.2	—	17.2	10.0	—	9.3	—
Diseases of the genito-urinary system (580-629)	5.1	9.4	—	7.2	7.0	9.9	—	14.2	10.0	—	7.6	—
Complications of pregnancy and childbirth (630-676)	6.2	7.1	—	4.8	5.3	6.7	—	9.1	5.0	—	—	—
Diseases of the skin and subcutaneous tissue (680-709)	6.9	11.9	—	9.5	9.5	11.1	—	20.5	9.0	—	8.1	—
Diseases of musculo-skeletal system and connective tissue (710-739)	9.6	16.9	—	12.5	14.5	14.2	—	23.4	14.0	—	15.5	—
Congenital anomalies (740-759)	16.0	—	—	10.2	7.2	8.7	—	16.1	11.0	—	9.9	—
Certain causes of perinatal morbidity and mortality (760-779)	10.6	15.7	—	14.9	9.9	10.1	—	19.9	12.0	—	—	—
Symptoms of ill-defined conditions (780-799)	7.2	—	—	9.4	7.0	9.5	—	16.4	7.0	—	7.7	—
Accidents, poisoning, and violence (800-999)	7.9	11.9	—	10.6	9.5	13.2	—	17.8	9.0	—	8.2	—
All other	5.0	14.5	—	11.5	5.0	5.2	—	—	7.0	—	7.7	—
All categories (001-999)	11.1	13.9	—	12.0	9.4	13.9	—	18.4	14.0	—	10.2	—

International Classification of Disease categories	Japan	Luxem-bourg	Nether-lands	New Zealand	Norway	Portugal	Spain	Sweden	Switzer-land	Turkey	United Kingdom	United States
Infectious and parasitic diseases (001-139)	117.6	—	18.2	—	—	33.7	21.0	11.5	13.9	16.8	9.6	6.9
Neoplasms (140-239)	51.7	—	18.5	—	—	27.3	17.0	15.4	18.4	13.6	12.2	10.5
Endocrine and metabolic diseases (240-279)	51.9	—	19.7	—	—	26.4	15.0	19.8	20.4	9.8	16.5	9.6
Diseases of the blood (280-289)	41.7	—	17.4	—	—	22.1	14.0	14.4	13.8	8.7	12.6	7.2
Mental disorders (290-319)	333.3	—	35.6	—	—	18.7	195.0	74.3	18.9	58.1	50.3	11.6
Diseases of the nervous system (320-389)	86.4	—	11.2	—	13.4	18.4	26.0	25.2	16.5	9.9	14.8	5.4
Diseases of the circulatory system (390-459)	100.4	—	17.5	—	8.4	23.7	16.0	37.4	22.7	9.7	24.5	10.0
Diseases of the respiratory system (460-519)	25.6	—	8.6	—	8.3	14.4	10.0	15.6	11.6	7.3	12.3	6.3
Diseases of the digestive system (520-579)	32.6	—	15.1	—	6.1	24.0	12.0	9.7	13.1	7.2	8.0	7.0
Diseases of the genito-urinary system (580-629)	31.0	—	10.2	—	7.3	20.3	9.0	9.0	10.8	8.4	6.3	7.0
Complications of pregnancy and childbirth (630-676)	8.7	—	8.8	—	—	5.3	4.0	5.9	9.1	2.7	2.9	5.6
Diseases of the skin and subcutaneous tissue (680-709)	22.6	—	18.0	—	14.2	36.5	11.0	14.5	13.3	8.8	12.5	2.5
Diseases of musculo-skeletal system and connective tissue (710-739)	72.6	—	14.9	—	12.5	42.9	15.0	20.2	17.0	13.3	17.7	8.0
Congenital anomalies (740-759)	37.7	—	11.5	—	—	22.5	14.0	8.7	11.8	12.2	9.0	8.3
Certain causes of perinatal morbidity and mortality (760-779)	12.5	—	15.1	—	9.4	18.0	13.0	10.6	13.3	4.6	8.8	6.6
Symptoms of ill-defined conditions (780-799)	17.5	—	12.7	—	—	17.1	10.0	8.4	10.6	7.4	10.3	8.7
Accidents, poisoning, and violence (800-999)	37.5	—	17.0	—	9.4	22.1	11.0	14.2	13.6	7.9	10.3	4.5
All other	0.9	—	7.6	—	—	—	11.0	7.2	8.3	—	7.7	3.7
All categories (001-999)	55.1	—	13.5	—	9.2	21.6	16.0	17.0	14.9	9.0	12.4	7.3

SOURCE: Organization for Economic Cooperation and Development: Health Data File, 1989.

Table 32

Mean length-of-stay in days for disease categories, by country: 1981

International Classification of Disease categories	Australia	Austria	Belgium	Canada	Denmark	Finland	France	Germany	Greece	Iceland	Ireland	Italy
Infectious and parasitic diseases (001-139)	4.7	18.5	—	9.8	8.5	13.1	—	—	23.0	—	12.5	—
Neoplasms (140-239)	10.4	15.3	—	16.1	10.9	13.0	—	—	14.0	—	14.9	—
Endocrine and metabolic diseases (240-279)	13.6	16.2	—	17.3	12.1	16.6	—	—	13.0	—	11.6	—
Diseases of the blood (280-289)	7.4	12.2	—	11.1	10.1	12.7	—	—	5.0	—	9.4	—
Mental disorders (290-319)	66.0	23.5	—	28.6	13.8	30.4	—	—	109.0	—	—	—
Diseases of the nervous system (320-389)	11.7	16.0	—	19.3	9.0	13.8	—	—	16.0	—	9.3	—
Diseases of the circulatory system (390-459)	20.5	17.9	—	25.0	15.4	23.4	—	—	13.0	—	16.3	—
Diseases of the respiratory system (460-519)	7.2	11.6	—	7.9	8.2	15.1	—	—	9.0	—	10.7	—
Diseases of the digestive system (520-579)	6.6	13.0	—	8.3	8.5	9.8	—	—	10.0	—	8.7	—
Diseases of the genito-urinary system (580-629)	4.9	9.6	—	7.0	6.7	8.4	—	—	9.0	—	7.1	—
Complications of pregnancy and childbirth (630-676)	6.0	7.0	—	4.8	5.2	7.3	—	—	5.0	—	—	—
Diseases of the skin and subcutaneous tissue (680-709)	7.0	12.0	—	9.6	9.8	11.2	—	—	10.0	—	7.4	—
Diseases of musculo-skeletal system and connective tissue (710-739)	7.0	16.6	—	12.7	14.2	13.5	—	—	14.0	—	13.4	—
Congenital anomalies (740-759)	10.3	—	—	10.7	7.1	11.2	—	—	11.0	—	10.2	—
Certain causes of perinatal morbidity and mortality (760-779)	13.9	15.6	—	13.5	10.0	9.9	—	—	11.0	—	—	—
Symptoms of ill-defined conditions (780-799)	8.8	—	—	9.9	7.1	9.0	—	—	7.0	—	6.2	—
Accidents, poisoning, and violence (800-999)	5.8	11.8	—	10.7	9.2	14.7	—	—	9.0	—	7.3	—
All other	7.9	14.6	—	12.1	5.0	6.5	—	—	—	—	—	—
All categories (001-999)	11.0	13.8	—	12.3	9.1	13.8	—	—	13.0	—	9.6	—

International Classification of Disease categories	Japan	Luxem-bourg	Nether-lands	New Zealand	Norway	Portugal	Spain	Sweden	Switzer-land	Turkey	United Kingdom	United States
Infectious and parasitic diseases (001-139)	95.5	—	17.3	7.7	—	24.1	26.0	11.1	14.9	—	9.3	7.0
Neoplasms (140-239)	50.4	—	17.6	13.6	—	20.4	16.0	14.0	18.2	—	12.2	10.3
Endocrine and metabolic diseases (240-279)	57.7	—	19.4	21.3	—	21.1	14.2	13.5	21.6	—	15.6	9.1
Diseases of the blood (280-289)	34.2	—	16.3	10.4	—	17.3	11.9	13.5	17.9	—	11.3	7.1
Mental disorders (290-319)	318.8	—	36.3	42.1	—	13.1	164.9	99.1	19.4	—	44.4	12.0
Diseases of the nervous system (320-389)	57.9	—	11.2	16.7	—	15.1	26.3	26.8	15.9	—	14.7	5.4
Diseases of the circulatory system (390-459)	78.5	—	16.8	30.9	—	18.9	15.6	40.6	21.9	—	23.0	9.6
Diseases of the respiratory system (460-519)	26.2	—	8.7	7.7	—	9.8	9.6	17.6	13.7	—	12.2	6.5
Diseases of the digestive system (520-579)	30.8	—	14.7	7.4	—	17.5	12.0	9.7	13.2	—	8.0	7.0
Diseases of the genito-urinary system (580-629)	31.0	—	9.9	5.9	—	15.6	9.3	8.8	10.2	—	6.2	5.6
Complications of pregnancy and childbirth (630-676)	8.5	—	8.2	5.9	6.7	5.1	4.4	5.8	8.9	—	3.1	2.5
Diseases of the skin and subcutaneous tissue (680-709)	19.5	—	17.7	7.8	10.2	23.2	10.1	15.3	13.5	—	12.7	7.9
Diseases of musculo-skeletal system and connective tissue (710-739)	61.4	—	14.2	15.3	—	31.3	15.8	18.9	17.6	—	16.9	7.9
Congenital anomalies (740-759)	28.0	—	10.7	9.3	6.6	17.1	12.1	8.1	12.5	—	9.3	5.9
Certain causes of perinatal morbidity and mortality (760-779)	16.8	—	13.8	10.2	10.2	14.2	12.7	10.9	13.0	—	9.0	11.8
Symptoms of ill-defined conditions (780-799)	14.0	—	12.2	15.1	—	21.2	9.6	9.4	10.7	—	9.8	4.2
Accidents, poisoning, and violence (800-999)	38.0	—	16.3	10.3	—	17.7	11.8	15.1	13.7	—	9.9	7.5
All other	3.4	—	7.0	5.4	—	—	9.9	7.5	8.0	—	8.1	3.7
All categories (001-999)	49.0	—	13.1	12.6	—	16.3	14.8	18.2	15.1	—	12.0	7.2

SOURCE: Organization for Economic Cooperation and Development: Health Data File, 1989.

Table 33
Mean length-of-stay for disease categories, by country: 1982

International Classification of Disease categories	Australia	Austria	Belgium	Canada	Denmark	Finland	France	Germany	Greece	Iceland	Ireland	Italy
Infectious and parasitic diseases (001-139)	—	17.8	—	10.0	8.1	14.3	14.5	16.4	22.0	—	10.9	16.5
Neoplasms (140-239)	—	14.5	—	15.8	10.0	19.0	13.0	17.4	14.0	—	14.4	15.0
Endocrine and metabolic diseases (240-279)	—	15.7	—	16.0	11.5	16.1	13.7	21.2	12.0	—	11.3	14.3
Diseases of the blood (280-289)	—	12.5	—	10.9	9.6	13.5	13.4	17.2	5.0	—	9.7	11.1
Mental disorders (290-319)	—	22.5	—	26.9	12.9	32.3	15.7	36.7	109.0	—	—	47.8
Diseases of the nervous system (320-389)	—	15.6	—	17.9	8.7	14.4	12.2	17.1	15.0	—	8.9	16.2
Diseases of the circulatory system (390-459)	—	17.5	—	23.3	14.7	23.1	14.2	22.3	9.0	—	14.6	14.9
Diseases of the respiratory system (460-519)	—	11.1	—	7.9	8.0	12.7	10.6	13.4	10.0	—	11.1	10.5
Diseases of the digestive system (520-579)	—	12.9	—	8.1	8.2	8.5	12.4	16.8	10.0	—	8.1	11.8
Diseases of the genito-urinary system (580-629)	—	9.3	—	7.1	6.5	7.1	9.8	13.6	10.0	—	7.0	10.0
Complications of pregnancy and childbirth (630-676)	—	7.0	—	4.7	5.0	6.6	7.2	7.5	5.0	—	—	5.9
Diseases of the skin and subcutaneous tissue (680-709)	—	11.7	—	9.7	9.3	10.2	10.9	18.8	9.0	—	7.7	9.2
Diseases of musculo-skeletal system and connective tissue (710-739)	—	16.1	—	12.5	13.3	14.7	14.8	22.4	14.0	—	11.8	12.6
Congenital anomalies (740-759)	—	—	—	10.0	6.9	9.4	11.9	14.8	10.0	—	9.7	8.7
Certain causes of perinatal morbidity and mortality (760-779)	—	15.0	—	13.3	10.2	9.7	15.9	19.9	10.0	—	—	10.2
Symptoms of ill-defined conditions (780-799)	—	—	—	9.2	7.0	9.6	8.6	16.1	6.0	—	5.9	8.8
Accidents, poisoning, and violence (800-999)	—	11.4	—	10.5	9.1	14.9	7.7	16.9	8.0	—	7.3	7.0
All other	—	14.4	—	11.8	4.5	6.0	7.8	—	—	—	—	6.8
All categories (001-999)	—	13.5	—	11.8	8.8	13.5	11.3	17.6	15.0	—	10.2	12.1

International Classification of Disease categories	Japan	Luxem-bourg	Nether-lands	New Zealand	Norway	Portugal	Spain	Sweden	Switzer-land	Turkey	United Kingdom	United States
Infectious and parasitic diseases (001-139)	65.9	—	16.9	6.8	—	23.4	21.4	9.3	15.4	—	8.6	6.7
Neoplasms (140-239)	53.1	—	17.0	14.4	—	23.5	15.1	14.2	17.9	—	11.9	9.9
Endocrine and metabolic diseases (240-279)	59.4	—	18.8	17.9	—	21.5	14.9	22.2	21.0	—	18.1	8.8
Diseases of the blood (280-289)	40.4	—	14.9	8.8	—	19.7	12.4	13.1	14.1	—	11.5	7.0
Mental disorders (290-319)	331.6	—	34.9	47.9	—	28.9	124.0	103.2	19.2	—	48.1	12.1
Diseases of the nervous system (320-389)	54.7	—	10.7	18.9	—	13.8	22.8	27.8	14.9	—	15.6	5.4
Diseases of the circulatory system (390-459)	82.2	—	16.2	30.9	—	18.5	14.8	39.4	21.1	—	22.8	9.4
Diseases of the respiratory system (460-519)	27.3	—	8.8	8.0	—	11.6	9.6	17.3	14.3	—	12.0	6.2
Diseases of the digestive system (520-579)	34.9	—	14.1	7.2	—	17.7	11.6	9.1	12.7	—	7.7	6.8
Diseases of the genito-urinary system (580-629)	34.4	—	9.5	5.8	—	15.8	9.4	8.7	10.2	—	6.1	5.6
Complications of pregnancy and childbirth (630-676)	8.8	—	7.9	5.6	—	5.3	4.4	5.7	8.5	—	2.7	2.5
Diseases of the skin and subcutaneous tissue (680-709)	23.7	—	17.2	7.5	—	23.7	10.2	15.1	13.3	—	13.2	8.3
Diseases of musculo-skeletal system and connective tissue (710-739)	59.1	—	13.7	14.7	—	29.2	14.6	18.8	16.8	—	16.2	7.7
Congenital anomalies (740-759)	30.5	—	10.2	8.6	—	16.0	11.9	7.4	12.1	—	8.6	6.1
Certain causes of perinatal morbidity and mortality (760-779)	15.5	—	12.9	10.2	—	6.6	12.0	13.2	13.3	—	9.8	12.7
Symptoms of ill-defined conditions (780-799)	18.8	—	11.5	16.4	—	14.6	9.2	9.8	9.9	—	9.3	4.1
Accidents, poisoning, and violence (800-999)	38.1	—	16.0	10.2	—	16.9	11.1	15.5	13.1	—	9.9	7.4
All other	3.0	—	6.6	5.8	—	—	9.6	—	13.1	—	9.3	3.6
All categories (001-999)	50.0	—	12.8	12.3	—	16.5	13.5	18.3	14.6	—	12.0	7.1

SOURCE: Organization for Economic Cooperation and Development: Health Data File, 1989.

Table 34

Mean length-of-stay in days for disease categories, by country: 1983

International Classification of Disease categories	Australia	Austria	Belgium	Canada	Denmark	Finland	France	Germany	Greece	Iceland	Ireland	Italy
Infectious and parasitic diseases (001-139)	—	17.2	—	9.3	7.5	14.4	14.4	15.9	12.0	6.8	9.8	—
Neoplasms (140-239)	—	13.7	—	15.5	9.5	12.4	12.5	17.1	12.0	9.7	11.2	—
Endocrine and metabolic diseases (240-279)	—	15.3	—	14.7	10.5	15.4	13.1	21.0	12.0	11.4	10.4	—
Diseases of the blood (280-289)	—	12.0	—	11.1	8.8	9.6	12.4	17.1	5.0	7.5	9.4	—
Mental disorders (290-319)	—	22.1	—	26.6	13.3	34.9	15.6	36.4	100.0	7.5	—	—
Diseases of the nervous system (320-389)	—	14.9	—	16.5	8.3	16.1	11.6	16.6	13.0	9.6	8.6	—
Diseases of the circulatory system (390-459)	—	17.1	—	20.1	14.4	23.4	14.0	22.0	9.0	10.2	14.8	—
Diseases of the respiratory system (460-519)	—	11.0	—	7.7	7.8	14.3	10.1	13.2	10.0	8.1	10.4	—
Diseases of the digestive system (520-579)	—	12.6	—	8.1	7.8	9.8	12.0	16.5	9.0	9.2	7.8	—
Diseases of the genito-urinary system (580-629)	—	9.0	—	7.0	6.2	8.2	9.5	13.5	9.0	5.2	6.6	—
Complications of pregnancy and childbirth (630-676)	—	6.9	—	4.7	5.0	6.9	7.1	7.4	5.0	6.1	—	—
Diseases of the skin and subcutaneous tissue (680-709)	—	11.3	—	9.8	9.3	12.7	9.5	18.5	9.0	11.1	7.3	—
Diseases of musculo-skeletal system and connective tissue (710-739)	—	16.1	—	11.7	12.8	14.0	14.1	22.3	14.0	11.4	11.2	—
Congenital anomalies (740-759)	—	—	—	10.4	6.5	8.4	11.3	14.3	9.0	7.4	9.7	—
Certain causes of perinatal morbidity and mortality (760-779)	—	14.2	—	14.3	10.2	10.2	16.0	19.2	9.0	4.7	—	—
Symptoms of ill-defined conditions (780-799)	—	—	—	7.9	6.5	10.0	8.2	15.8	7.0	6.2	5.9	—
Accidents, poisoning, and violence (800-999)	—	11.1	—	10.6	8.9	14.9	7.7	16.6	9.0	7.7	7.0	—
All other	—	14.3	—	11.8	4.3	5.2	8.1	—	—	3.5	5.3	—
All categories (001-999)	—	13.2	—	11.3	8.6	13.9	10.9	17.4	12.0	8.0	9.0	—

International Classification of Disease categories	Japan	Luxem-bourg	Nether-lands	New Zealand	Norway	Portugal	Spain	Sweden	Switzer-land	Turkey	United Kingdom	United States
Infectious and parasitic diseases (001-139)	58.1	—	15.6	7.3	—	13.4	18.0	10.1	15.6	—	8.8	6.6
Neoplasms (140-239)	51.4	—	16.4	13.1	—	18.6	14.9	14.1	17.4	—	11.4	9.6
Endocrine and metabolic diseases (240-279)	51.4	—	18.1	20.5	—	19.0	14.9	22.1	15.9	—	16.1	8.7
Diseases of the blood (280-289)	41.6	—	14.3	8.5	—	20.7	12.0	13.0	14.2	—	10.4	6.7
Mental disorders (290-319)	308.8	—	36.1	51.9	—	27.6	135.8	111.3	19.9	—	47.8	12.4
Diseases of the nervous system (320-389)	44.0	—	10.6	18.6	—	13.7	16.5	27.9	15.0	—	14.8	5.0
Diseases of the circulatory system (390-459)	82.7	—	15.5	31.5	—	18.2	14.6	37.3	20.5	—	21.9	9.1
Diseases of the respiratory system (460-519)	27.4	—	9.1	7.8	—	9.0	9.6	17.8	13.6	—	11.8	6.2
Diseases of the digestive system (520-579)	31.4	—	13.6	7.2	—	15.7	11.5	9.3	12.6	—	7.5	6.6
Diseases of the genito-urinary system (580-629)	30.8	—	9.3	5.5	—	12.3	9.8	8.5	10.4	—	5.8	5.6
Complications of pregnancy and childbirth (630-676)	8.8	—	7.6	5.8	—	5.3	4.5	5.6	8.1	—	2.6	2.5
Diseases of the skin and subcutaneous tissue (680-709)	20.6	—	16.5	7.5	—	20.5	9.8	15.6	13.2	—	11.8	8.1
Diseases of musculo-skeletal system and connective tissue (710-739)	61.9	—	13.1	15.3	—	25.5	13.7	18.1	16.4	—	14.6	7.3
Congenital anomalies (740-759)	29.6	—	10.2	8.7	—	15.7	12.5	7.7	11.3	—	8.0	5.9
Certain causes of perinatal morbidity and mortality (760-779)	15.2	—	11.9	9.6	—	8.3	11.3	11.6	12.9	—	9.8	12.8
Symptoms of ill-defined conditions (780-799)	15.8	—	11.1	16.4	—	11.4	9.9	9.8	9.1	—	9.1	4.2
Accidents, poisoning, and violence (800-999)	38.0	—	15.4	9.8	—	15.0	11.4	15.8	13.2	—	9.5	7.2
All other	2.7	—	6.6	6.9	—	—	9.2	—	13.2	—	8.5	3.5
All categories (001-999)	49.1	—	12.5	12.4	—	14.3	13.6	18.3	14.3	—	11.5	6.9

SOURCE: Organization for Economic Cooperation and Development: Health Data File, 1989.

162

Table 35
Mean length-of-stay in days for disease categories, by country: 1984

International Classification of Disease categories	Australia	Austria	Belgium	Canada	Denmark	Finland	France	Germany	Greece	Iceland	Ireland	Italy
Infectious and parasitic diseases (001-139)	4.4	16.3	—	9.4	7.2	13.1	14.2	17.4	11.0	—	9.4	—
Neoplasms (140-239)	9.2	13.3	—	15.6	9.3	13.3	12.1	16.7	13.0	—	13.1	—
Endocrine and metabolic diseases (240-279)	11.0	15.0	—	14.6	10.5	14.6	12.5	20.6	11.0	—	9.9	—
Diseases of the blood (280-289)	5.3	11.4	—	13.7	9.1	9.9	11.5	17.1	5.0	—	8.5	—
Mental disorders (290-319)	61.6	22.2	—	23.1	12.3	48.6	15.6	34.6	92.0	—	—	—
Diseases of the nervous system (320-389)	8.1	14.7	—	16.7	8.0	17.6	11.0	16.2	13.0	—	7.6	—
Diseases of the circulatory system (390-459)	14.2	16.6	—	20.7	13.6	24.3	13.5	21.7	9.0	—	12.9	—
Diseases of the respiratory system (460-519)	6.1	10.8	—	8.0	7.8	15.3	10.1	13.1	10.0	—	11.0	—
Diseases of the digestive system (520-579)	5.9	12.3	—	8.0	7.4	9.5	11.4	16.1	9.0	—	7.4	—
Diseases of the genito-urinary system (580-629)	4.5	8.7	—	7.0	6.1	7.5	8.6	13.3	9.0	—	6.4	—
Complications of pregnancy and childbirth (630-676)	5.5	6.9	—	4.6	4.8	6.8	6.8	7.5	5.0	—	—	—
Diseases of the skin and subcutaneous tissue (680-709)	6.7	10.9	—	9.9	8.8	11.1	9.8	18.6	9.0	—	7.0	—
Diseases of musculo-skeletal system and connective tissue (710-739)	8.0	15.8	—	11.5	12.3	13.3	13.2	21.9	14.0	—	10.0	—
Congenital anomalies (740-759)	16.0	—	—	9.7	6.3	7.9	11.1	13.7	9.0	—	8.6	—
Certain causes of perinatal morbidity and mortality (760-779)	9.7	13.7	—	13.8	10.7	12.9	15.1	20.9	9.0	—	9.6	—
Symptoms of ill-defined conditions (780-799)	4.7	—	—	7.9	6.4	9.8	8.0	16.1	6.0	—	5.6	—
Accidents, poisoning, and violence (800-999)	8.0	11.2	—	10.7	8.5	16.0	7.8	16.5	8.0	—	6.6	—
All other	2.5	14.0	—	11.3	4.3	5.6	8.2	—	—	—	6.8	—
All categories (001-999)	9.4	12.9	—	11.4	8.3	14.5	10.6	17.2	12.0	—	8.6	—

International Classification of Disease categories	Japan	Luxembourg	Netherlands	New Zealand	Norway	Portugal	Spain	Sweden	Switzerland	Turkey	United Kingdom	United States
Infectious and parasitic diseases (001-139)	47.5	—	—	8.3	—	10.3	20.6	—	13.9	—	7.7	6.6
Neoplasms (140-239)	53.2	—	—	12.7	—	15.7	14.9	—	17.0	—	11.2	9.0
Endocrine and metabolic diseases (240-279)	61.1	—	—	20.4	—	15.9	14.1	—	20.4	—	15.9	7.6
Diseases of the blood (280-289)	42.7	—	—	9.4	—	15.6	12.8	—	12.8	—	9.9	6.2
Mental disorders (290-319)	305.4	—	—	50.1	—	18.8	156.9	—	18.0	—	46.6	11.9
Diseases of the nervous system (320-389)	45.6	—	—	18.0	—	10.8	21.3	—	14.8	—	14.3	4.8
Diseases of the circulatory system (390-459)	84.2	—	—	29.5	—	15.4	14.9	—	20.6	—	19.9	8.2
Diseases of the respiratory system (460-519)	23.4	—	—	8.0	—	7.9	9.6	—	13.2	—	11.5	6.0
Diseases of the digestive system (520-579)	33.0	—	—	6.9	—	13.0	11.3	—	12.2	—	7.3	6.3
Diseases of the genito-urinary system (580-629)	25.4	—	—	5.4	—	10.9	9.5	—	10.0	—	5.6	5.4
Complications of pregnancy and childbirth (630-676)	10.2	—	7.2	5.7	—	4.3	4.4	—	7.9	—	2.5	2.6
Diseases of the skin and subcutaneous tissue (680-709)	21.9	—	—	6.9	—	17.6	19.2	—	13.8	—	12.4	8.0
Diseases of musculo-skeletal system and connective tissue (710-739)	71.4	—	—	14.1	—	22.7	14.9	—	16.3	—	15.0	7.0
Congenital anomalies (740-759)	33.9	—	—	8.2	—	14.3	11.6	—	11.2	—	7.3	6.0
Certain causes of perinatal morbidity and mortality (760-779)	12.7	—	—	9.8	—	6.9	10.3	—	13.1	—	10.6	12.2
Symptoms of ill-defined conditions (780-799)	16.4	—	—	10.1	—	10.5	9.6	—	8.9	—	9.4	4.1
Accidents, poisoning, and violence (800-999)	37.2	—	—	10.4	—	12.1	11.0	—	13.1	—	9.1	6.8
All other	6.3	—	—	7.2	—	—	9.1	—	8.2	—	8.4	3.4
All categories (001-999)	40.9	—	—	12.0	—	12.1	14.4	—	14.6	—	11.2	6.6

SOURCE: Organization for Economic Cooperation and Development: Health Data File, 1989.

Table 36
Mean length-of-stay in days for disease categories, by country: 1985

International Classification of Disease categories	Australia	Austria	Belgium	Canada	Denmark	Finland	France	Germany	Greece	Iceland	Ireland	Italy
Infectious and parasitic diseases (001-139)	–	15.7	–	–	7.3	11.3	9.7	17.9	9.0	–	10.3	–
Neoplasms (140-239)	–	12.8	–	–	9.0	11.8	12.1	16.2	12.0	–	13.4	–
Endocrine and metabolic diseases (240-279)	–	14.9	–	–	10.0	14.1	11.5	20.3	11.0	–	10.1	–
Diseases of the blood (280-289)	–	10.6	–	–	8.8	9.0	9.0	16.3	4.0	–	8.9	–
Mental disorders (290-319)	–	21.4	–	–	11.2	48.7	9.8	35.6	97.0	–	–	–
Diseases of the nervous system (320-389)	–	14.3	–	–	7.9	13.7	10.5	16.0	11.0	–	7.6	–
Diseases of the circulatory system (390-459)	–	15.8	–	–	13.2	23.3	12.7	21.1	8.0	–	13.6	–
Diseases of the respiratory system (460-519)	–	10.8	–	–	7.8	14.7	9.5	13.2	9.0	–	9.9	–
Diseases of the digestive system (520-579)	–	11.9	–	–	7.2	8.3	9.6	15.5	9.0	–	7.1	–
Diseases of the genito-urinary system (580-629)	–	8.1	–	–	5.9	7.2	7.4	13.2	9.0	–	6.1	–
Complications of pregnancy and childbirth (630-676)	–	6.8	–	–	4.8	6.4	6.9	7.4	5.0	–	–	–
Diseases of the skin and subcutaneous tissue (680-709)	–	10.1	–	–	8.7	10.9	10.4	18.5	9.0	–	7.1	–
Diseases of musculo-skeletal system and connective tissue (710-739)	–	15.1	–	–	12.0	11.1	10.6	21.4	14.0	–	9.7	–
Congenital anomalies (740-759)	–	–	–	–	6.0	7.8	8.0	14.3	9.0	–	8.4	–
Certain causes of perinatal morbidity and mortality (760-779)	–	13.4	–	–	10.7	10.5	13.7	20.4	9.0	–	11.7	–
Symptoms of ill-defined conditions (780-799)	–	–	–	–	6.4	9.2	7.1	15.7	6.0	–	5.4	–
Accidents, poisoning, and violence (800-999)	–	10.7	–	–	8.7	12.9	7.0	16.2	8.0	–	6.3	–
All other	–	13.6	–	–	4.2	5.5	5.8	–	–	–	6.3	–
All categories (001-999)	–	12.5	–	–	8.1	13.3	9.1	17.0	12.0	–	8.4	–

International Classification of Disease categories	Japan	Luxem-bourg	Nether-lands	New Zealand	Norway	Portugal	Spain	Sweden	Switzer-land	Turkey	United Kingdom	United States
Infectious and parasitic diseases (001-139)	–	–	14.7	7.0	–	13.0	15.0	9.7	13.0	–	7.4	7.0
Neoplasms (140-239)	–	–	15.6	12.0	–	14.8	14.7	13.6	16.7	–	10.6	8.2
Endocrine and metabolic diseases (240-279)	–	–	17.0	21.0	–	15.3	14.0	21.0	20.4	–	15.6	7.3
Diseases of the blood (280-289)	–	–	13.0	7.9	–	14.8	11.6	13.0	12.1	–	10.1	6.0
Mental disorders (290-319)	–	–	35.1	63.9	–	25.5	146.0	86.1	20.0	–	44.9	12.3
Diseases of the nervous system (320-389)	–	–	10.3	19.2	–	10.5	16.4	26.5	14.7	–	13.3	5.4
Diseases of the circulatory system (390-459)	–	–	14.6	32.0	–	13.7	14.6	37.1	19.7	–	19.6	7.9
Diseases of the respiratory system (460-519)	–	–	10.1	8.8	–	8.1	9.8	18.4	13.1	–	11.1	6.0
Diseases of the digestive system (520-579)	–	–	12.6	6.6	–	12.5	11.0	9.3	12.1	–	7.1	6.2
Diseases of the genito-urinary system (580-629)	–	–	9.2	5.3	–	10.2	9.3	8.1	9.6	–	5.3	5.2
Complications of pregnancy and childbirth (630-676)	–	–	7.0	5.5	–	4.6	4.5	5.3	7.8	–	2.4	2.5
Diseases of the skin and subcutaneous tissue (680-709)	–	–	15.9	8.0	–	15.2	9.7	15.4	13.3	–	12.3	7.9
Diseases of musculo-skeletal system and connective tissue (710-739)	–	–	12.2	15.0	–	20.5	13.6	18.2	16.5	–	13.3	6.7
Congenital anomalies (740-759)	–	–	9.4	8.2	–	13.7	11.3	7.8	10.8	–	7.5	5.6
Certain causes of perinatal morbidity and mortality (760-779)	–	–	11.2	10.1	–	6.3	10.6	12.2	13.2	–	10.8	13.0
Symptoms of ill-defined conditions (780-799)	–	–	10.5	13.0	–	10.0	9.2	10.5	8.8	–	8.5	3.8
Accidents, poisoning, and violence (800-999)	–	–	14.7	9.8	–	11.6	11.0	15.5	13.5	–	9.2	6.6
All other	–	–	6.3	7.3	–	–	8.8	–	8.2	–	8.0	3.3
All categories (001-999)	–	–	12.0	12.7	–	11.9	13.6	22.6	14.5	–	10.7	6.5

SOURCE: Organization for Economic Cooperation and Development: Health Data File, 1989.

Table 37

Mean length-of-stay in days for disease categories, by country: 1986

International Classification of Disease categories	Australia	Austria	Belgium	Canada	Denmark	Finland	France	Germany	Greece	Iceland	Ireland	Italy
Infectious and parasitic diseases (001-139)	4.5	15.6	—	—	6.8	11.2	13.1	—	10.0	—	8.6	—
Neoplasms (140-239)	8.5	12.4	—	—	8.6	11.6	11.3	—	11.0	—	11.8	—
Endocrine and metabolic diseases (240-279)	9.3	14.5	—	—	10.2	15.3	12.3	—	10.0	—	8.9	—
Diseases of the blood (280-289)	5.0	12.3	—	—	8.4	9.6	10.8	—	4.0	—	8.6	—
Mental disorders (290-319)	63.7	23.5	—	—	11.1	48.2	16.3	—	112.0	—	—	—
Diseases of the nervous system (320-389)	5.8	14.8	—	—	7.3	13.6	11.1	—	11.0	—	7.1	—
Diseases of the circulatory system (390-459)	11.8	15.3	—	—	12.5	22.2	12.9	—	7.0	—	13.0	—
Diseases of the respiratory system (460-519)	5.6	10.2	—	—	7.5	14.4	10.3	—	9.0	—	9.0	—
Diseases of the digestive system (520-579)	5.0	11.6	—	—	6.9	8.2	10.6	—	8.0	—	6.8	—
Diseases of the genito-urinary system (580-629)	4.1	7.8	—	—	5.6	7.5	7.7	—	8.0	—	6.0	—
Complications of pregnancy and childbirth (630-676)	5.2	6.8	—	—	4.7	6.0	6.6	—	5.0	—	—	—
Diseases of the skin and subcutaneous tissue (680-709)	7.0	9.7	—	—	8.7	9.9	9.6	—	8.0	—	6.4	—
Diseases of musculo-skeletal system and connective tissue (710-739)	7.3	14.6	—	—	11.9	11.5	12.7	—	13.0	—	9.3	—
Congenital anomalies (740-759)	11.5	—	—	—	5.6	7.5	10.4	—	9.0	—	8.0	—
Certain causes of perinatal morbidity and mortality (760-779)	9.9	13.0	—	—	10.5	9.3	14.6	—	9.0	—	11.7	—
Symptoms of ill-defined conditions (780-799)	4.7	—	—	—	6.3	7.6	7.6	—	5.0	—	5.0	—
Accidents, poisoning, and violence (800-999)	6.9	10.6	—	—	8.5	11.5	8.2	—	8.0	—	5.9	—
All other	4.0	13.3	—	—	4.2	4.3	7.7	—	—	—	6.0	—
All categories (001-999)	7.3	12.2	—	—	7.8	12.9	10.2	—	12.0	—	7.9	—

International Classification of Disease categories	Japan	Luxembourg	Netherlands	New Zealand	Norway	Portugal	Spain	Sweden	Switzerland	Turkey	United Kingdom	United States
Infectious and parasitic diseases (001-139)	—	—	14.3	—	7.7	12.2	14.7	9.6	12.5	—	—	7.0
Neoplasms (140-239)	—	—	15.4	—	10.4	17.4	14.6	12.9	16.6	—	—	8.4
Endocrine and metabolic diseases (240-279)	—	—	16.4	—	8.6	14.5	14.2	20.0	19.8	—	—	7.2
Diseases of the blood (280-289)	—	—	13.1	—	7.1	14.1	11.8	12.1	12.2	—	—	5.8
Mental disorders (290-319)	—	—	35.5	—	23.8	27.0	129.5	72.1	19.2	—	—	12.3
Diseases of the nervous system (320-389)	—	—	10.2	—	7.6	9.1	14.8	24.5	14.3	—	—	5.6
Diseases of the circulatory system (390-459)	—	—	14.5	—	11.0	12.2	13.6	33.3	20.1	—	—	7.5
Diseases of the respiratory system (460-519)	—	—	10.0	—	7.6	8.0	9.9	18.3	12.8	—	—	6.0
Diseases of the digestive system (520-579)	—	—	12.2	—	7.1	12.2	10.8	8.8	12.1	—	—	6.1
Diseases of the genito-urinary system (580-629)	—	—	9.0	—	5.2	8.5	9.0	8.0	9.5	—	—	5.2
Complications of pregnancy and childbirth (630-676)	—	—	0.7	—	5.4	4.6	4.5	5.1	7.8	—	—	2.5
Diseases of the skin and subcutaneous tissue (680-709)	—	—	15.2	—	11.2	17.1	10.2	14.2	13.0	—	—	7.9
Diseases of musculo-skeletal system and connective tissue (710-739)	—	—	11.8	—	10.9	14.7	13.1	15.8	15.8	—	—	6.6
Congenital anomalies (740-759)	—	—	9.3	—	6.7	12.5	13.6	7.4	10.7	—	—	5.5
Certain causes of perinatal morbidity and mortality (760-779)	—	—	10.6	—	11.4	6.6	10.7	13.6	11.4	—	—	9.0
Symptoms of ill-defined conditions (780-799)	—	—	10.4	—	4.7	8.0	9.1	10.9	8.8	—	—	3.4
Accidents, poisoning, and violence (800-999)	—	—	14.6	—	8.3	11.0	11.2	16.1	12.9	—	—	6.4
All other	—	—	6.1	—	—	—	8.5	—	8.1	—	—	3.3
All categories (001-999)	—	—	11.8	—	8.2	11.3	13.0	20.7	14.2	—	—	6.4

SOURCE: Organization for Economic Cooperation and Development: Health Data File, 1989.

Table 38

Mean length-of-stay in days for selected disease subcategories, by country: 1980

International Classification of Disease categories	Australia	Austria	Belgium	Canada	Denmark	Finland	France	Germany	Greece	Iceland	Ireland	Italy
Pulmonary tuberculosis (011)	49.1	40.4	—	43.6	—	29.8	—	19.4	64.0	—	64.1	85.8
Malignant neoplasm of trachea, bronchus, and lung (162,197.0,197.3)	—	—	—	—	—	—	—	—	—	—	—	—
Breast cancer (174)	14.5	—	—	19.6	—	15.4	—	16.8	19.0	—	19.8	18.0
Prostate cancer (185)	15.2	—	—	15.9	—	14.1	9.0	25.2	13.0	—	10.7	—
Diabetes mellitus (250)	20.1	—	—	19.8	—	18.0	16.0	24.9	16.0	—	11.3	18.0
Alcoholic psychoses (291)	15.2	—	—	—	—	16.3	—	15.4	13.0	—	—	—
Alcohol dependence syndrome (303)	18.7	—	—	11.7	—	14.0	—	—	50.0	—	—	—
Inflammatory disease of the eye (360,363,364.0,370,372-373,375-377)	5.3	—	—	5.9	—	7.0	—	11.8	10.0	—	8.4	13.6
Cataract (366)	—	—	—	—	—	16.4	—	21.0	—	—	—	—
Otitis (380-382)	2.4	—	—	3.5	—	8.1	—	23.4	8.0	—	—	10.8
Rheumatic fever (390-398)	13.3	—	—	14.5	—	15.2	—	28.9	12.0	—	13.7	17.8
Hypertension (401-405)	—	—	—	15.1	—	12.5	—	21.3	10.0	—	11.3	15.7
Acute myocardial infarction (410)	26.7	—	—	—	—	20.4	—	21.3	12.0	—	—	—
Pneumonia (480-486)	11.5	—	—	14.8	—	39.6	—	11.2	—	—	10.9	16.8
Pneumococcal pneumonia (481)	—	—	—	—	—	18.4	—	23.3	13.0	—	—	—
Bronchitis (490-491)	7.4	—	—	9.6	—	16.9	—	17.2	—	—	9.3	—
Asthma (493)	7.4	—	—	6.0	—	10.6	—	16.2	11.0	—	—	11.3
Ulcers of stomach and small intestine (531-534)	10.0	—	—	11.1	—	10.8	—	21.8	—	—	7.8	—
Appendicitis (540-543)	5.7	—	—	5.7	—	9.0	—	28.4	8.0	—	—	9.2
Hernia of abdominal cavity (550-553)	—	—	—	—	—	6.4	—	—	—	—	—	—
Cholelithiasis (574)	10.7	—	—	10.1	—	12.3	16.0	—	14.0	—	—	18.7
Nephritis (580-583)	7.4	—	—	16.3	—	15.3	—	—	13.0	—	12.8	19.1
Calculus of kidney and ureter (592)	7.6	—	—	6.9	—	5.2	—	—	11.0	—	—	—
Cystitis (595)	—	—	—	—	—	7.9	—	—	—	—	—	—
Normal delivery (650)	—	—	—	—	—	6.9	—	—	—	—	—	—
Major puerperal infection (670)	—	—	—	—	—	6.4	—	—	—	—	—	—
Infections of the skin (680-686)	7.5	—	—	7.3	—	10.5	—	—	9.0	—	8.2	11.3
Other inflammatory diseases of the skin (690-698)	6.6	—	—	11.9	—	11.2	—	—	10.0	—	16.0	11.3
Osteoarthrosis (715)	20.0	—	—	23.8	—	19.4	—	—	16.0	—	21.5	13.9
Intervertebral disc disorders (722)	6.7	—	—	10.6	—	7.4	—	—	13.0	—	—	—
Respiratory distress syndrome (769)	—	—	—	—	—	10.8	—	—	—	—	—	—
Hemolytic diseases and jaundice (773-774)	—	—	—	—	—	7.2	—	—	—	—	—	—
Fracture of neck of femur (820)	—	—	—	—	—	35.6	—	—	—	—	—	—
Sprains and strains of back (846-847)	30.8	—	—	6.4	—	5.2	—	—	9.0	—	—	—

See source note at end of table.

Table 38 – Continued
Mean length-of-stay in days for selected disease subcategories, by country: 1980

International Classification of Disease categories	Japan	Luxem-bourg	Nether-lands	New Zealand	Norway	Portugal	Spain	Sweden	Switzer-land	Turkey	United Kingdom	United States
Pulmonary tuberculosis (011)	330.0	—	44.7	33.5	20.7	30.6	72.1	31.5	32.0	—	33.0	15.1
Malignant neoplasm of trachea, bronchus, and lung (162,197.0,197.3)	—	—	20.8	13.8	11.2	27.6	23.3	12.4	20.3	—	12.4	12.8
Breast cancer (174)	—	—	21.8	17.9	15.9	39.2	19.4	20.4	22.4	—	13.2	11.0
Prostate cancer (185)	—	—	20.3	22.8	13.2	25.0	27.2	27.1	19.7	—	15.3	10.9
Diabetes mellitus (250)	63.8	—	—	—	—	9.6	16.7	—	25.8	—	18.2	10.5
Alcoholic psychoses (291)	—	—	—	—	—	—	53.3	—	16.5	—	—	—
Alcohol dependence syndrome (303)	—	—	—	—	—	—	—	—	16.4	—	10.7	10.1
Inflammatory disease of the eye (360,363,364.0,370,372-373,375-377)	—	—	11.8	9.2	11.7	13.1	11.3	7.8	13.5	—	6.8	4.5
Cataract (366)	27.0	—	—	—	—	21.2	11.7	—	14.3	—	8.4	3.6
Otitis (380-382)	45.2	—	5.6	3.2	6.5	24.3	7.8	5.7	6.2	—	9.0	2.6
Rheumatic fever (390-398)	75.8	—	16.2	18.3	12.7	17.8	17.5	11.8	14.8	—	13.1	10.6
Hypertension (401-405)	—	—	17.8	14.0	9.2	18.6	12.7	14.0	16.8	—	13.3	8.1
Acute myocardial infarction (410)	19.3	—	—	—	—	11.6	14.0	—	20.7	—	13.1	12.6
Pneumonia (480-486)	67.9	—	19.9	16.2	14.1	9.8	14.7	44.7	17.6	—	40.9	8.3
Pneumococcal pneumonia (481)	—	—	—	—	—	—	—	—	19.1	—	11.5	7.7
Bronchitis (490-491)	44.1	—	20.2	13.7	9.3	23.1	15.3	10.1	17.9	—	15.4	6.9
Asthma (493)	—	—	16.1	4.5	9.3	32.6	12.9	10.1	13.8	—	5.9	6.0
Ulcers of stomach and small intestine (531-534)	10.1	—	—	—	—	18.5	14.8	—	15.2	—	12.0	8.6
Appendicitis (540-543)	—	—	11.1	5.9	5.9	27.7	8.9	5.4	9.8	—	6.2	5.5
Hernia of abdominal cavity (550-553)	—	—	—	—	—	61.7	13.1	—	—	—	6.9	4.7
Cholelithiasis (574)	69.1	—	20.5	10.6	—	35.1	15.6	10.6	15.5	—	11.3	9.3
Nephritis (580-583)	—	—	25.5	12.7	4.5	25.0	17.4	14.5	15.3	—	17.1	11.1
Calculus of kidney and ureter (592)	—	—	—	—	—	20.6	14.7	—	10.6	—	8.8	5.0
Cystitis (595)	—	—	—	—	—	3.2	—	—	12.3	—	4.9	5.5
Normal delivery (650)	—	—	—	—	—	32.9	4.0	—	9.2	—	3.8	3.0
Major puerperal infection (670)	—	—	—	—	—	17.3	—	—	10.3	—	4.8	3.7
Infections of the skin (680-686)	—	—	12.1	7.2	—	—	10.2	8.4	11.9	—	9.2	7.3
Other inflammatory diseases of the skin (690-698)	—	—	13.4	11.5	11.9	—	18.2	15.3	15.1	—	13.3	10.2
Osteoarthrosis (715)	—	—	27.8	16.0	—	—	22.8	25.0	22.3	—	31.6	11.9
Intervertebral disc disorders (722)	—	—	—	—	—	—	17.4	—	18.5	—	14.9	9.9
Respiratory distress syndrome (769)	—	—	—	—	—	—	—	—	22.6	—	12.3	19.3
Hemolytic diseases and jaundice (773-774)	—	—	—	—	—	—	—	—	9.4	—	5.8	7.8
Fracture of neck of femur (820)	—	—	—	—	—	—	23.3	—	36.4	—	37.6	20.6
Sprains and strains of back (846-847)	—	—	—	—	—	—	5.6	—	7.0	—	10.1	7.1

SOURCE: Organization for Economic Cooperation and Development: Health Data File, 1989.

Table 39
Mean length-of-stay in days for selected disease subcategories, by country: 1981

International Classification of Disease categories	Australia	Austria	Belgium	Canada	Denmark	Finland	France	Germany	Greece	Iceland	Ireland	Italy
Pulmonary tuberculosis (011)	—	40.0	—	40.7	—	27.4	—	—	59.0	—	68.3	—
Malignant neoplasm of trachea, bronchus, and lung (162,197.0,197.3)	14.9	—	—	—	—	—	—	—	—	—	—	—
Breast cancer (174)	—	—	—	19.6	—	14.8	—	—	18.0	—	18.8	—
Prostate cancer (185)	—	—	—	17.0	—	13.2	8.0	—	13.0	—	17.8	—
Diabetes mellitus (250)	—	—	—	20.3	—	15.7	—	—	16.0	—	11.2	—
Alcoholic psychoses (291)	—	—	—	20.0	—	19.8	15.0	—	14.0	—	—	—
Alcohol dependence syndrome (303)	17.7	—	—	11.1	—	16.8	—	—	55.0	—	9.0	—
Inflammatory disease of the eye (360,363,364.0,370,372-373,375-377)	—	—	—	5.9	—	7.3	—	—	10.0	—	7.2	—
Cataract (366)	—	—	—	—	—	9.8	—	—	—	—	10.0	—
Otitis (380-382)	—	—	—	3.3	—	7.4	—	—	8.0	—	3.9	—
Rheumatic fever (390-398)	—	—	—	13.1	—	13.0	—	—	12.0	—	11.8	—
Hypertension (401-405)	—	—	—	13.6	—	10.4	—	—	11.0	—	12.2	—
Acute myocardial infarction (410)	—	—	—	—	—	22.5	—	—	—	—	14.9	—
Pneumonia (480-486)	—	—	—	15.6	—	43.9	—	—	12.0	—	22.6	—
Pneumococcal pneumonia (481)	—	—	—	—	—	19.4	—	—	—	—	19.6	—
Bronchitis (490-491)	—	—	—	9.8	—	17.6	—	—	13.0	—	14.4	—
Asthma (493)	—	—	—	5.8	—	11.1	—	—	—	—	7.2	—
Ulcers of stomach and small intestine (531-534)	9.2	—	—	11.1	—	11.0	—	—	11.0	—	9.4	—
Appendicitis (540-543)	—	—	—	5.7	—	5.6	—	—	8.0	—	7.4	—
Hernia of abdominal cavity (550-553)	—	—	—	—	—	6.1	—	—	—	—	7.7	—
Cholelithiasis (574)	—	—	—	9.9	—	11.8	16.0	—	13.0	—	13.5	—
Nephritis (580-583)	—	—	—	15.9	—	13.6	—	—	12.0	—	16.3	—
Calculus of kidney and ureter (592)	6.3	—	—	6.7	—	7.8	—	—	10.0	—	8.8	—
Cystitis (595)	—	—	—	—	—	6.7	—	—	—	—	4.7	—
Normal delivery (650)	—	—	—	—	—	7.5	—	—	—	—	—	—
Major puerperal infection (670)	—	—	—	—	—	6.3	—	—	—	—	—	—
Infections of the skin (680-686)	—	—	—	7.2	—	8.6	—	—	9.0	—	7.6	—
Other inflammatory diseases of the skin (690-698)	—	—	—	11.3	—	11.5	—	—	12.0	—	14.2	—
Osteoarthrosis (715)	23.9	—	—	24.3	—	18.6	—	—	16.0	—	22.6	—
Intervertebral disc disorders (722)	6.6	—	—	10.6	—	7.5	—	—	13.0	—	13.9	—
Respiratory distress syndrome (769)	—	—	—	—	—	8.9	—	—	—	—	18.8	—
Hemolytic diseases and jaundice (773-774)	—	—	—	—	—	4.6	—	—	—	—	8.9	—
Fracture of neck of femur (820)	—	—	—	—	—	35.3	—	—	—	—	22.1	—
Sprains and strains of back (846-847)	35.9	—	—	6.5	—	5.9	—	—	5.0	—	7.2	—

See source note at end of table.

Table 39 – Continued
Mean length-of-stay in days for selected disease subcategories, by country: 1981

International Classification of Disease categories	Japan	Luxem-bourg	Nether-lands	New Zealand	Norway	Portugal	Spain	Sweden	Switzer-land	Turkey	United Kingdom	United States
Pulmonary tuberculosis (011)	–	–	–	–	–	25.3	93.8	–	41.7	–	28.9	17.6
Malignant neoplasm of trachea, bronchus, and lung (162,197.0,197.3)	–	–	–	–	–	16.2	22.4	–	19.8	–	12.1	12.1
Breast cancer (174)	–	–	–	–	–	35.2	15.7	–	20.3	–	12.5	10.6
Prostate cancer (185)	–	–	–	–	–	23.2	24.4	–	19.1	–	15.7	10.8
Diabetes mellitus (250)	67.3	–	–	–	–	7.1	15.6	–	27.9	–	16.8	9.7
Alcoholic psychoses (291)	–	–	–	–	–	–	–	–	15.4	–	–	–
Alcohol dependence syndrome (303)	–	–	–	–	–	–	62.1	–	14.9	–	10.8	10.4
Inflammatory disease of the eye (360,363,364.0,370,372-373,375-377)	–	–	–	–	–	10.8	9.1	–	10.2	–	6.9	4.0
Cataract (366)	–	–	–	–	–	22.0	11.3	–	14.3	–	7.6	3.3
Otitis (380-382)	18.1	–	–	–	–	15.8	8.6	–	6.9	–	10.9	2.6
Rheumatic fever (390-398)	40.6	–	–	–	–	12.8	16.0	–	16.6	–	13.2	10.8
Hypertension (401-405)	70.1	–	–	–	–	15.2	12.0	–	22.7	–	12.4	7.7
Acute myocardial infarction (410)	–	–	–	–	–	5.9	14.0	–	19.8	–	12.7	11.9
Pneumonia (480-486)	22.8	–	–	–	–	8.7	13.6	–	22.0	–	40.3	8.6
Pneumococcal pneumonia (481)	–	–	–	–	–	–	–	–	18.2	–	11.6	8.6
Bronchitis (490-491)	89.2	–	–	–	–	18.7	14.4	–	20.5	–	17.2	7.4
Asthma (493)	33.9	–	–	–	–	19.2	11.7	–	16.0	–	5.2	5.8
Ulcers of stomach and small intestine (531-534)	9.7	–	–	–	–	13.5	14.2	–	16.2	–	11.1	8.2
Appendicitis (540-543)	–	–	–	–	–	24.3	8.6	–	9.7	–	6.0	5.7
Hernia of abdominal cavity (550-553)	–	–	–	–	–	48.4	12.8	–	–	–	6.5	4.6
Cholelithiasis (574)	–	–	–	–	–	28.6	15.8	–	15.4	–	11.4	9.6
Nephritis (580-583)	70.8	–	–	–	–	14.4	16.1	–	17.7	–	14.3	10.8
Calculus of kidney and ureter (592)	–	–	–	–	–	18.5	16.3	–	9.6	–	9.2	5.0
Cystitis (595)	–	–	–	–	–	2.0	–	–	10.6	–	8.6	5.4
Normal delivery (650)	–	–	–	–	–	23.8	4.0	–	9.0	–	3.5	2.9
Major puerperal infection (670)	–	–	–	–	–	17.0	–	–	10.2	–	6.0	4.9
Infections of the skin (680-686)	–	–	–	–	–	–	10.1	–	10.2	–	8.7	7.7
Other inflammatory diseases of the skin (690-698)	–	–	–	–	–	–	15.2	–	14.1	–	12.2	7.4
Osteoarthrosis (715)	–	–	–	–	–	–	24.0	–	25.1	–	30.5	11.9
Intervertebral disc disorders (722)	–	–	–	–	–	–	16.2	–	19.9	–	13.9	9.2
Respiratory distress syndrome (769)	–	–	–	–	–	–	–	–	21.5	–	12.5	18.8
Hemolytic diseases and jaundice (773-774)	–	–	–	–	–	–	–	–	9.1	–	7.5	7.3
Fracture of neck of femur (820)	–	–	–	–	–	–	24.5	–	36.3	–	37.8	19.6
Sprains and strains of back (846-847)	–	–	–	–	–	–	5.2	–	10.3	–	13.3	7.4

SOURCE: Organization for Economic Cooperation and Development: Health Data File, 1989.

169

Table 40
Mean length-of-stay in days for selected disease subcategories, by country: 1982

International Classification of Disease categories	Australia	Austria	Belgium	Canada	Denmark	Finland	France	Germany	Greece	Iceland	Ireland	Italy
Pulmonary tuberculosis (011)	–	37.8	–	41.4	–	27.9	–	–	56.0	–	50.9	–
Malignant neoplasm of trachea, bronchus, and lung (162,197.0,197.3)	–	–	–	–	–	–	–	–	–	–	–	–
Breast cancer (174)	–	–	–	18.8	–	16.9	–	–	14.0	–	16.9	–
Prostate cancer (185)	–	–	–	15.5	–	11.4	8.0	–	13.0	–	16.3	–
Diabetes mellitus (250)	–	–	–	19.0	–	16.3	–	–	14.0	–	16.5	–
Alcoholic psychoses (291)	–	–	–	17.9	–	18.9	15.0	–	13.0	–	10.7	–
Alcohol dependence syndrome (303)	–	–	–	19.5	–	13.9	–	–	48.0	–	7.9	–
Inflammatory disease of the eye (360,363,364.0,370,372-373,375-377)	–	–	–	11.3	–	6.9	–	–	–	–	6.9	–
Cataract (366)	–	–	–	5.4	–	9.5	–	–	9.0	–	9.7	–
Otitis (380-382)	–	–	–	5.3	–	6.0	–	–	–	–	3.9	–
Rheumatic fever (390-398)	–	–	–	3.4	–	13.0	–	–	8.0	–	12.4	–
Hypertension (401-405)	–	–	–	14.0	–	9.6	–	–	11.0	–	10.5	–
Acute myocardial infarction (410)	–	–	–	13.6	–	18.8	–	–	10.0	–	14.0	–
Pneumonia (480-486)	–	–	–	16.1	–	37.8	–	–	–	–	28.7	–
Pneumococcal pneumonia (481)	–	–	–	15.2	–	14.9	–	–	10.0	–	21.7	–
Bronchitis (490-491)	–	–	–	10.7	–	15.7	–	–	–	–	11.2	–
Asthma (493)	–	–	–	9.0	–	9.5	–	–	12.0	–	6.7	–
Ulcers of stomach and small intestine (531-534)	–	–	–	11.1	–	10.5	–	–	–	–	8.9	–
Appendicitis (540-543)	–	–	–	5.6	–	5.6	–	–	11.0	–	7.3	–
Hernia of abdominal cavity (550-553)	–	–	–	5.8	–	5.8	–	–	7.0	–	7.0	–
Cholelithiasis (574)	–	–	–	9.8	–	9.9	–	–	7.0	–	12.2	–
Nephritis (580-583)	–	–	–	17.6	–	13.4	15.0	–	13.0	–	16.2	–
Calculus of kidney and ureter (592)	–	–	–	6.6	–	6.0	–	–	12.0	–	8.3	–
Cystitis (595)	–	–	–	6.4	–	5.6	–	–	11.0	–	4.6	–
Normal delivery (650)	–	–	–	4.4	–	6.9	–	–	–	–	–	–
Major puerperal infection (670)	–	–	–	4.9	–	6.1	–	–	–	–	–	–
Infections of the skin (680-686)	–	–	–	7.2	–	7.2	–	–	9.0	–	7.3	–
Other inflammatory diseases of the skin (690-698)	–	–	–	11.6	–	10.6	–	–	10.0	–	14.5	–
Osteoarthrosis (715)	–	–	–	23.7	–	22.7	–	–	17.0	–	17.6	–
Intervertebral disc disorders (722)	–	–	–	10.0	–	7.1	–	–	14.0	–	12.7	–
Respiratory distress syndrome (769)	–	–	–	21.5	–	10.9	–	–	–	–	22.0	–
Hemolytic diseases and jaundice (773-774)	–	–	–	5.4	–	4.6	–	–	–	–	–	–
Fracture of neck of femur (820)	–	–	–	31.6	–	39.3	–	–	–	–	22.3	–
Sprains and strains of back (846-847)	–	–	–	6.4	–	5.0	–	–	7.0	–	5.6	–

See source note at end of table.

Table 40 – Continued
Mean length-of-stay in days for selected disease subcategories, by country: 1982

International Classification of Disease categories	Japan	Luxembourg	Netherlands	New Zealand	Norway	Portugal	Spain	Sweden	Switzerland	Turkey	United Kingdom	United States
Pulmonary tuberculosis (011)	237.0	–	–	–	–	28.0	51.9	–	45.5	–	25.2	13.4
Malignant neoplasm of trachea, bronchus, and lung (162,197.0,197.3)	–	–	–	–	–	13.5	18.0	–	18.4	–	12.3	10.9
Breast cancer (174)	–	–	–	–	–	25.4	16.9	–	20.0	–	11.7	10.0
Prostate cancer (185)	–	–	–	–	–	22.7	22.2	–	19.5	–	14.9	9.9
Diabetes mellitus (250)	66.3	–	–	–	–	10.4	15.9	–	26.7	–	20.7	9.5
Alcoholic psychoses (291)	–	–	–	–	–	–	–	–	17.2	–	–	–
Alcohol dependence syndrome (303)	–	–	–	–	–	–	48.7	–	13.8	–	9.4	11.2
Inflammatory disease of the eye (360,363,364.0,370,372-373,375-377)	–	–	–	–	–	9.5	9.8	–	11.0	–	6.6	3.8
Cataract (366)	25.0	–	–	–	–	–	10.5	–	13.6	–	7.6	2.9
Otitis (380-382)	58.0	–	–	–	–	16.3	7.9	–	7.1	–	12.2	2.8
Rheumatic fever (390-398)	75.4	–	–	–	–	14.1	14.7	–	16.9	–	13.3	10.6
Hypertension (401-405)	–	–	–	–	–	27.6	12.6	–	17.1	–	13.0	7.5
Acute myocardial infarction (410)	23.6	–	–	–	–	8.7	–	–	18.5	–	14.3	11.2
Pneumonia (480-486)	–	–	–	–	–	7.7	14.6	–	19.2	–	36.5	8.0
Pneumococcal pneumonia (481)	72.0	–	–	–	–	–	–	–	18.9	–	12.0	8.6
Bronchitis (490-491)	26.8	–	–	–	–	20.2	14.9	–	21.6	–	15.6	6.9
Asthma (493)	–	–	–	–	–	21.8	11.4	–	16.5	–	5.1	5.5
Ulcers of stomach and small intestine (531-534)	10.0	–	–	–	–	17.5	13.5	–	16.9	–	11.1	7.9
Appendicitis (540-543)	–	–	–	–	–	27.6	8.3	–	9.8	–	6.0	5.3
Hernia of abdominal cavity (550-553)	–	–	–	–	–	40.6	12.3	–	–	–	6.3	4.5
Cholelithiasis (574)	–	–	–	–	–	28.6	15.5	–	14.9	–	10.7	8.9
Nephritis (580-583)	89.5	–	–	–	–	16.7	17.4	–	15.5	–	16.5	10.9
Calculus of kidney and ureter (592)	–	–	–	–	–	16.3	14.2	–	9.4	–	8.3	4.8
Cystitis (595)	–	–	–	–	–	1.9	–	–	11.1	–	4.5	5.4
Normal delivery (650)	–	–	–	–	–	26.8	–	–	9.1	–	2.5	2.9
Major puerperal infection (670)	–	–	–	–	–	17.1	–	–	10.9	–	6.5	3.8
Infections of the skin (680-686)	–	–	–	–	–	–	9.7	–	10.5	–	9.2	7.9
Other inflammatory diseases of the skin (690-698)	–	–	–	–	–	–	16.1	–	14.3	–	11.3	8.0
Osteoarthrosis (715)	–	–	–	–	–	–	24.7	–	24.4	–	27.9	10.9
Intervertebral disc disorders (722)	–	–	–	–	–	–	16.6	–	18.8	–	13.7	9.5
Respiratory distress syndrome (769)	–	–	–	–	–	–	–	–	13.4	–	16.5	21.3
Hemolytic diseases and jaundice (773-774)	–	–	–	–	–	–	–	–	8.7	–	7.8	7.0
Fracture of neck of femur (820)	–	–	–	–	–	–	22.8	–	34.9	–	35.8	18.6
Sprains and strains of back (846-847)	–	–	–	–	–	–	8.5	–	11.1	–	5.1	7.4

Source: Organization for Economic Cooperation and Development: Health Data File, 1989

171

Table 41
Mean length-of-stay in days for selected disease subcategories, by country: 1983

International Classification of Disease categories	Australia	Austria	Belgium	Canada	Denmark	Finland	France	Germany	Greece	Iceland	Ireland	Italy
Pulmonary tuberculosis (011)	22.8	39.4	—	37.1	—	25.6	—	—	36.0	15.8	48.2	—
Malignant neoplasm of trachea, bronchus, and lung (162,197.0,197.3)	12.6	—	—	18.3	—	14.0	—	—	12.0	15.6	16.6	—
Breast cancer (174)	14.2	—	—	15.1	—	12.7	7.0	—	12.0	7.1	15.2	—
Prostate cancer (185)	16.9	—	—	17.1	—	16.7	—	—	16.0	9.2	14.5	—
Diabetes mellitus (250)	16.2	—	—	15.9	—	16.9	14.0	—	14.0	13.8	10.2	—
Alcoholic psychoses (291)	—	—	—	19.1	—	—	—	—	—	—	—	—
Alcohol dependence syndrome (303)	18.4	—	—	11.0	—	16.9	—	—	35.0	6.0	7.4	—
Inflammatory disease of the eye (360,363,364.0,370,372-373,375-377)	5.0	—	—	5.3	—	7.3	—	—	9.0	9.8	6.6	—
Cataract (366)	—	—	—	4.9	—	9.2	—	—	—	10.7	8.7	—
Otitis (380-382)	2.0	—	—	3.3	—	5.5	—	—	8.0	5.0	3.5	—
Rheumatic fever (390-398)	10.8	—	—	12.8	—	10.7	—	—	10.0	12.7	10.7	—
Hypertension (401-405)	46.3	—	—	14.3	—	10.8	—	—	10.0	9.3	9.2	—
Acute myocardial infarction (410)	—	—	—	14.8	—	21.5	—	—	—	14.5	15.5	—
Pneumonia (480-486)	16.1	—	—	14.7	—	42.0	—	—	12.0	11.2	26.0	—
Pneumococcal pneumonia (481)	—	—	—	12.2	—	37.1	—	—	—	16.6	18.2	—
Bronchitis (490-491)	5.6	—	—	9.3	—	15.2	—	—	12.0	9.8	10.3	—
Asthma (493)	5.6	—	—	5.7	—	8.9	—	—	—	12.0	6.3	—
Ulcers of stomach and small intestine (531-534)	7.6	—	—	10.8	—	11.2	—	—	10.0	6.7	8.3	—
Appendicitis (540-543)	5.5	—	—	5.6	—	8.8	—	—	7.0	7.2	7.0	—
Hernia of abdominal cavity (550-553)	—	—	—	5.8	—	6.0	—	—	—	12.6	6.9	—
Cholelithiasis (574)	9.9	—	—	9.6	—	10.4	14.0	—	13.0	10.4	12.4	—
Nephritis (580-583)	12.7	—	—	16.7	—	14.5	—	—	12.0	6.1	15.3	—
Calculus of kidney and ureter (592)	5.2	—	—	6.4	—	6.7	—	—	11.0	6.6	8.1	—
Cystitis (595)	—	—	—	7.2	—	9.1	—	—	—	—	4.5	—
Normal delivery (650)	—	—	—	4.4	—	7.2	—	—	—	—	—	—
Major puerperal infection (670)	—	—	—	4.9	—	5.6	—	—	—	8.3	—	—
Infections of the skin (680-686)	7.3	—	—	7.4	—	7.1	—	—	8.0	15.7	7.0	—
Other inflammatory diseases of the skin (690-698)	5.7	—	—	11.8	—	11.0	—	—	10.0	16.9	13.8	—
Osteoarthrosis (715)	17.2	—	—	20.9	—	18.0	—	—	17.0	14.0	14.7	—
Intervertebral disc disorders (722)	6.6	—	—	10.0	—	7.0	—	—	14.0	—	13.2	—
Respiratory distress syndrome (769)	—	—	—	22.5	—	10.9	—	—	—	—	18.2	—
Hemolytic diseases and jaundice (773-774)	—	—	—	3.8	—	2.9	—	—	—	6.2	6.7	—
Fracture of neck of femur (820)	—	—	—	33.0	—	35.9	—	—	—	20.6	22.0	—
Sprains and strains of back (846-847)	35.9	—	—	6.1	—	4.7	—	—	7.0	8.6	6.5	—

See source note at end of table.

Table 41 – Continued
Mean length-of-stay in days for selected disease subcategories, by country: 1983

International Classification of Disease categories	Japan	Luxem-bourg	Nether-lands	New Zealand	Norway	Portugal	Spain	Sweden	Switzer-land	Turkey	United Kingdom	United States
Pulmonary tuberculosis (011)	227.0	–	–	–	–	28.1	48.2	–	43.4	–	27.0	17.7
Malignant neoplasm of trachea, bronchus, and lung (162,197.0,197.3)	–	–	–	–	–	9.2	18.7	–	18.7	–	11.7	10.5
Breast cancer (174)	–	–	–	–	–	34.0	16.7	–	19.3	–	12.2	9.4
Prostate cancer (185)	–	–	–	–	–	20.1	17.2	–	18.8	–	13.6	10.1
Diabetes mellitus (250)	62.3	–	–	–	–	11.9	16.4	–	23.7	–	18.0	9.5
Alcoholic psychoses (291)	–	–	–	–	–	–	–	–	15.2	–	–	–
Alcohol dependence syndrome (303)	–	–	–	–	–	–	98.0	–	14.5	–	10.5	11.5
Inflammatory disease of the eye (360,363,364.0,370,372-373,375-377)	–	–	–	–	–	14.6	9.3	–	11.9	–	6.7	4.3
Cataract (366)	–	–	–	–	–	14.3	10.3	–	12.8	–	7.1	2.5
Otitis (380-382)	20.3	–	–	–	–	15.5	7.1	–	7.3	–	8.3	2.5
Rheumatic fever (390-398)	70.0	–	–	–	–	14.0	16.1	–	15.4	–	14.1	10.3
Hypertension (401-405)	56.2	–	–	–	–	14.0	13.9	–	21.0	–	11.6	7.2
Acute myocardial infarction (410)	–	–	–	–	–	4.2	13.0	–	17.8	–	13.5	10.9
Pneumonia (480-486)	23.2	–	–	–	–	7.7	13.7	–	17.8	–	40.4	8.0
Pneumococcal pneumonia (481)	–	–	–	–	–	–	–	–	17.8	–	12.0	8.0
Bronchitis (490-491)	55.3	–	–	–	–	20.2	13.2	–	19.5	–	18.1	6.6
Asthma (493)	34.4	–	–	–	–	18.8	9.4	–	17.0	–	5.8	5.5
Ulcers of stomach and small intestine (531-534)	–	–	–	–	–	15.6	13.3	–	15.8	–	11.1	7.7
Appendicitis (540-543)	9.8	–	–	–	–	25.9	8.1	–	9.5	–	5.7	5.4
Hernia of abdominal cavity (550-553)	–	–	–	–	–	37.7	12.1	–	–	–	6.0	4.1
Cholelithiasis (574)	–	–	–	–	–	21.1	15.3	–	15.2	–	10.4	8.7
Nephritis (580-583)	71.1	–	–	–	–	16.0	17.2	–	15.5	–	13.3	11.0
Calculus of kidney and ureter (592)	–	–	–	–	–	13.6	14.3	–	9.4	–	8.4	4.5
Cystitis (595)	–	–	–	–	–	1.7	–	–	12.3	–	4.7	5.4
Normal delivery (650)	–	–	–	–	–	21.9	4.0	–	8.9	–	4.0	2.8
Major puerperal infection (670)	–	–	–	–	–	–	–	–	8.3	–	4.1	4.0
Infections of the skin (680-686)	–	–	–	–	–	–	9.7	–	11.0	–	8.4	7.8
Other inflammatory diseases of the skin (690-698)	–	–	–	–	–	–	13.2	–	15.1	–	10.3	7.5
Osteoarthrosis (715)	–	–	–	–	–	–	20.8	–	23.2	–	25.5	10.9
Intervertebral disc disorders (722)	–	–	–	–	–	–	16.5	–	18.8	–	13.0	8.2
Respiratory distress syndrome (769)	–	–	–	–	–	–	–	–	12.4	–	15.5	26.6
Hemolytic diseases and jaundice (773-774)	–	–	–	–	–	–	–	–	9.2	–	7.8	8.0
Fracture of neck of femur (820)	–	–	–	–	–	–	24.6	–	34.6	–	33.0	18.0
Sprains and strains of back (846-847)	–	–	–	–	–	–	5.6	–	7.1	–	9.0	6.6

SOURCE: Organization for Economic Cooperation and Development: Health Data File, 1989.

173

Table 42

Mean length-of-stay in days for selected disease subcategories, by country: 1984

International Classification of Disease categories	Australia	Austria	Belgium	Canada	Denmark	Finland	France	Germany	Greece	Iceland	Ireland	Italy
Pulmonary tuberculosis (011)	19.3	37.6	—	32.0	—	25.2	—	—	36.0	—	45.2	—
Malignant neoplasm of trachea, bronchus, and lung (162,197.0,197.3)	—	—	—	—	—	—	—	—	—	—	—	—
Breast cancer (174)	13.1	—	—	18.6	—	14.3	—	—	12.0	—	16.1	—
Prostate cancer (185)	14.5	—	—	15.7	—	17.6	—	—	11.0	—	14.6	—
Diabetes mellitus (250)	16.8	—	—	17.0	—	21.8	—	—	14.0	—	13.6	—
Alcoholic psychoses (291)	13.3	—	—	15.9	—	16.6	—	—	12.0	—	9.7	—
Alcohol dependence syndrome (303)	15.6	—	—	21.8	—	13.0	—	—	42.0	—	—	—
Inflammatory disease of the eye (360,363,364.0,370,372-373,375-377)	7.4	—	—	11.6	—	6.7	—	—	9.0	—	7.3	—
Cataract (366)	—	—	—	4.8	—	10.6	—	—	—	—	6.2	—
Otitis (380-382)	1.9	—	—	4.3	—	5.2	—	—	8.0	—	7.9	—
Rheumatic fever (390-398)	15.9	—	—	3.2	—	12.9	—	—	12.0	—	2.6	—
Hypertension (401-405)	14.6	—	—	13.2	—	13.5	—	—	10.0	—	11.2	—
Acute myocardial infarction (410)	—	—	—	14.2	—	21.3	—	—	—	—	8.7	—
Pneumonia (480-486)	10.2	—	—	14.7	—	51.7	—	—	12.0	—	14.4	—
Pneumococcal pneumonia (481)	—	—	—	15.1	—	16.0	—	—	—	—	31.1	—
Bronchitis (490-491)	5.1	—	—	11.6	—	14.4	—	—	—	—	23.4	—
Asthma (493)	5.1	—	—	9.0	—	8.4	—	—	5.0	—	14.0	—
Ulcers of stomach and small intestine (531-534)	6.2	—	—	10.7	—	10.7	—	—	10.0	—	5.9	—
Appendicitis (540-543)	5.4	—	—	5.5	—	5.1	—	—	7.0	—	8.4	—
Hernia of abdominal cavity (550-553)	—	—	—	5.7	—	8.2	—	—	—	—	6.7	—
Cholelithiasis (574)	9.6	—	—	9.5	—	9.5	—	—	13.0	—	6.9	—
Nephritis (580-583)	9.4	—	—	14.6	—	14.3	—	—	12.0	—	11.5	—
Calculus of kidney and ureter (592)	5.0	—	—	6.3	—	5.3	—	—	10.0	—	12.7	—
Cystitis (595)	—	—	—	6.8	—	7.0	—	—	—	—	8.0	—
Normal delivery (650)	—	—	—	4.3	—	6.7	—	—	—	—	4.8	—
Major puerperal infection (670)	—	—	—	5.1	—	8.9	—	—	—	—	—	—
Infections of the skin (680-686)	6.8	—	—	7.4	—	7.5	—	—	8.0	—	6.8	—
Other inflammatory diseases of the skin (690-698)	6.6	—	—	11.9	—	11.0	—	—	10.0	—	12.6	—
Osteoarthrosis (715)	15.5	—	—	20.0	—	18.5	—	—	16.0	—	14.1	—
Intervertebral disc disorders (722)	6.6	—	—	9.8	—	6.7	—	—	13.0	—	12.6	—
Respiratory distress syndrome (769)	—	—	—	21.8	—	8.9	—	—	—	—	18.4	—
Hemolytic diseases and jaundice (773-774)	—	—	—	3.8	—	3.3	—	—	—	—	6.4	—
Fracture of neck of femur (820)	29.9	—	—	33.4	—	39.6	—	—	7.0	—	21.1	—
Sprains and strains of back (846-847)	—	—	—	6.0	—	4.5	—	—	—	—	6.4	—

See source note at end of table.

Table 42 – Continued
Mean length-of-stay in days for selected disease subcategories, by country: 1984

International Classification of Disease categories	Japan	Luxem-bourg	Nether-lands	New Zealand	Norway	Portugal	Spain	Sweden	Switzer-land	Turkey	United Kingdom	United States
Pulmonary tuberculosis (011)	204.0	—	—	27.8	—	21.7	50.1	—	41.4	—	24.4	15.9
Malignant neoplasm of trachea, bronchus, and lung (162,197.0,197.3)	—	—	—	—	—	—	—	—	—	—	—	9.5
Breast cancer (174)	—	—	—	12.5	—	8.2	17.6	—	17.8	—	11.4	8.3
Prostate cancer (185)	—	—	—	16.6	—	21.4	14.9	—	18.9	—	13.0	9.1
Diabetes mellitus (250)	71.0	—	—	19.9	—	17.0	16.4	—	19.5	—	12.9	8.2
Alcoholic psychoses (291)	—	—	—	25.9	—	9.9	15.3	—	25.5	—	17.8	10.6
Alcohol dependence syndrome (303)	185.1	—	—	—	—	—	61.4	—	16.5	—	—	—
Inflammatory disease of the eye (360,363,364.0,370,372-373,375-377)	—	—	—	12.5	—	—	—	—	13.7	—	8.0	4.3
Cataract (366)	—	—	—	4.8	—	8.0	10.8	—	11.0	—	5.9	2.4
Otitis (380-382)	20.9	—	—	1.5	—	18.3	10.0	—	12.4	—	6.9	2.8
Rheumatic fever (390-398)	65.6	—	—	15.4	—	13.3	7.4	—	7.3	—	9.5	8.5
Hypertension (401-405)	74.7	—	—	17.7	—	11.2	15.1	—	15.3	—	11.7	6.5
Acute myocardial infarction (410)	—	—	—	—	—	14.2	10.6	—	18.7	—	13.3	10.0
Pneumonia (480-486)	20.7	—	—	20.3	—	9.6	13.0	—	17.5	—	12.5	7.8
Pneumococcal pneumonia (481)	—	—	—	—	—	6.7	13.9	—	17.3	—	42.9	7.9
Bronchitis (490-491)	93.1	—	—	17.5	—	17.7	11.6	—	17.5	—	12.4	6.6
Asthma (493)	23.0	—	—	5.1	—	17.9	9.8	—	19.3	—	16.9	5.2
Ulcers of stomach and small intestine (531-534)	—	—	—	6.2	—	12.7	12.9	—	17.2	—	4.8	7.4
Appendicitis (540-543)	10.2	—	—	5.4	—	22.9	7.8	—	15.2	—	11.6	5.1
Hernia of abdominal cavity (550-553)	—	—	—	—	—	34.8	11.8	—	8.4	—	5.5	3.8
Cholelithiasis (574)	—	—	—	10.0	—	22.0	15.2	—	14.3	—	5.8	7.6
Nephritis (580-583)	58.2	—	—	14.6	—	14.6	15.6	—	15.6	—	10.0	10.8
Calculus of kidney and ureter (592)	—	—	—	6.8	—	14.0	14.4	—	8.4	—	12.5	4.2
Cystitis (595)	—	—	—	—	—	1.7	—	—	12.2	—	7.5	5.2
Normal delivery (650)	—	—	—	—	—	18.3	4.0	—	8.6	—	4.8	2.7
Major puerperal infection (670)	—	—	—	—	—	19.6	—	—	9.5	—	5.6	5.7
Infections of the skin (680-686)	—	—	—	7.0	—	—	10.1	—	9.8	—	7.7	7.5
Other inflammatory diseases of the skin (690-698)	—	—	—	10.9	—	—	16.0	—	16.8	—	8.5	9.3
Osteoarthrosis (715)	83.0	—	—	30.1	—	—	21.3	—	23.1	—	27.8	10.3
Intervertebral disc disorders (722)	—	—	—	10.3	—	—	16.2	—	17.8	—	12.0	7.6
Respiratory distress syndrome (769)	—	—	—	—	—	—	—	—	13.0	—	15.1	24.1
Hemolytic diseases and jaundice (773-774)	—	—	—	—	—	—	—	—	8.6	—	7.5	7.1
Fracture of neck of femur (820)	—	—	—	—	—	—	23.0	—	35.0	—	32.2	15.8
Sprains and strains of back (846-847)	—	—	—	—	—	—	8.6	—	9.0	—	6.9	6.4

SOURCE: Organization for Economic Cooperation and Development: Health Data File, 1989.

175

Table 43
Mean length-of-stay in days for selected disease subcategories, by country: 1985

International Classification of Disease categories	Australia	Austria	Belgium	Canada	Denmark	Finland	France	Germany	Greece	Iceland	Ireland	Italy
Pulmonary tuberculosis (011)	—	36.5	—	32.6	20.6	25.4	19.5	—	25.0	—	46.6	—
Malignant neoplasm of trachea, bronchus, and lung (162,197.0,197.3)	—	—	—	17.8	11.7	13.8	13.9	—	12.0	—	15.8	—
Breast cancer (174)	—	—	—	14.5	8.7	13.7	7.1	—	10.0	—	15.1	—
Prostate cancer (185)	—	—	—	17.0	12.5	15.2	13.4	—	15.0	—	15.1	—
Diabetes mellitus (250)	—	—	—	17.2	10.9	16.1	12.9	—	12.0	—	10.3	—
Alcoholic psychoses (291)	—	—	—	19.4	—	—	16.3	—	—	—	—	—
Alcohol dependence syndrome (303)	—	—	—	11.4	5.3	11.9	13.1	—	43.0	—	7.0	—
Inflammatory disease of the eye (360,363,364.0,370,372-373,375-377)	—	—	—	4.3	5.7	5.3	7.5	—	9.0	—	8.1	—
Cataract (366)	—	—	—	4.0	4.0	10.9	8.2	—	—	—	7.5	—
Otitis (380-382)	—	—	—	3.1	9.4	4.9	5.4	—	11.0	—	3.0	—
Rheumatic fever (390-398)	—	—	—	13.3	9.1	12.5	12.1	—	11.0	—	10.2	—
Hypertension (401-405)	—	—	—	13.5	10.7	11.3	10.1	—	9.0	—	8.4	—
Acute myocardial infarction (410)	—	—	—	14.7	11.6	23.7	12.8	—	—	—	15.9	—
Pneumonia (480-486)	—	—	—	16.8	11.7	47.5	13.5	—	9.0	—	23.0	—
Pneumococcal pneumonia (481)	—	—	—	11.4	11.6	17.7	14.5	—	—	—	16.2	—
Bronchitis (490-491)	—	—	—	8.7	6.8	13.6	13.5	—	10.0	—	9.2	—
Asthma (493)	—	—	—	5.5	7.3	8.4	8.4	—	—	—	5.7	—
Ulcers of stomach and small intestine (531-534)	—	—	—	10.5	4.7	11.9	13.6	—	10.0	—	7.9	—
Appendicitis (540-543)	—	—	—	5.5	—	5.0	8.0	—	7.0	—	6.3	—
Hernia of abdominal cavity (550-553)	—	—	—	5.5	10.9	5.6	6.3	—	—	—	6.3	—
Cholelithiasis (574)	—	—	—	9.2	8.7	9.8	12.3	—	13.0	—	11.2	—
Nephritis (580-583)	—	—	—	13.1	6.7	10.0	11.8	—	12.0	—	12.5	—
Calculus of kidney and ureter (592)	—	—	—	6.0	7.5	6.4	7.1	—	10.0	—	7.5	—
Cystitis (595)	—	—	—	6.9	4.7	6.7	11.1	—	—	—	4.8	—
Normal delivery (650)	—	—	—	4.2	—	6.8	6.3	—	—	—	—	—
Major puerperal infection (670)	—	—	—	4.9	—	5.6	6.4	—	—	—	—	—
Infections of the skin (680-686)	—	—	—	7.2	5.5	8.0	5.4	—	8.0	—	6.8	—
Other inflammatory diseases of the skin (690-698)	—	—	—	12.0	13.6	10.7	13.9	—	9.0	—	12.5	—
Osteoarthrosis (715)	—	—	—	19.9	16.7	14.8	18.1	—	16.0	—	14.2	—
Intervertebral disc disorders (722)	—	—	—	9.7	7.3	5.9	11.4	—	13.0	—	11.4	—
Respiratory distress syndrome (769)	—	—	—	18.5	—	13.9	18.1	—	—	—	15.9	—
Hemolytic diseases and jaundice (773-774)	—	—	—	3.7	—	6.7	6.2	—	—	—	6.4	—
Fracture of neck of femur (820)	—	—	—	32.9	—	34.4	19.4	—	—	—	19.9	—
Sprains and strains of back (846-847)	—	—	—	5.7	6.4	4.3	8.1	—	8.0	—	5.6	—

See source note at end of table.

Table 43 – Continued

Mean length-of-stay in days for selected disease subcategories, by country: 1985

International Classification of Disease categories	Japan	Luxem-bourg	Nether-lands	New Zealand	Norway	Portugal	Spain	Sweden	Switzer-land	Turkey	United Kingdom	United States
Pulmonary tuberculosis (011)	–	–	–	20.6	–	22.2	40.0	24.8	36.6	–	19.6	12.9
Malignant neoplasm of trachea, bronchus, and lung (162,197.0,197.3)	–	–	–	11.9	–	7.6	16.9	–	16.2	–	11.4	9.2
Breast cancer (174)	–	–	–	14.7	–	17.7	14.7	14.0	18.7	–	12.0	7.2
Prostate cancer (185)	–	–	–	18.7	–	15.7	18.2	14.5	19.3	–	13.0	7.4
Diabetes mellitus (250)	–	–	–	28.4	–	8.2	15.5	–	25.5	–	17.9	8.1
Alcoholic psychoses (291)	–	–	–	–	–	–	–	21.8	18.1	–	–	–
Alcohol dependence syndrome (303)	–	–	–	15.5	–	–	61.6	10.3	13.6	–	8.6	10.7
Inflammatory disease of the eye (360,363,364.0,370,372-373,375-377)	–	–	–	7.1	–	6.6	21.9	–	11.1	–	5.7	4.0
Cataract (366)	–	–	–	–	–	14.3	9.4	–	12.0	–	6.4	2.0
Otitis (380-382)	–	–	–	1.4	–	13.4	6.6	–	6.7	–	7.7	2.5
Rheumatic fever (390-398)	–	–	–	14.4	–	10.4	15.3	13.3	16.2	–	11.8	9.2
Hypertension (401-405)	–	–	–	22.8	–	12.5	11.8	13.2	15.8	–	13.5	5.9
Acute myocardial infarction (410)	–	–	–	–	–	4.7	13.0	11.9	17.3	–	11.2	9.5
Pneumonia (480-486)	–	–	–	22.3	–	6.6	13.6	13.0	16.9	–	39.9	7.9
Pneumococcal pneumonia (481)	–	–	–	–	–	–	–	–	17.1	–	15.7	8.2
Bronchitis (490-491)	–	–	–	15.3	–	16.2	12.6	13.2	19.6	–	15.8	6.9
Asthma (493)	–	–	–	5.0	–	16.6	9.1	7.7	15.1	–	4.9	4.9
Ulcers of stomach and small intestine (531-534)	–	–	–	10.1	–	11.0	12.9	–	14.1	–	10.7	7.1
Appendicitis (540-543)	–	–	–	5.2	–	19.5	7.6	49.8	9.1	–	5.6	5.0
Hernia of abdominal cavity (550-553)	–	–	–	–	–	28.7	11.6	8.2	–	–	5.5	3.2
Cholelithiasis (574)	–	–	–	9.0	–	21.8	14.3	10.3	14.2	–	9.9	7.5
Nephritis (580-583)	–	–	–	13.2	–	14.9	15.4	15.3	16.3	–	11.7	10.4
Calculus of kidney and ureter (592)	–	–	–	6.7	–	12.6	11.8	8.5	7.4	–	7.4	3.7
Cystitis (595)	–	–	–	–	–	1.5	–	–	11.6	–	3.8	4.8
Normal delivery (650)	–	–	–	–	–	16.6	4.0	39.5	8.5	–	4.3	2.5
Major puerperal infection (670)	–	–	–	–	–	29.0	–	6.9	24.8	–	4.4	3.0
Infections of the skin (680-686)	–	–	–	7.1	–	–	9.3	7.7	10.1	–	8.1	7.3
Other inflammatory diseases of the skin (690-698)	–	–	–	12.0	–	–	15.8	16.3	14.6	–	9.4	6.7
Osteoarthrosis (715)	–	–	–	34.9	–	–	20.2	4.5	24.3	–	25.7	10.5
Intervertebral disc disorders (722)	–	–	–	9.8	–	–	16.0	–	18.0	–	12.0	7.3
Respiratory distress syndrome (769)	–	–	–	–	–	–	–	–	14.3	–	19.7	26.5
Hemolytic diseases and jaundice (773-774)	–	–	–	–	–	–	–	–	8.4	–	6.7	7.6
Fracture of neck of femur (820)	–	–	–	–	–	–	22.6	14.7	35.9	–	29.7	14.7
Sprains and strains of back (846-847)	–	–	–	5.2	–	–	7.6	–	7.9	–	5.9	6.0

SOURCE: Organization for Economic Cooperation and Development: Health Data File, 1989.

Table 44
Mean length-of-stay in days for selected disease subcategories, by country: 1986

International Classification of Disease categories	Australia	Austria	Belgium	Canada	Denmark	Finland	France	Germany	Greece	Iceland	Ireland	Italy
Pulmonary tuberculosis (011)	20.4	34.1	–	–	18.5	24.8	20.3	–	32.0	–	43.6	–
Malignant neoplasm of trachea, bronchus, and lung (162,197.0,197.3)	12.0	–	–	–	11.1	13.6	13.8	–	17.0	–	14.6	–
Breast cancer (174)	11.8	–	–	–	8.2	12.5	7.0	–	9.0	–	13.8	–
Prostate cancer (185)	12.4	–	–	–	12.3	15.6	12.7	–	13.0	–	14.5	–
Diabetes mellitus (250)	11.7	–	–	–	11.1	17.3	12.6	–	11.0	–	8.7	–
Alcoholic psychoses (291)	–	–	–	–	–	–	17.0	–	–	–	–	–
Alcohol dependence syndrome (303)	12.6	–	–	–	4.9	11.3	12.3	–	53.0	–	7.4	–
Inflammatory disease of the eye (360,363,364.0,370,372-373,375-377)	4.6	–	–	–	5.3	5.1	7.0	–	8.0	–	7.6	–
Cataract (366)	3.8	–	–	–	–	12.4	8.4	–	–	–	7.5	–
Otitis (380-382)	1.7	–	–	–	3.6	4.7	5.2	–	8.0	–	2.4	–
Rheumatic fever (390-398)	10.2	–	–	–	8.9	14.4	12.6	–	10.0	–	10.6	–
Hypertension (401-405)	8.2	–	–	–	9.0	10.5	10.2	–	8.0	–	7.5	–
Acute myocardial infarction (410)	10.9	–	–	–	9.5	24.4	12.8	–	–	–	13.2	–
Pneumonia (480-486)	11.6	–	–	–	11.0	49.4	13.4	–	11.0	–	18.2	–
Pneumococcal pneumonia (481)	–	–	–	–	9.9	28.2	14.5	–	–	–	15.4	–
Bronchitis (490-491)	4.6	–	–	–	11.0	13.9	13.2	–	9.0	–	10.9	–
Asthma (493)	5.1	–	–	–	6.6	7.3	8.3	–	–	–	5.4	–
Ulcers of stomach and small intestine (531-534)	4.9	–	–	–	6.6	10.8	13.1	–	9.0	–	7.5	–
Appendicitis (540-543)	5.0	–	–	–	4.7	5.1	7.6	–	7.0	–	6.2	–
Hernia of abdominal cavity (550-553)	8.6	–	–	–	–	5.6	6.0	–	–	–	6.1	–
Cholelithiasis (574)	10.6	–	–	–	10.5	9.8	11.5	–	12.0	–	11.5	–
Nephritis (580-583)	5.9	–	–	–	8.7	9.3	11.0	–	11.0	–	13.5	–
Calculus of kidney and ureter (592)	2.3	–	–	–	6.1	6.6	7.1	–	8.0	–	7.4	–
Cystitis (595)	5.1	–	–	–	7.1	7.1	8.2	–	–	–	4.6	–
Normal delivery (650)	4.9	–	–	–	4.6	6.3	6.3	–	–	–	–	–
Major puerperal infection (670)	–	–	–	–	–	5.4	9.3	–	–	–	–	–
Infections of the skin (680-686)	6.5	–	–	–	5.4	7.2	5.2	–	8.0	–	6.6	–
Other inflammatory diseases of the skin (690-698)	6.6	–	–	–	14.0	10.1	13.9	–	9.0	–	11.9	–
Osteoarthrosis (715)	14.1	–	–	–	16.3	15.3	17.5	–	17.0	–	12.6	–
Intervertebral disc disorders (722)	7.6	–	–	–	7.2	5.9	11.2	–	13.0	–	10.4	–
Respiratory distress syndrome (769)	6.2	–	–	–	–	8.8	19.2	–	–	–	15.7	–
Hemolytic diseases and jaundice (773-774)	7.0	–	–	–	–	4.3	7.4	–	–	–	6.6	–
Fracture of neck of femur (820)	25.2	–	–	–	–	31.4	18.9	–	–	–	18.1	–
Sprains and strains of back (846-847)	–	–	–	–	6.8	5.3	9.8	–	8.0	–	5.2	–

See source note at end of table.

Table 44 – Continued

Mean length-of-stay in days for selected disease subcategories, by country: 1986

International Classification of Disease categories	Japan	Luxem-bourg	Nether-lands	New Zealand	Norway	Portugal	Spain	Sweden	Switzer-land	Turkey	United Kingdom	United States
Pulmonary tuberculosis (011)	–	–	–	–	10.5	26.4	34.9	18.9	32.5	–	–	13.9
Malignant neoplasm of trachea, bronchus, and lung (162,197.0,197.3)	–	–	–	–	–	15.6	15.9	–	16.1	–	–	8.8
Breast cancer (174)	–	–	–	–	10.2	13.4	16.0	16.6	19.3	–	–	7.1
Prostate cancer (185)	–	–	–	–	11.8	13.1	17.4	13.6	18.4	–	–	7.2
Diabetes mellitus (250)	–	–	–	–	9.4	12.1	15.5	–	25.6	–	–	7.6
Alcoholic psychoses (291)	–	–	–	–	–	–	–	19.6	19.6	–	–	–
Alcohol dependence syndrome (303)	–	–	–	–	–	–	35.9	9.5	13.6	–	–	10.7
Inflammatory disease of the eye (360,363,364.0,370,372-373,375-377)	–	–	–	–	5.8	4.7	11.2	–	11.1	–	–	3.9
Cataract (366)	–	–	–	–	–	15.9	9.3	–	11.1	–	–	1.7
Otitis (380-382)	–	–	–	–	5.3	11.5	6.5	–	6.4	–	–	2.6
Rheumatic fever (390-398)	–	–	–	–	9.1	10.0	14.3	–	16.3	–	–	9.1
Hypertension (401-405)	–	–	–	–	9.0	12.9	10.4	–	19.6	–	–	5.6
Acute myocardial infarction (410)	–	–	–	–	–	4.3	13.0	10.7	17.8	–	–	8.9
Pneumonia (480-486)	–	–	–	–	11.5	6.6	13.5	10.8	16.9	–	–	7.8
Pneumococcal pneumonia (481)	–	–	–	–	–	–	–	–	17.9	–	–	7.7
Bronchitis (490-491)	–	–	–	–	11.2	14.3	11.7	15.3	18.7	–	–	6.6
Asthma (493)	–	–	–	–	6.6	14.7	8.4	–	14.4	–	–	4.8
Ulcers of stomach and small intestine (531-534)	–	–	–	–	–	13.4	12.3	–	14.1	–	–	7.1
Appendicitis (540-543)	–	–	–	–	4.4	19.3	7.8	49.5	8.5	–	–	4.8
Hernia of abdominal cavity (550-553)	–	–	–	–	–	15.1	11.3	7.6	–	–	–	3.0
Cholelithiasis (574)	–	–	–	–	8.7	22.3	14.1	–	14.2	–	–	6.9
Nephritis (580-583)	–	–	–	–	7.7	12.6	14.8	14.2	17.6	–	–	11.0
Calculus of kidney and ureter (592)	–	–	–	–	–	11.6	10.9	6.3	7.3	–	–	3.6
Cystitis (595)	–	–	–	–	–	1.4	–	–	10.4	–	–	6.0
Normal delivery (650)	–	–	–	–	–	11.6	4.0	42.4	8.5	–	–	2.4
Major puerperal infection (670)	–	–	–	–	–	–	–	7.0	6.8	–	–	4.3
Infections of the skin (680-686)	–	–	–	–	5.9	–	10.0	7.4	10.1	–	–	7.3
Other inflammatory diseases of the skin (690-698)	–	–	–	–	14.0	–	15.4	12.6	15.2	–	–	6.7
Osteoarthrosis (715)	–	–	–	–	–	–	21.1	4.4	22.2	–	–	10.2
Intervertebral disc disorders (722)	–	–	–	–	–	–	14.5	–	17.9	–	–	6.9
Respiratory distress syndrome (769)	–	–	–	–	–	–	–	–	11.5	–	–	23.6
Hemolytic diseases and jaundice (773-774)	–	–	–	–	–	–	–	–	7.4	–	–	7.0
Fracture of neck of femur (820)	–	–	–	–	–	–	24.6	15.3	33.6	–	–	14.2
Sprains and strains of back (846-847)	–	–	–	–	–	–	6.0	–	9.4	–	–	5.6

SOURCE: Organization for Economic Cooperation and Development: Health Data File, 1989.

Table 45
Hospital staffing ratio, by country: 1960-87

Number of personnel per occupied bed

Country	1960	1961	1962	1963	1964	1965	1966	1967	1968	1969	1970	1971	1972	1973
Australia	—	—	—	—	—	—	—	—	—	—	0.40	0.40	0.40	0.40
Austria	—	—	—	—	—	—	—	—	—	—	—	—	—	—
Belgium	—	—	—	—	—	—	—	—	—	—	—	—	—	—
Canada	1.38	—	—	—	—	—	—	—	—	—	—	—	—	—
Denmark	—	—	—	—	—	1.81	—	—	—	—	1.99	—	—	—
Finland	1.07	—	1.06	1.10	1.11	1.17	1.24	1.24	1.32	1.35	1.37	1.40	1.44	1.58
France	—	—	—	—	—	1.32	—	—	—	—	1.59	—	—	—
Germany	0.62	—	0.62	0.65	0.68	0.69	0.72	0.74	0.75	0.77	0.80	0.85	0.87	0.91
Greece	—	—	—	—	—	—	—	0.63	0.62	0.61	0.64	0.66	0.69	0.70
Iceland	—	—	—	—	—	—	—	—	—	—	—	—	—	—
Ireland	—	—	—	—	—	—	—	—	—	—	—	—	—	—
Italy	0.39	—	—	—	—	0.47	—	—	—	—	0.58	—	—	—
Japan	0.54	—	—	—	—	0.57	—	—	—	0.59	0.60	0.61	0.62	0.63
Luxembourg	—	—	—	—	—	—	—	—	—	—	—	—	—	—
Netherlands	1.14	—	—	—	—	1.25	—	—	—	—	1.52	—	—	—
New Zealand	1.36	—	—	—	—	1.63	—	—	—	—	1.78	—	—	—
Norway	0.24	—	—	—	—	0.55	—	—	—	—	0.67	—	—	—
Portugal	—	—	—	—	—	—	—	—	—	—	—	—	—	—
Spain	—	—	—	—	—	—	—	—	—	—	—	—	—	—
Sweden	0.71	—	—	—	—	0.75	—	—	—	—	0.98	—	0.76	0.88
Switzerland	—	—	—	—	—	—	—	—	—	—	—	—	—	—
Turkey	—	—	—	—	—	—	—	—	—	—	—	—	—	—
United Kingdom	—	—	—	—	—	—	—	—	—	—	—	—	—	—
United States	0.96	—	—	1.08	1.11	1.15	1.25	1.32	1.39	1.47	1.57	1.66	1.72	1.80

Country	1974	1975	1976	1977	1978	1979	1980	1981	1982	1983	1984	1985	1986	1987
Australia	0.40	0.50	0.50	0.50	0.60	0.60	0.60	0.60	0.60	0.60	0.60	0.70	0.70	0.70
Austria	—	3.15	—	—	—	—	3.27	—	—	—	—	—	3.75	—
Belgium	—	0.85	—	0.92	—	0.99	—	1.03	—	1.07	—	1.11	—	1.25
Canada	—	2.12	—	—	—	—	2.09	2.11	2.13	—	—	—	—	—
Denmark	—	1.86	—	—	—	—	2.08	2.12	2.24	2.36	2.30	2.30	2.40	—
Finland	1.63	1.66	1.74	1.66	1.71	1.75	1.80	1.83	1.86	1.84	1.83	1.86	1.90	1.88
France	—	0.99	—	—	—	—	1.25	1.29	1.34	1.37	—	—	—	—
Germany	0.96	0.97	0.97	0.98	1.01	1.04	1.08	1.11	1.14	1.16	1.18	1.21	1.23	1.25
Greece	0.70	0.74	0.70	0.70	0.70	0.70	0.88	0.92	0.77	0.82	0.88	1.00	1.09	1.17
Iceland	—	—	—	—	—	—	—	—	—	—	—	—	—	—
Ireland	—	—	—	—	—	—	1.07	1.13	1.17	1.20	1.21	1.25	1.50	1.50
Italy	—	0.83	—	—	—	—	—	—	—	—	—	1.32	1.32	1.37
Japan	0.65	0.67	0.69	0.71	0.72	0.74	0.75	0.76	0.77	0.77	0.78	0.79	0.80	0.77
Luxembourg	—	—	—	—	—	—	—	—	—	—	—	—	—	—
Netherlands	—	1.96	—	—	—	—	1.74	1.80	1.86	1.86	1.89	1.91	1.89	2.00
New Zealand	—	1.97	—	—	—	—	1.98	2.03	2.11	—	—	—	—	—
Norway	—	—	—	—	—	—	1.18	1.31	1.38	—	—	—	—	—
Portugal	—	0.95	—	—	—	—	1.35	1.34	1.52	1.37	1.40	1.70	1.70	1.70
Spain	0.93	1.03	1.11	1.18	1.23	1.29	—	—	1.74	1.60	1.58	1.85	—	1.70
Sweden	—	1.27	—	—	—	—	1.64	1.68	1.60	—	—	—	1.70	—
Switzerland	—	—	—	—	—	—	—	—	—	1.65	1.66	1.67	1.73	1.75
Turkey	—	—	—	—	—	—	—	—	—	—	—	—	—	—
United Kingdom	1.60	1.74	1.84	1.88	1.94	2.02	2.10	2.20	2.30	2.30	2.30	2.40	2.40	—
United States	1.93	2.06	2.17	2.28	2.38	2.47	2.56	2.69	2.91	2.75	2.71	2.75	—	2.60

SOURCE: Organisation for Economic Cooperation and Development, Health Data File, 1989.

Table 3
Nurse staffing ratio, by country: 1960-87

Number of nurses per occupied bed

Country	1960	1961	1962	1963	1964	1965	1966	1967	1968	1969	1970	1971	1972	1973
Australia	—	—	—	—	—	—	—	—	—	—	—	—	—	—
Austria	0.21	0.23	0.24	0.24	0.24	0.24	0.24	0.25	0.26	0.27	0.27	0.28	0.29	0.31
Belgium	—	—	—	—	—	—	—	—	—	—	—	—	—	—
Canada	0.27	—	—	—	—	0.38	—	—	—	—	0.46	—	—	—
Denmark	—	—	—	—	—	0.33	—	—	—	—	0.37	—	—	—
Finland	0.28	0.26	0.26	0.28	0.28	0.30	0.30	0.30	0.31	0.32	0.34	0.35	0.35	0.38
France	—	—	—	—	—	—	—	—	—	—	0.13	—	—	—
Germany	0.16	0.16	0.16	0.16	0.16	0.17	0.18	0.19	0.19	0.20	0.21	0.23	0.24	0.26
Greece	—	—	—	—	—	0.22	—	0.26	0.27	0.29	0.29	0.29	0.29	0.29
Iceland	—	—	—	—	—	—	—	—	—	—	—	—	—	—
Ireland	—	—	—	—	—	—	—	—	—	—	—	—	—	—
Italy	0.13	—	—	—	—	0.16	—	—	—	—	0.21	—	—	—
Japan	0.23	—	—	—	0.30	0.23	0.23	0.23	0.24	0.25	0.26	0.26	0.27	0.28
Luxembourg	—	—	—	—	—	—	—	—	—	—	—	—	—	—
Netherlands	—	—	—	—	—	—	—	—	—	—	—	—	—	—
New Zealand	0.25	—	—	—	—	0.31	—	—	—	—	0.39	—	—	—
Norway	—	—	—	—	—	0.34	—	—	—	—	0.39	—	—	—
Portugal	0.12	—	—	—	—	0.14	—	—	—	—	0.23	—	—	—
Spain	—	—	—	—	—	—	—	—	—	—	—	0.21	0.21	0.25
Sweden	—	—	—	—	—	—	—	—	—	—	—	—	—	—
Switzerland	—	—	—	—	—	—	—	—	—	—	0.51	—	—	—
Turkey	—	—	—	—	—	—	—	—	—	—	—	—	—	—
United Kingdom	—	—	—	—	—	—	—	—	—	—	—	—	—	—
United States	—	—	—	—	—	—	—	—	—	—	—	—	—	—

Country	1974	1975	1976	1977	1978	1979	1980	1981	1982	1983	1984	1985	1986	1987
Australia	—	1.36	—	—	—	—	1.67	1.76	1.84	—	—	—	1.69	—
Austria	0.33	0.35	0.38	0.40	0.42	0.43	0.44	0.46	0.46	0.47	0.49	0.52	0.54	0.54
Belgium	—	—	—	0.25	—	0.28	—	0.40	—	0.41	—	0.75	—	0.68
Canada	—	0.54	—	—	—	—	0.56	0.57	0.58	—	—	—	—	—
Denmark	—	0.38	—	—	—	—	0.42	0.44	0.47	—	—	—	—	—
Finland	0.42	0.42	0.43	0.44	0.43	0.43	0.43	0.44	0.45	0.46	0.50	0.51	0.54	0.55
France	—	0.17	—	—	—	—	0.24	0.25	0.25	0.26	—	—	—	—
Germany	0.28	0.28	0.29	0.31	0.32	0.34	0.35	0.36	0.38	0.39	0.41	0.42	0.43	0.45
Greece	0.30	0.26	0.30	0.30	0.30	0.30	0.31	0.33	0.33	0.35	0.35	0.41	0.43	0.49
Iceland	—	—	—	—	—	—	—	—	—	—	—	—	—	—
Ireland	—	0.53	—	—	—	—	0.76	—	—	—	—	—	—	1.20
Italy	—	0.34	—	—	—	—	0.45	0.47	0.49	0.51	0.52	0.54	0.58	0.60
Japan	0.29	0.30	0.31	0.32	0.33	0.34	0.35	0.35	0.36	0.36	0.37	0.38	0.38	0.39
Luxembourg	—	—	—	—	—	—	—	—	—	—	—	—	—	—
Netherlands	—	—	—	—	—	—	—	—	—	—	—	—	—	—
New Zealand	—	0.55	—	—	—	—	0.58	0.62	0.62	0.67	0.76	0.80	0.81	0.91
Norway	—	0.40	—	—	—	—	0.56	0.57	0.61	—	—	0.68	0.67	—
Portugal	—	0.34	—	—	—	—	0.30	0.34	0.37	0.36	0.37	0.43	0.46	0.47
Spain	0.28	0.32	0.35	0.39	0.42	0.45	0.46	0.46	0.47	—	—	—	—	—
Sweden	—	—	—	—	—	—	—	—	—	—	—	—	—	—
Switzerland	—	0.72	—	—	—	—	0.78	—	0.78	0.80	0.81	0.82	0.83	0.79
Turkey	—	—	—	—	—	—	—	—	—	—	—	—	—	—
United Kingdom	0.34	0.36	0.38	0.41	0.43	0.45	0.47	0.51	0.53	0.55	0.57	0.61	0.64	0.69
United States	—	—	—	—	—	—	—	—	—	—	—	—	—	—

SOURCE: Organization for Economic Cooperation and Development: Health Data File, 1989.

Table 47
Number of patients treated for end stage renal disease failure, by country: 1970-87

Number per million population

Country	1970	1971	1972	1973	1974	1975	1976	1977	1978	1979	1980	1981	1982	1983	1984	1985	1986	1987
Australia	–	–	–	–	–	–	–	–	–	–	–	–	–	243.0	263.0	275.0	294.0	311.0
Austria	13.0	19.3	24.1	31.2	41.6	55.5	65.8	84.0	92.9	119.6	133.9	157.5	161.6	191.6	209.6	255.5	292.0	–
Belgium	30.1	44.0	58.5	66.1	87.1	102.7	128.5	140.8	167.6	205.9	233.1	263.4	256.1	304.8	393.7	332.5	392.0	–
Canada	–	–	–	–	–	–	121.1	–	–	–	–	237.0	242.4	273.8	287.3	306.6	336.4	–
Denmark	55.7	71.5	88.4	104.6	126.8	132.4	146.2	176.2	167.6	181.2	202.0	227.5	163.3	190.0	252.0	189.8	262.0	–
Finland	24.5	31.3	48.3	52.6	55.6	71.0	82.5	85.7	106.0	118.3	134.6	155.4	170.0	180.0	231.9	253.0	262.0	–
France	26.0	36.6	51.7	64.4	80.2	102.2	125.0	147.2	154.9	187.9	228.6	259.7	222.0	255.1	285.7	291.3	303.0	–
Germany	17.7	24.7	37.8	52.7	68.2	87.7	105.2	119.8	126.8	160.9	208.0	250.4	228.2	258.3	301.4	304.5	333.0	–
Greece	5.2	8.7	17.0	24.1	37.1	48.4	59.9	58.7	72.0	77.2	118.6	115.9	100.5	136.2	142.3	153.7	228.0	229.5
Iceland	20.0	24.6	28.6	27.3	40.9	41.5	50.0	63.6	55.0	68.6	75.0	85.0	105.0	100.0	105.0	66.7	158.0	–
Ireland	19.7	23.1	30.3	33.7	37.3	44.7	53.2	59.5	69.4	68.6	99.4	115.5	118.2	118.5	160.9	178.6	193.0	–
Italy	6.2	16.3	27.4	46.3	64.8	81.2	102.1	114.1	131.0	158.2	197.0	239.0	214.2	229.2	237.9	265.4	305.0	–
Japan	9.2	17.5	34.3	51.9	84.5	117.4	160.2	198.9	236.2	280.0	312.9	360.3	403.9	446.3	500.4	551.4	608.0	662.8
Luxembourg	6.6	14.7	35.3	42.9	51.4	90.6	88.9	105.6	80.0	163.9	177.5	165.0	187.5	225.0	225.0	276.7	383.0	–
Netherlands	36.0	45.8	58.8	71.7	86.8	90.2	108.9	126.0	130.7	148.5	185.5	211.7	179.5	189.8	292.8	288.6	318.0	–
New Zealand	–	35.0	49.0	56.0	64.0	79.0	87.0	100.0	112.0	128.0	145.0	170.0	187.0	199.0	199.0	251.0	–	–
Norway	9.2	22.5	40.9	44.1	57.2	67.4	79.4	92.3	104.4	117.2	133.7	164.4	171.5	194.4	201.2	226.7	234.0	–
Portugal	2.0	3.3	4.6	4.4	5.2	4.4	5.3	7.6	6.1	15.0	27.8	54.7	53.6	132.7	158.0	197.4	269.0	–
Spain	3.8	4.9	6.3	11.3	17.2	26.9	39.9	62.1	83.5	114.4	144.5	184.9	175.4	236.2	284.2	281.8	337.0	–
Sweden	54.2	54.1	65.5	66.2	73.5	85.4	99.1	118.9	131.9	149.5	178.1	208.6	202.0	189.9	197.6	318.7	283.0	–
Switzerland	49.2	62.2	78.1	91.0	112.6	136.1	150.2	172.3	198.3	220.8	259.7	272.5	275.1	265.5	357.3	383.1	405.0	–
Turkey	–	–	–	0.4	0.2	0.8	1.6	1.9	2.5	3.4	3.9	6.0	6.7	7.9	20.1	20.1	26.0	–
United Kingdom	23.0	30.0	38.2	46.1	53.2	62.0	71.3	79.5	94.2	111.2	127.8	151.7	122.9	153.1	200.2	215.8	242.0	–
United States	–	–	–	–	76.0	106.0	135.0	160.0	221.8	258.3	292.7	326.0	364.7	407.4	445.9	484.5	522.0	561.8

SOURCE: Organization for Economic Cooperation and Development: Health Data File, 1989.

Table 48
Percent of end stage renal disease patients with functioning transplants, by country: 1970-87

Country	1970	1971	1972	1973	1974	1975	1976	1977	1978	1979	1980	1981	1982	1983	1984	1985	1986	1987
									Percent of patients									
Australia	-	-	-	-	-	-	-	52.4	50.7	49.4	48.6	47.6	48.3	47.4	47.4	49.9	51.0	51.1
Austria	18.8	19.6	26.1	34.5	37.0	32.7	27.9	24.7	38.3	20.4	19.3	18.5	18.3	19.4	22.8	24.0	29.6	-
Belgium	34.3	33.0	32.7	26.5	26.2	27.1	25.4	24.7	26.9	29.0	27.8	28.2	28.3	30.1	35.8	23.7	33.0	-
Canada	-	-	-	-	-	-	37.1	-	-	-	-	41.3	40.5	43.1	43.8	45.0	48.3	-
Denmark	61.9	57.4	54.5	60.6	58.0	52.6	49.4	47.6	52.4	50.2	46.6	43.6	38.2	36.5	48.6	22.4	45.8	-
Finland	41.7	46.3	44.2	55.1	69.9	60.2	61.5	63.7	66.0	66.1	65.2	61.7	51.9	58.1	65.3	63.3	58.3	-
France	15.1	15.3	13.6	13.5	14.2	12.7	12.7	12.0	13.8	12.3	13.0	11.5	13.8	14.0	17.2	18.5	30.6	-
Germany	7.2	7.1	6.4	5.1	5.1	5.5	6.6	6.4	8.1	8.5	8.4	8.7	11.5	12.0	13.5	16.2	17.2	-
Greece	39.1	26.3	17.4	23.6	20.9	15.7	14.6	12.8	16.3	10.8	12.5	12.3	18.7	12.2	12.5	8.9	14.1	-
Iceland	25.0	20.0	16.6	50.0	55.6	44.4	45.5	57.1	54.5	52.9	53.3	41.2	33.3	35.0	-	24.0	47.2	-
Ireland	17.5	17.6	20.0	19.6	24.8	26.8	28.0	29.8	35.0	60.0	45.0	51.0	62.0	49.0	82.0	72.0	100.0	87.0
Italy	1.5	2.0	6.0	6.1	6.7	6.3	7.0	7.8	8.1	7.3	7.1	7.5	8.1	9.7	4.9	8.9	12.3	-
Japan	-	-	-	-	-	-	-	-	-	-	-	-	-	-	-	-	-	-
Luxembourg	-	-	8.3	-	-	9.7	0.0	2.6	0.0	1.7	2.8	3.0	5.3	5.6	7.8	12.9	16.2	-
Netherlands	17.7	19.6	21.4	23.9	27.1	24.7	28.4	31.5	29.9	31.6	30.1	29.7	30.0	22.7	42.1	40.7	43.6	-
New Zealand	-	66.0	63.0	62.0	61.0	62.0	57.0	43.0	51.0	50.0	48.6	45.4	43.5	47.9	47.7	-	-	-
Norway	51.4	60.5	60.6	65.5	73.5	73.7	72.7	60.8	70.0	68.7	66.4	69.7	66.0	73.0	70.1	75.3	78.1	14.2
Portugal	0.5	3.1	2.5	2.6	-	2.6	4.3	3.0	3.3	2.7	2.9	3.2	3.4	5.2	6.8	9.3	8.5	-
Spain	9.8	9.1	12.4	12.2	9.5	4.3	7.5	6.3	6.6	6.7	8.2	9.6	12.0	12.0	16.8	19.3	23.4	25.3
Sweden	49.8	46.0	49.9	49.5	51.7	47.6	47.4	45.5	50.7	47.7	47.1	44.5	49.9	49.1	46.5	56.7	55.3	-
Switzerland	31.3	29.5	31.2	35.6	37.2	35.0	36.2	35.1	35.8	33.1	34.1	33.7	34.6	26.9	40.4	42.0	34.7	-
Turkey	-	-	-	12.5	-	9.7	47.7	43.6	35.5	33.6	29.2	32.6	22.1	37.3	19.2	10.7	25.8	-
United Kingdom	27.2	39.0	32.0	33.3	33.9	36.0	37.7	39.4	44.0	43.4	44.0	41.7	45.5	44.4	49.8	47.5	49.7	-
United States	-	-	-	-	-	-	-	-	12.7	13.3	13.9	14.9	16.2	17.4	19.3	21.4	23.9	25.6

SOURCE: Organization for Economic Cooperation and Development: Health Data File, 1989.

Table 49
Number of end stage renal disease patients with new grafts, by country: 1970-87

Country	1970	1971	1972	1973	1974	1975	1976	1977	1978	1979	1980	1981	1982	1983	1984	1985	1986	1987
							Number per million population											
Australia	—	—	—	19.8	19.4	20.9	18.7	21.6	21.2	21.8	25.9	24.1	27.3	24.0	27.0	26.0	27.0	25.0
Austria	—	—	—	—	12.7	11.6	8.1	10.4	8.3	11.1	8.8	9.5	11.5	11.1	29.9	22.2	35.8	—
Belgium	—	—	—	—	10.2	9.6	9.4	9.8	11.4	18.4	18.6	16.4	15.7	11.9	28.5	29.4	30.0	—
Canada	—	—	—	—	—	—	15.1	—	—	—	—	20.0	20.3	26.1	26.3	29.1	33.9	—
Denmark	—	—	—	—	29.0	24.3	22.7	25.9	25.9	22.9	24.3	22.9	16.7	12.9	38.4	40.7	44.4	—
Finland	2.0	7.0	13.0	18.0	19.4	16.3	19.2	23.8	24.2	27.9	29.2	28.1	19.2	12.5	29.6	28.8	28.1	27.4
France	—	—	—	—	4.9	5.4	6.8	6.8	8.9	9.0	10.4	9.6	11.5	6.8	22.8	21.0	23.8	—
Germany	—	—	—	—	2.2	3.5	4.2	5.9	6.2	7.1	7.9	8.1	9.5	6.4	16.4	20.8	26.6	—
Greece	—	—	—	—	4.1	1.7	2.9	3.1	3.9	5.2	5.8	4.8	4.7	2.6	2.4	3.1	6.2	—
Iceland	—	—	—	—	10.0	0.0	10.0	25.0	0.0	10.0	0.0	10.0	5.0	0.0	0.0	0.0	0.0	—
Ireland	—	—	—	—	8.2	6.4	6.1	9.1	10.6	17.9	13.0	15.2	19.1	6.1	24.9	20.4	40.0	—
Italy	0.2	—	—	—	2.6	2.6	3.8	4.7	3.1	3.3	4.6	5.2	5.9	6.6	5.0	6.6	4.4	—
Japan	—	0.4	0.4	0.8	1.1	1.2	1.4	1.7	2.2	2.0	2.5	3.1	3.4	4.4	4.7	4.6	5.2	4.7
Luxembourg	—	—	—	—	0.0	0.0	7.5	0.0	0.0	0.0	12.5	0.0	2.5	7.5	7.5	24.7	13.6	—
Netherlands	—	—	—	—	7.9	9.4	11.4	14.2	14.9	13.1	12.2	15.0	12.5	9.9	25.9	22.4	29.5	—
New Zealand	—	—	—	17.0	16.0	27.0	21.0	19.0	19.0	22.0	25.0	20.0	20.0	30.0	—	—	—	—
Norway	—	—	—	—	21.0	25.6	19.8	23.9	22.4	21.2	21.0	29.3	27.1	41.0	38.1	43.1	41.0	—
Portugal	—	—	—	—	0.2	0.2	0.2	0.2	0.0	0.0	0.8	1.7	2.6	3.7	5.5	12.0	13.0	14.0
Spain	—	—	—	—	0.7	1.0	1.3	1.9	2.9	5.2	7.1	9.8	9.9	12.1	21.4	21.2	22.8	—
Sweden	—	—	—	—	19.9	21.8	19.0	24.8	25.9	24.3	27.0	24.7	24.6	18.6	41.1	39.7	41.5	—
Switzerland	—	—	—	—	16.9	16.2	18.3	20.2	20.2	17.1	22.9	22.5	18.3	13.8	30.9	32.4	30.9	—
Turkey	—	—	—	—	0.1	0.1	1.0	0.5	0.4	0.3	0.3	0.7	1.0	1.5	1.1	1.3	2.9	—
United Kingdom	—	—	—	—	10.7	12.2	12.2	14.1	17.2	15.3	18.4	16.4	19.8	16.4	28.3	27.6	28.6	—
United States	—	—	—	—	15.1	17.5	16.3	18.3	17.7	19.0	20.6	21.3	23.1	26.1	29.5	32.2	37.3	36.9

SOURCE: Organization for Economic Cooperation and Development: Health Data File, 1989.

Table 50

Female life expectancy at birth, by country: 1960-87

Life expectancy in years

Country	1960	1961	1962	1963	1964	1965	1966	1967	1968	1969	1970	1971	1972	1973
Australia	74.0	74.2	–	–	–	–	74.2	–	–	–	74.2	–	–	–
Austria	71.9	72.8	72.5	72.7	73.2	73.0	73.4	73.4	73.5	73.3	73.4	73.7	74.0	74.6
Belgium	72.7	73.5	–	–	–	–	–	–	–	–	74.2	–	–	–
Canada	–	74.3	–	–	–	75.2	75.2	–	–	–	–	76.4	–	–
Denmark	74.1	–	–	–	–	–	–	75.4	75.6	75.7	76.1	76.1	–	76.6
Finland	72.4	74.5	74.1	72.6	–	–	–	–	73.6	–	74.5	74.2	74.9	75.5
France	73.6	72.4	74.1	74.1	75.1	75.0	75.5	75.4	75.2	75.1	76.1	75.9	76.2	76.3
Germany	71.9	–	–	–	–	–	–	73.6	–	–	73.6	73.8	–	–
Greece	70.4	–	–	–	–	–	–	–	–	–	–	–	–	–
Iceland	75.0	–	–	76.2	–	–	–	–	76.3	–	–	–	–	77.5
Ireland	71.8	–	–	–	–	–	–	–	–	–	73.2	–	–	–
Italy	71.8	72.3	71.2	72.3	72.9	73.0	73.6	74.2	74.3	74.7	74.6	74.9	75.9	76.0
Japan	70.3	70.8	71.2	72.3	72.9	73.0	73.6	74.2	74.3	74.7	74.7	75.6	75.9	76.0
Luxembourg	71.9	–	–	–	–	–	–	–	–	–	73.9	–	–	74.5
Netherlands	75.5	–	–	–	–	–	–	–	–	–	76.6	76.7	76.8	77.2
New Zealand	73.9	–	–	–	–	–	–	–	–	–	74.4	–	–	–
Norway	75.9	–	–	76.0	–	–	–	–	76.8	–	77.5	77.4	–	77.8
Portugal	67.2	–	–	–	–	69.3	–	69.7	–	70.0	71.0	–	71.7	–
Spain	72.2	–	–	–	–	–	–	–	–	–	75.1	–	–	–
Sweden	74.9	75.4	75.4	75.6	75.9	76.1	76.5	76.5	76.3	76.5	77.1	77.3	77.4	77.7
Switzerland	74.2	–	–	–	–	–	–	–	–	–	76.3	–	–	–
Turkey	–	–	–	–	–	–	–	–	–	–	60.9	–	–	–
United Kingdom	74.2	73.8	73.4	73.4	73.7	73.7	73.8	74.2	74.6	74.8	75.2	75.0	75.1	75.3
United States	73.3	73.6	73.4	73.4	73.7	73.7	73.8	74.2	74.6	74.8	74.7	75.0	75.1	75.3

Country	1974	1975	1976	1977	1978	1979	1980	1981	1982	1983	1984	1985	1986	1987
Australia	75.4	76.2	76.3	76.8	77.2	77.8	78.0	78.4	78.2	78.7	78.9	78.8	79.1	79.5
Austria	74.6	74.7	75.0	75.5	75.7	76.0	76.1	76.4	76.6	76.6	77.2	77.4	77.7	78.1
Belgium	75.1	75.1	75.5	75.8	76.1	76.7	76.8	76.8	76.8	–	–	–	–	–
Canada	–	–	77.5	77.5	–	–	–	78.9	–	–	79.8	–	–	–
Denmark	–	76.8	77.1	77.5	77.4	77.3	77.6	77.4	77.5	77.5	77.5	77.5	77.5	77.6
Finland	75.4	75.9	76.7	77.1	77.1	77.2	77.6	77.8	78.1	78.0	78.8	78.5	78.7	78.7
France	76.7	76.9	77.2	77.8	77.9	78.3	78.4	78.5	78.9	78.8	79.3	79.4	79.7	80.3
Germany	74.5	75.2	75.6	76.1	76.4	76.7	76.5	76.9	77.2	77.5	77.8	–	78.4	–
Greece	–	–	–	–	–	–	76.6	–	–	–	–	–	–	–
Iceland	–	–	79.2	–	79.3	–	79.7	–	79.4	–	80.2	80.2	80.4	80.0
Ireland	–	–	–	–	–	–	75.0	75.6	75.6	–	–	–	–	–
Italy	–	–	–	–	–	77.2	77.4	77.8	78.2	78.1	78.1	–	–	–
Japan	76.3	76.9	78.0	78.3	78.3	78.9	78.7	79.1	79.7	79.8	80.2	80.5	80.9	81.4
Luxembourg	–	77.0	77.4	78.0	78.3	78.9	78.7	79.1	79.4	79.5	79.5	79.6	77.9	80.1
Netherlands	77.6	77.6	78.0	78.4	78.5	78.9	79.2	79.3	79.4	79.5	79.5	79.6	79.6	80.1
New Zealand	–	–	–	75.1	78.5	78.9	76.4	76.7	76.9	76.9	77.7	76.7	77.1	–
Norway	78.0	78.1	78.4	78.7	78.7	79.2	79.0	79.4	79.4	79.6	79.5	79.4	79.7	79.6
Portugal	72.0	–	73.0	74.3	–	75.2	–	75.8	–	76.2	–	76.7	–	76.9
Spain	–	76.2	78.4	78.7	78.6	78.7	78.6	78.8	79.3	79.1	79.7	80.0	80.0	–
Sweden	77.8	77.9	77.9	78.5	78.6	78.7	78.8	79.1	79.4	79.6	79.9	79.7	80.0	80.2
Switzerland	–	78.2	78.2	78.5	78.7	78.8	79.1	79.0	79.2	79.5	79.7	80.0	80.3	–
Turkey	–	–	–	–	–	–	62.3	–	–	65.5	–	–	–	–
United Kingdom	–	–	–	77.2	77.3	77.8	76.7	76.2	–	77.2	77.4	77.4	77.5	77.6
United States	75.9	76.6	76.8	77.2	77.3	77.8	77.4	77.9	78.2	78.3	78.3	78.2	78.3	78.3

SCURCE: Organization for Economic Cooperation and Development: Health Data File, 1989.

Table 51

Male life expectancy at birth, by country: 1960-87

Life expectancy in years

Country	1960	1961	1962	1963	1964	1965	1966	1967	1968	1969	1970	1971	1972	1973
Australia	67.9	67.9	–	–	–	–	67.6	–	–	–	67.4	–	–	–
Austria	65.4	66.5	66.3	66.4	66.8	66.6	66.8	66.6	66.8	66.5	66.5	66.6	66.9	67.5
Belgium	66.7	66.7	–	–	–	–	–	–	–	–	67.8	–	–	–
Canada	–	68.4	–	–	–	–	68.8	–	–	–	–	69.3	–	–
Denmark	72.3	–	–	–	–	–	–	70.6	70.7	70.8	71.0	70.7	70.8	70.8
Finland	65.4	–	–	65.4	–	–	–	68.0	65.9	–	66.2	65.9	66.6	66.9
France	67.0	67.6	67.3	67.1	68.0	67.8	68.1	67.6	67.8	67.4	68.6	68.3	68.5	68.7
Germany	66.5	66.9	–	–	–	–	–	–	–	–	67.3	67.4	–	–
Greece	67.3	–	–	70.8	–	–	–	–	70.7	–	70.1	–	–	–
Iceland	70.7	–	–	–	–	–	–	–	–	–	–	–	–	71.6
Ireland	68.5	–	–	–	–	–	–	–	–	–	68.5	–	–	–
Italy	66.8	67.2	66.2	67.2	67.7	67.7	68.4	68.9	69.1	69.2	68.6	69.0	70.5	70.7
Japan	65.4	66.0	–	–	–	–	–	–	–	–	69.3	70.2	–	–
Luxembourg	66.1	–	–	–	–	–	–	–	–	–	67.0	–	–	67.3
Netherlands	71.6	–	–	–	–	–	–	–	–	–	70.9	71.0	70.8	71.2
New Zealand	68.7	–	–	–	–	–	–	–	–	–	68.1	–	–	–
Norway	71.4	–	–	–	–	–	–	–	–	–	71.0	71.2	–	71.5
Portugal	61.7	–	–	–	–	65.3	–	64.0	–	64.2	65.3	–	65.3	–
Spain	67.4	–	–	–	–	–	–	–	–	–	69.6	–	–	–
Sweden	71.2	71.6	71.3	71.6	71.7	71.7	71.9	71.9	71.7	71.7	72.2	72.0	72.0	72.1
Switzerland	68.7	–	–	–	–	–	–	–	–	–	70.1	–	–	–
Turkey	–	–	–	–	–	–	–	–	–	–	55.2	–	–	–
United Kingdom	68.3	67.9	–	–	–	–	–	–	–	–	68.8	68.8	–	–
United States	66.7	67.0	66.8	66.6	66.9	66.8	66.7	67.0	66.6	67.1	67.2	67.4	67.4	67.6

Country	1974	1975	1976	1977	1978	1979	1980	1981	1982	1983	1984	1985	1986	1987
Australia	68.4	69.2	69.3	69.9	70.2	70.8	70.9	71.4	71.2	72.1	72.4	72.3	72.8	73.0
Austria	67.5	67.7	68.2	68.5	68.5	68.8	69.0	69.3	69.4	69.4	70.1	70.4	71.0	71.5
Belgium	68.6	68.6	68.7	69.1	69.4	69.9	70.0	70.0	70.0	–	–	–	–	–
Canada	–	–	70.2	–	–	–	–	71.9	–	–	73.0	–	–	–
Denmark	–	71.1	71.2	71.5	71.3	71.2	71.4	71.4	71.5	71.5	71.6	71.6	71.6	71.8
Finland	66.9	67.4	67.9	68.5	68.5	68.9	69.2	69.5	70.1	70.2	70.4	70.1	70.5	70.7
France	68.9	69.0	69.2	69.7	69.8	70.1	70.2	70.4	70.7	70.7	71.2	71.3	71.5	72.0
Germany	68.1	68.6	69.0	69.1	69.4	69.9	69.7	70.2	70.5	70.8	71.2	–	71.8	–
Greece	–	–	–	–	–	–	72.2	–	73.9	–	–	–	–	–
Iceland	–	–	73.0	–	73.4	–	73.7	–	–	–	74.0	74.7	75.0	75.1
Ireland	–	–	–	–	–	–	69.5	70.1	70.1	–	–	–	–	–
Italy	–	69.7	70.1	70.3	70.5	70.6	70.7	71.1	71.5	71.4	–	–	–	–
Japan	71.2	71.8	72.2	72.7	73.0	73.5	73.3	73.8	74.2	74.2	74.5	74.8	75.2	75.6
Luxembourg	–	–	–	68.0	–	–	68.0	70.0	–	–	–	–	70.6	–
Netherlands	71.6	–	–	72.0	71.9	–	72.4	72.7	72.7	72.8	73.0	73.1	73.1	73.5
New Zealand	–	–	–	–	–	–	69.7	70.5	70.7	70.8	71.2	–	–	–
Norway	71.7	71.9	72.1	72.3	72.3	–	72.5	72.6	72.7	72.9	72.8	72.7	72.9	72.8
Portugal	65.3	–	65.4	–	67.0	–	68.9	68.9	–	69.3	–	69.7	70.6	69.9
Spain	–	70.4	–	72.3	72.3	72.3	72.5	72.6	73.2	73.0	73.2	74.0	74.0	–
Sweden	72.2	72.1	72.1	72.4	72.4	72.5	72.8	73.1	73.4	73.6	73.8	73.8	74.0	74.2
Switzerland	–	71.8	71.9	72.0	72.1	–	72.4	72.5	72.7	72.8	73.1	73.5	73.6	–
Turkey	–	–	–	–	–	–	58.3	–	–	60.8	–	–	–	–
United Kingdom	–	–	–	–	70.5	70.6	70.7	71.1	71.5	71.4	71.5	71.5	71.7	71.9
United States	68.2	68.8	69.1	69.5	69.6	70.0	69.6	70.4	70.9	71.0	71.1	71.2	71.3	71.5

Table 42

Female life expectancy at age 40, by country: 1960-87

Life expectancy in years

Country	1960	1961	1962	1963	1964	1965	1966	1967	1968	1969	1970	1971	1972	1973	1974	1975	1976	1977	1978	1979	1980	1981	1982	1983	1984	1985	1986	1987
Australia	36.9	37.0	—	—	—	—	36.9	—	—	—	36.8	—	—	—	37.7	38.4	38.4	38.8	39.2	39.7	39.9	40.1	39.9	40.3	40.5	40.4	40.7	41.0
Austria	36.2	36.6	36.3	36.3	36.7	36.3	36.7	36.5	36.6	36.3	36.5	36.7	37.0	37.4	37.4	37.4	37.5	37.8	37.8	38.2	38.2	38.4	38.6	38.5	39.1	39.0	39.4	39.7
Belgium	36.1	36.3	—	—	—	—	—	—	—	—	36.9	38.9	—	—	37.5	—	39.7	—	—	—	38.8	38.8	—	—	41.3	—	—	—
Canada	—	37.5	—	—	—	—	38.2	—	—	—	—	38.2	38.3	—	—	—	—	—	—	—	—	40.7	—	—	—	—	—	—
Denmark	36.7	—	—	35.2	—	—	—	37.6	37.8	37.9	38.2	—	38.3	37.3	—	38.6	38.8	38.8	38.6	38.7	39.2	39.0	39.1	39.1	39.1	39.1	39.0	39.1
Finland	35.3	—	—	—	—	37.7	—	—	35.8	—	36.5	38.5	36.8	—	37.3	37.7	38.3	38.6	40.0	40.1	39.0	39.0	39.4	39.3	40.0	39.7	39.9	40.0
France	37.2	—	—	—	—	—	—	—	38.1	37.8	38.4	36.8	38.7	37.3	—	39.1	39.3	38.0	—	40.3	40.3	40.4	40.7	40.6	41.1	41.1	41.4	—
Germany	35.8	36.1	—	—	—	—	36.5	36.5	—	—	36.6	36.8	—	—	—	37.4	37.7	—	—	38.5	38.6	38.8	38.9	39.2	39.4	—	39.9	—
Greece	36.4	—	—	—	—	—	—	—	38.2	—	37.8	—	—	39.4	—	—	—	—	—	—	39.0	—	—	—	—	—	—	—
Iceland	38.0	—	—	38.7	—	—	—	—	—	—	—	—	—	—	—	—	40.8	—	41.1	—	41.0	—	40.8	—	41.5	41.4	41.7	41.6
Ireland	35.4	—	—	—	—	—	—	—	—	—	35.8	—	—	—	—	—	—	—	—	36.8	36.2	37.3	37.3	—	—	—	—	—
Italy	36.7	37.0	35.2	35.9	36.1	35.9	36.6	36.8	36.9	37.2	37.9	38.1	38.1	38.1	38.3	38.4	—	—	39.2	—	39.5	39.6	39.9	39.8	39.8	—	—	—
Japan	34.9	35.1	—	—	—	—	—	—	—	—	37.0	37.9	—	36.5	38.3	38.8	39.1	39.6	40.0	40.4	40.2	40.6	41.0	41.1	41.5	41.7	42.1	42.5
Luxembourg	35.8	—	—	—	—	—	—	—	—	—	36.4	—	—	—	—	—	—	—	37.1	—	37.1	38.4	—	—	—	—	39.4	—
Netherlands	37.8	—	—	—	—	—	—	—	—	—	38.7	—	—	—	—	—	—	—	—	—	40.7	40.8	40.9	41.0	41.0	—	41.5	41.9
New Zealand	37.0	—	—	—	—	—	—	—	—	—	37.0	—	—	—	—	—	—	—	—	—	38.5	—	38.9	39.0	—	—	39.1	—
Norway	38.3	—	—	—	—	—	—	—	—	—	39.3	39.2	—	39.5	39.7	—	40.0	—	40.2	—	40.4	40.8	40.9	41.0	41.0	41.0	41.1	40.9
Portugal	36.2	—	—	—	—	—	—	—	—	—	36.6	—	—	—	—	—	36.9	—	37.9	—	—	39.8	—	38.9	—	42.5	—	39.3
Spain	36.6	—	—	—	—	—	—	—	—	—	37.8	—	—	—	—	38.6	—	—	—	—	40.5	40.6	—	—	—	41.0	—	—
Sweden	37.2	37.6	37.6	37.8	38.0	38.1	38.4	38.5	38.3	38.3	38.9	39.1	39.2	39.4	39.5	39.5	39.6	40.0	40.1	40.2	40.4	40.4	40.7	41.0	41.1	41.0	41.2	41.4
Switzerland	36.9	—	—	—	—	—	—	—	—	—	38.4	—	—	—	—	—	—	—	—	—	40.7	—	—	41.2	—	—	41.7	—
Turkey	—	—	—	—	—	—	—	—	—	—	—	—	—	—	—	—	—	—	—	—	—	—	—	—	—	—	—	—
United Kingdom	36.9	36.5	—	—	—	—	—	—	—	—	37.5	37.3	—	—	—	—	—	—	—	—	38.2	38.0	—	38.8	39.9	38.9	39.0	39.1
United States	36.7	—	—	—	—	—	—	—	—	—	37.7	—	—	—	—	—	—	—	—	—	39.8	—	40.2	40.2	40.1	40.1	40.2	40.3

SOURCE: Organization for Economic Cooperation and Development: Health Data File, 1989.

Table 53
Male life expectancy at age 40, by country: 1960-87

Life expectancy in years

Country	1960	1961	1962	1963	1964	1965	1966	1967	1968	1969	1970	1971	1972	1973
Australia	31.9	31.8	—	—	—	—	—	—	—	—	31.2	—	—	—
Austria	31.2	31.8	31.4	31.5	31.7	31.3	31.4	31.4	31.5	31.2	31.2	31.5	31.6	32.1
Belgium	31.4	31.7	—	—	—	—	31.7	—	—	—	31.6	—	—	—
Canada	—	33.0	—	—	—	—	33.0	—	—	—	—	33.2	—	—
Denmark	34.2	—	—	—	—	—	—	33.8	33.9	—	34.0	33.8	—	—
Finland	29.8	—	—	29.5	—	—	—	—	29.4	—	29.8	29.3	30.1	30.2
France	31.7	—	—	—	—	31.6	—	—	31.7	31.4	32.3	32.1	—	—
Germany	31.8	31.9	—	—	—	—	—	31.8	—	—	31.7	31.8	—	—
Greece	34.0	—	—	—	—	—	—	—	—	—	—	—	—	—
Iceland	35.2	—	—	34.9	—	—	—	—	34.6	—	35.1	—	—	35.0
Ireland	32.8	33.1	—	—	—	—	—	—	—	—	31.8	—	—	—
Italy	31.1	31.4	31.2	31.8	32.0	—	—	—	—	—	32.9	33.2	—	—
Japan	31.7	—	—	—	—	31.7	32.3	32.6	32.6	32.7	32.7	33.4	33.7	33.7
Luxembourg	—	—	—	—	—	—	—	—	—	—	30.8	—	—	31.1
Netherlands	34.8	—	—	—	—	—	—	—	—	—	33.7	—	—	—
New Zealand	32.7	—	—	—	—	—	—	—	—	—	31.9	—	—	—
Norway	35.1	—	—	—	—	—	—	—	—	—	34.1	34.3	—	34.4
Portugal	31.9	—	—	—	—	—	—	—	—	—	32.0	—	—	—
Spain	33.1	—	—	—	—	—	—	—	—	—	33.4	—	—	—
Sweden	34.5	34.9	34.5	34.7	34.8	34.8	34.8	34.7	34.7	34.6	35.0	34.7	34.7	34.7
Switzerland	32.9	—	—	—	—	—	—	—	—	—	33.6	—	—	—
Turkey	—	—	—	—	—	—	—	—	—	—	—	—	—	—
United Kingdom	31.9	31.5	—	—	—	—	—	—	—	—	31.8	31.9	—	34.0
United States	31.3	—	—	—	—	—	—	—	—	—	31.6	—	—	34.7

Country	1974	1975	1976	1977	1978	1979	1980	1981	1982	1983	1984	1985	1986	1987
Australia	31.9	32.6	32.5	33.1	33.4	33.8	33.9	34.1	34.1	34.7	35.0	35.0	35.4	35.6
Austria	31.9	31.8	32.0	32.3	32.2	32.4	32.5	32.6	32.8	32.7	33.2	33.4	33.9	34.2
Belgium	32.0	—	—	—	—	—	33.0	33.0	—	—	—	—	—	—
Canada	—	—	38.6	—	—	—	33.0	34.7	—	—	35.5	—	—	—
Denmark	—	33.8	33.6	33.8	33.8	—	33.9	33.8	33.9	33.9	34.0	34.0	34.0	34.1
Finland	30.1	30.6	30.7	31.1	31.1	31.5	31.8	32.3	32.4	32.5	—	32.4	32.9	33.1
France	—	32.4	32.5	33.0	33.0	33.1	33.3	33.4	33.7	33.7	34.0	34.0	34.3	34.1
Germany	32.0	32.1	32.3	32.5	—	32.8	32.9	33.1	33.2	33.5	33.6	34.0	34.0	33.1
Greece	—	—	—	—	—	—	35.6	—	—	—	—	—	—	—
Iceland	—	—	35.9	—	36.6	—	36.4	—	36.2	—	36.2	37.1	37.1	37.2
Ireland	—	—	—	—	—	—	32.0	—	32.6	—	—	—	—	—
Italy	—	—	—	—	—	—	33.7	—	34.1	—	—	—	—	—
Japan	34.0	34.4	34.7	35.1	35.3	35.7	35.5	35.9	36.2	36.2	36.5	—	37.0	37.4
Luxembourg	—	—	—	31.3	—	—	31.3	—	—	—	—	—	—	—
Netherlands	—	—	—	—	—	—	34.6	—	34.8	34.8	35.0	35.1	35.4	35.8
New Zealand	—	—	—	—	—	—	33.1	—	33.7	33.8	—	—	—	—
Norway	34.5	—	—	—	34.7	—	34.7	—	—	—	—	35.1	35.2	35.1
Portugal	—	—	31.0	31.3	32.1	32.6	—	—	—	33.5	—	33.7	34.2	33.8
Spain	—	33.8	—	—	—	—	35.4	35.5	—	—	—	—	—	—
Sweden	34.7	34.7	34.7	34.5	34.8	34.8	34.8	35.1	35.4	35.6	35.8	35.7	36.0	36.1
Switzerland	—	—	—	—	—	—	35.1	—	—	35.7	—	—	36.0	—
Turkey	—	—	—	—	—	—	—	—	—	—	—	—	—	—
United Kingdom	—	—	—	—	—	—	32.7	—	—	—	—	33.7	33.8	34.0
United States	—	—	—	—	—	—	33.3	—	34.0	34.1	34.3	34.3	34.5	34.7

SOURCE: [illegible]

Table 54
Female life expectancy at age 60, by country: 1960-87

Life expectancy in years

Country	1960	1961	1962	1963	1964	1965	1966	1967	1968	1969	1970	1971	1972	1973	1974	1975	1976	1977	1978	1979	1980	1981	1982	1983	1984	1985	1986	1987
Australia	19.5	19.5	–	–	–	–	–	–	–	–	19.5	–	–	–	20.2	20.8	20.7	21.1	21.4	21.8	22.0	22.1	22.1	21.9	22.4	22.3	22.5	22.8
Austria	18.6	19.0	–	18.7	19.0	18.7	19.0	18.8	18.9	18.7	18.8	19.0	19.3	19.6	19.6	19.6	19.7	20.0	20.0	20.3	20.3	20.4	20.6	20.6	21.1	21.0	21.3	21.6
Belgium	18.5	18.7	–	–	–	–	–	–	–	–	19.2	19.0	–	–	19.7	–	–	–	–	–	20.9	20.9	–	–	–	–	–	–
Canada	–	19.9	–	–	–	–	20.6	–	–	–	–	21.4	–	–	–	–	22.0	–	–	–	20.9	–	–	–	23.3	–	–	–
Denmark	19.1	–	–	–	–	–	–	20.0	20.2	20.4	20.7	20.7	20.8	–	–	21.1	21.3	21.3	21.5	21.5	21.7	21.6	21.6	21.6	21.6	21.6	21.6	21.7
Finland	17.7	–	–	17.5	–	–	–	18.0	–	–	–	18.3	18.8	–	19.4	19.7	20.1	20.4	20.4	20.5	20.7	20.7	21.0	21.1	21.6	21.3	21.6	21.7
France	19.5	–	–	–	–	20.1	–	–	20.4	–	20.8	20.9	21.1	–	–	21.3	21.5	–	22.1	22.2	22.4	22.3	22.7	22.6	23.0	23.0	23.2	23.7
Germany	18.1	18.5	–	–	–	–	–	18.9	–	–	19.0	19.1	–	19.2	19.5	19.7	19.9	20.2	–	20.6	20.7	20.8	–	21.2	21.4	–	21.7	–
Greece	18.6	–	–	–	–	–	–	–	–	–	–	–	–	–	–	–	–	–	–	–	20.6	–	–	–	–	–	–	–
Iceland	20.4	–	–	20.9	–	–	–	–	20.5	–	–	–	–	21.7	–	–	22.7	–	23.0	–	23.0	–	22.5	–	23.1	22.9	23.2	23.3
Ireland	18.3	–	–	–	–	–	–	–	–	–	18.5	–	–	–	–	–	–	–	–	–	18.8	19.5	19.5	–	–	–	–	–
Italy	19.0	19.3	–	18.5	18.7	18.5	19.0	19.2	19.2	19.5	–	–	–	–	20.3	20.8	21.5	21.4	21.7	22.2	22.4	22.3	21.7	21.5	21.5	–	–	–
Japan	17.9	17.9	–	–	–	18.5	–	19.2	19.2	19.5	–	20.2	20.2	–	–	20.8	21.0	–	–	22.1	–	22.2	22.6	22.7	23.0	23.2	23.6	24.0
Luxembourg	18.3	–	–	–	–	19.2	–	–	–	–	20.0	–	19.2	–	–	–	19.8	19.8	–	–	19.8	20.7	20.7	–	–	–	–	–
Netherlands	19.9	–	–	–	–	–	–	20.7	20.7	–	20.7	–	–	–	–	–	–	–	–	–	22.5	–	22.7	22.8	22.8	–	23.3	23.6
New Zealand	19.5	–	–	–	–	–	–	–	–	–	–	–	–	–	–	–	–	–	–	–	21.2	–	21.5	21.3	–	–	21.4	–
Norway	20.1	–	–	–	–	–	–	–	–	–	21.1	21.0	–	21.3	21.4	–	21.9	–	21.9	–	22.1	22.5	22.6	22.7	22.7	22.7	22.9	22.7
Portugal	18.6	–	–	–	–	–	–	–	–	–	–	–	–	–	–	–	19.1	–	19.9	20.6	–	21.9	–	20.9	–	21.1	–	–
Spain	19.0	–	–	–	–	–	–	–	–	–	–	–	–	–	–	20.5	–	–	–	–	–	22.3	–	–	–	23.5	–	–
Sweden	19.3	19.6	19.6	19.8	20.0	–	20.3	–	20.2	20.3	20.9	21.0	21.1	21.3	21.4	21.4	21.4	21.9	21.9	22.0	22.1	22.2	22.5	22.7	22.8	22.7	22.9	23.1
Switzerland	19.1	–	–	19.9	20.0	20.1	20.3	20.4	20.2	20.3	20.5	21.0	–	–	–	21.4	–	–	–	–	22.6	–	22.5	–	22.8	22.9	23.3	23.1
Turkey	–	–	–	–	–	–	–	–	–	–	–	–	–	–	–	–	–	–	–	–	–	–	–	–	–	–	–	–
United Kingdom	19.3	–	–	–	–	–	–	–	–	–	19.9	19.8	–	–	–	20.0	–	–	–	–	–	20.6	–	21.0	21.0	21.0	21.1	21.2
United States	19.6	20.0	19.9	19.9	20.1	20.1	20.2	20.4	20.2	20.5	20.7	–	–	–	–	–	–	–	–	22.3	22.4	–	22.6	22.6	22.5	22.4	22.5	22.5

SOURCE: Organization for Economic Cooperation and Development: Health Data File, 1989.

189

Table 55
Male life expectancy at age 60, by country: 1960-87

Life expectancy in years

Country	1960	1961	1962	1963	1964	1965	1966	1967	1968	1969	1970	1971	1972	1973
Australia	15.6	15.6	–	–	–	–	15.7	–	–	–	15.0	–	–	–
Austria	15.0	15.5	15.1	15.0	15.3	14.9	15.4	15.0	15.0	14.8	14.8	15.2	15.4	15.7
Belgium	15.4	15.5	–	–	–	–	–	–	–	–	15.2	–	–	–
Canada	–	16.8	–	–	–	–	16.8	–	–	–	–	17.0	17.0	–
Denmark	17.2	–	–	–	–	–	–	16.9	17.0	17.1	17.3	17.0	17.0	–
Finland	14.5	–	–	14.3	–	–	–	–	14.2	–	14.5	14.3	14.9	14.9
France	15.6	–	–	–	–	15.8	–	–	15.9	–	16.2	16.2	16.3	–
Germany	15.3	15.5	–	–	–	–	–	15.3	–	–	15.2	15.3	–	–
Greece	16.9	–	–	–	–	–	–	–	–	–	17.5	–	–	–
Iceland	18.6	–	–	18.6	–	–	–	–	18.0	–	–	–	–	18.6
Ireland	16.3	–	–	–	–	–	–	–	–	–	15.4	–	–	–
Italy	16.4	16.7	–	–	–	–	–	–	–	–	16.4	16.7	16.8	16.8
Japan	14.9	15.2	14.9	15.4	15.5	15.2	15.7	15.9	15.9	16.0	15.9	16.6	16.8	15.0
Luxembourg	15.9	–	–	–	–	–	–	–	–	–	14.7	–	–	–
Netherlands	17.8	–	–	–	–	–	–	–	–	–	16.9	–	–	–
New Zealand	16.3	–	–	–	–	–	–	–	–	–	15.6	–	–	–
Norway	18.0	–	–	–	–	–	–	–	–	–	17.3	17.4	–	17.5
Portugal	15.9	–	–	–	–	–	–	–	–	–	15.7	–	–	–
Spain	16.5	–	–	–	–	–	–	–	–	–	16.7	–	–	–
Sweden	17.3	17.6	17.3	17.4	17.6	17.5	17.6	17.6	17.5	17.4	17.8	17.6	17.7	17.6
Switzerland	16.2	–	–	–	–	–	–	–	–	–	16.8	–	–	–
Turkey	–	–	–	–	–	–	–	–	–	–	–	–	–	–
United Kingdom	15.3	15.0	–	–	–	–	–	–	–	–	15.2	15.3	–	–
United States	15.9	–	–	–	–	–	–	–	–	–	16.1	–	–	–

Country	1974	1975	1976	1977	1978	1979	1980	1981	1982	1983	1984	1985	1986	1987
Australia	15.7	16.3	16.1	16.6	16.7	17.1	17.2	17.3	17.2	17.7	17.8	17.8	18.1	18.3
Austria	15.6	15.6	15.8	16.1	15.9	16.2	16.3	16.4	16.6	16.5	17.0	17.0	17.4	17.6
Belgium	15.5	–	–	–	–	–	16.3	16.3	–	–	–	–	–	–
Canada	–	–	–	–	–	–	–	18.0	–	–	18.4	–	–	–
Denmark	–	17.1	17.2	17.2	17.1	17.1	17.2	17.1	17.2	17.2	17.2	17.2	17.3	17.4
Finland	14.9	15.0	15.2	15.4	15.4	15.7	15.6	16.0	16.2	16.1	16.5	16.1	16.7	16.7
France	15.6	16.5	16.7	16.0	17.1	17.1	17.3	17.3	17.6	17.6	17.9	17.9	18.0	18.4
Germany	15.5	15.6	15.8	–	–	16.3	16.4	16.5	16.6	16.8	16.9	–	17.3	–
Greece	–	–	–	–	–	–	18.2	–	18.9	–	–	–	–	–
Iceland	–	–	19.4	–	19.7	–	19.4	–	–	–	19.2	19.5	19.7	19.9
Ireland	–	–	–	–	–	–	15.5	15.9	–	–	–	–	–	–
Italy	–	–	–	–	–	–	17.1	17.0	17.2	17.0	17.1	–	–	–
Japan	17.0	17.4	17.6	18.0	18.2	18.5	18.3	18.6	19.0	19.0	19.2	19.4	19.7	19.9
Luxembourg	–	–	–	14.1	–	–	15.1	16.0	–	–	17.6	–	16.4	–
Netherlands	–	–	–	–	–	–	17.4	17.5	17.5	17.5	17.6	–	18.0	18.3
New Zealand	17.6	–	–	–	17.7	–	16.6	–	16.8	17.0	17.6	–	17.2	17.4
Norway	17.6	–	17.7	–	17.7	–	17.7	17.9	18.0	18.0	17.9	17.9	18.0	17.9
Portugal	–	17.1	15.1	–	15.9	16.3	–	17.7	–	17.1	–	17.3	–	17.4
Spain	–	–	–	–	–	–	18.4	18.6	–	18.3	–	19.5	–	–
Sweden	17.7	17.6	17.5	17.8	17.8	17.8	17.9	18.0	18.2	18.3	18.5	18.3	18.5	18.7
Switzerland	–	–	–	–	–	–	18.0	–	–	18.4	–	–	18.6	–
Turkey	–	–	–	–	–	–	–	–	–	–	–	–	–	–
United Kingdom	–	–	–	–	–	–	15.9	15.6	–	16.5	16.6	16.6	16.7	16.8
United States	–	–	–	–	–	–	17.2	–	17.7	17.8	17.9	17.9	18.0	18.2

SOURCE: Organization for Economic Cooperation and Development: Health Data File, 1989.

Table 56

Female life expectancy at age 80, by country: 1960-87

Life expectancy in years

Country	1960	1961	1962	1963	1964	1965	1966	1967	1968	1969	1970	1971	1972	1973
Australia	5.9	-	-	-	-	-	-	-	-	-	-	-	-	-
Austria	-	6.2	5.9	6.0	6.2	6.0	6.2	6.1	6.1	6.1	6.1	6.1	6.3	6.4
Belgium	-	6.1	-	-	-	-	-	-	-	-	6.3	-	-	-
Canada	-	7.0	-	-	-	-	7.4	-	-	-	-	7.9	-	-
Denmark	6.3	-	-	-	-	-	-	-	-	-	-	-	-	-
Finland	-	-	-	-	-	-	-	-	-	-	-	5.6	5.6	5.9
France	-	-	-	-	-	-	-	-	-	-	7.1	-	-	-
Germany	6.2	5.9	-	-	-	-	-	-	-	-	6.2	-	-	-
Greece	-	-	-	-	-	-	-	-	6.5	-	6.2	-	-	-
Iceland	7.1	-	-	7.1	-	-	-	-	-	-	-	-	-	7.7
Ireland	-	-	-	-	-	-	-	-	-	-	-	-	-	-
Italy	6.0	-	5.5	6.0	6.1	5.8	6.3	6.3	6.2	6.4	6.3	6.7	6.7	6.5
Japan	-	-	-	-	-	-	-	-	-	-	6.3	6.7	6.7	6.5
Luxembourg	-	-	-	-	-	-	-	-	-	-	-	-	-	-
Netherlands	-	-	-	-	-	-	-	-	-	-	-	-	-	-
New Zealand	-	-	-	-	-	-	6.7	-	-	-	-	6.8	-	-
Norway	-	-	-	-	-	-	-	-	-	-	-	-	-	-
Portugal	-	-	-	-	-	-	-	-	-	-	-	-	-	-
Spain	-	-	-	-	-	-	-	-	-	-	6.6	-	-	-
Sweden	6.2	6.4	6.2	6.4	6.6	6.6	6.7	6.8	6.4	6.6	6.9	7.0	7.1	7.2
Switzerland	-	-	-	-	-	-	-	-	-	-	-	-	-	-
Turkey	-	-	-	-	-	-	-	-	-	-	-	-	-	-
United Kingdom	-	6.3	-	-	-	-	-	-	-	-	-	6.9	-	-
United States	6.8	7.0	6.9	6.8	7.0	7.0	7.1	7.3	7.2	7.8	8.0	7.9	7.9	7.9

Country	1974	1975	1976	1977	1978	1979	1980	1981	1982	1983	1984	1985	1986	1987
Australia	7.0	7.4	7.3	7.5	7.6	7.8	8.0	8.1	7.9	8.2	8.2	8.1	8.3	8.4
Austria	6.4	6.3	6.2	6.5	6.4	6.6	6.6	6.6	6.8	6.7	7.0	6.9	7.1	7.3
Belgium	6.5	-	-	-	-	-	7.1	7.1	-	-	-	-	-	-
Canada	-	-	8.2	-	-	-	-	8.8	-	-	9.3	-	-	-
Denmark	-	7.5	7.6	7.6	-	7.7	7.7	7.7	-	7.9	7.6	7.9	8.0	8.1
Finland	5.9	6.1	6.2	6.4	6.4	6.6	6.5	6.5	6.7	6.7	-	7.2	7.5	7.5
France	-	7.2	-	-	-	-	7.7	7.6	7.9	7.7	8.0	8.0	8.1	8.4
Germany	-	-	-	-	-	-	-	-	-	-	7.3	-	7.5	-
Greece	-	-	-	-	-	-	7.6	-	-	-	-	-	-	-
Iceland	-	-	8.4	-	8.4	-	8.9	-	8.4	-	8.9	8.8	8.7	8.9
Ireland	-	-	-	-	-	-	-	-	-	-	-	-	-	-
Italy	6.5	-	-	-	-	-	-	7.3	-	-	-	-	-	-
Japan	6.5	6.9	6.9	7.2	7.4	7.7	7.3	7.5	7.7	7.7	7.9	8.0	8.3	8.5
Luxembourg	-	-	-	-	-	-	-	-	-	-	-	-	-	-
Netherlands	-	7.0	-	-	7.6	-	8.1	8.1	8.2	8.1	8.2	-	8.4	8.8
New Zealand	-	-	7.3	-	-	-	-	7.2	-	-	-	-	-	-
Norway	-	-	7.3	-	-	-	-	-	7.9	8.1	8.1	8.0	7.9	8.1
Portugal	-	-	-	-	-	-	-	-	-	-	-	-	-	6.9
Spain	-	6.6	-	-	-	-	7.6	-	-	-	-	8.3	8.2	-
Sweden	7.4	7.3	7.2	-	7.5	7.6	7.6	-	8.0	-	-	8.0	8.1	8.3
Switzerland	-	-	-	-	-	-	-	-	-	-	-	-	-	-
Turkey	-	-	-	-	-	-	-	-	-	-	-	-	-	-
United Kingdom	-	-	-	-	-	-	-	7.4	-	-	-	7.6	7.7	7.8
United States	8.2	8.7	8.7	9.0	8.9	9.2	8.6	8.9	9.1	8.9	8.9	8.8	8.8	8.8

SOURCE: Organization for Economic Cooperation and Development: Health Data File, 1989.

Table 57
Male life expectancy at age 80, by country: 1960-87

Life expectancy in years

Country	1960	1961	1962	1963	1964	1965	1966	1967	1968	1969	1970	1971	1972	1973
Australia	5.1	—	—	—	—	—	—	—	—	—	—	—	—	—
Austria	—	5.4	5.1	5.2	5.4	5.2	5.4	5.2	5.2	5.3	5.2	5.2	5.4	5.5
Belgium	—	5.3	—	—	—	—	—	—	—	—	5.4	—	—	—
Canada	—	6.2	—	—	—	—	6.5	—	—	—	—	6.4	—	—
Denmark	—	—	—	—	—	—	—	—	—	—	—	—	—	—
Finland	—	—	—	—	—	—	—	—	—	—	—	4.9	5.1	5.3
France	5.1	—	—	—	—	—	—	—	—	—	5.8	—	—	—
Germany	—	5.2	—	—	—	—	—	—	—	—	—	5.4	—	—
Greece	5.6	—	—	—	—	—	—	—	—	—	5.8	—	—	—
Iceland	6.2	—	—	6.3	—	—	—	—	6.0	—	—	—	—	6.6
Ireland	—	—	—	—	—	—	—	—	—	—	—	—	—	—
Italy	—	5.7	—	—	—	—	—	—	—	—	—	5.8	—	—
Japan	4.9	4.8	4.4	5.0	5.1	4.7	5.2	5.2	5.1	5.2	5.2	5.5	5.5	5.4
Luxembourg	—	—	—	—	—	—	—	—	—	—	—	—	—	—
Netherlands	—	—	—	—	—	—	—	—	—	—	—	—	—	—
New Zealand	—	—	—	—	—	—	5.6	—	—	—	—	—	—	—
Norway	—	—	—	—	—	—	—	—	—	—	—	5.5	—	—
Portugal	—	—	—	—	—	—	—	—	—	—	—	—	—	—
Spain	—	—	—	—	—	—	—	—	—	—	5.8	—	—	—
Sweden	5.7	5.9	5.7	5.7	5.9	5.9	6.0	6.1	5.9	6.0	6.1	6.0	6.0	6.0
Switzerland	—	—	—	—	—	—	—	—	—	—	—	—	—	—
Turkey	—	5.2	6.0	—	—	—	—	—	—	—	—	5.5	—	—
United Kingdom	—	—	—	—	—	—	—	—	—	—	—	—	—	—
United States	6.0	6.1	6.0	5.9	6.2	6.2	6.2	6.4	6.3	6.5	6.6	6.4	6.4	6.4

Country	1974	1975	1976	1977	1978	1979	1980	1981	1982	1983	1984	1985	1986	1987
Australia	5.5	5.8	5.7	6.0	6.1	6.3	6.4	6.3	6.2	6.4	6.5	6.3	6.6	6.6
Austria	5.4	5.2	5.4	5.5	5.3	5.5	5.5	5.4	5.6	5.6	5.9	5.8	6.0	6.2
Belgium	5.5	—	—	—	—	—	—	5.7	—	—	—	—	—	—
Canada	—	—	6.4	—	—	—	5.7	6.9	—	—	7.0	—	—	—
Denmark	—	6.2	—	6.3	6.3	6.3	—	6.2	—	6.3	6.3	6.3	6.4	6.5
Finland	5.1	5.3	5.3	5.2	5.3	5.6	5.4	5.6	5.7	5.6	6.2	5.7	6.1	6.1
France	—	5.8	—	—	—	—	6.1	—	6.2	6.1	6.3	6.2	6.4	6.6
Germany	—	—	—	—	—	—	—	—	—	—	5.9	—	6.0	—
Greece	—	—	—	—	—	—	—	—	—	—	—	—	—	—
Iceland	—	—	7.4	—	7.6	—	6.7	—	7.1	—	7.5	7.6	7.4	7.5
Ireland	—	—	—	—	—	—	7.0	—	—	—	—	—	—	—
Italy	—	—	—	—	—	—	—	5.9	6.0	5.9	6.0	6.2	6.7	6.9
Japan	5.4	5.8	5.8	6.0	6.0	6.3	6.1	6.2	6.5	6.4	6.5	6.5	6.5	6.7
Luxembourg	—	—	—	—	—	—	—	—	—	—	—	—	—	—
Netherlands	—	5.9	—	—	6.3	—	6.5	6.5	6.5	6.4	6.4	—	6.2	6.5
New Zealand	—	—	5.7	—	—	—	—	5.5	—	—	—	—	—	—
Norway	—	—	—	—	—	—	—	—	6.4	6.5	6.5	6.5	6.5	6.4
Portugal	—	—	—	—	—	—	—	—	—	—	—	—	—	—
Spain	—	5.9	—	—	—	—	6.6	—	—	—	—	7.0	—	5.8
Sweden	6.1	6.1	6.0	6.1	6.1	6.1	6.1	6.2	6.3	6.3	6.5	6.3	6.4	6.5
Switzerland	—	—	—	—	—	—	—	—	—	—	—	—	—	—
Turkey	—	—	—	—	—	—	—	—	—	—	—	—	—	—
United Kingdom	—	—	—	—	—	—	—	5.7	—	—	5.9	5.9	5.9	6.0
United States	6.6	6.8	6.8	6.9	6.9	7.1	6.7	6.9	7.0	6.9	6.9	6.8	6.9	6.9

Table 58

Infant mortality, by country: 1960-87

Percent of live births

Country	1960	1961	1962	1963	1964	1965	1966	1967	1968	1969	1970	1971	1972	1973
Australia	2.01	1.95	2.04	1.95	1.91	1.35	1.82	1.83	1.78	1.79	1.79	1.73	1.67	1.65
Austria	3.75	3.27	3.28	3.13	2.92	2.33	2.81	2.64	2.55	2.55	2.59	2.61	2.52	2.38
Belgium	3.12	2.81	2.75	2.72	2.54	2.37	2.47	2.29	2.17	2.12	2.11	2.04	1.88	1.77
Canada	2.73	2.72	2.76	2.63	2.47	2.36	2.31	2.20	2.08	1.93	1.88	1.75	1.71	1.55
Denmark	2.15	2.18	2.01	1.91	1.87	1.87	1.69	1.58	1.64	1.48	1.42	1.35	1.22	1.15
Finland	2.10	2.08	2.05	1.82	1.70	1.76	1.50	1.48	1.44	1.43	1.32	1.27	1.20	1.06
France	2.74	2.57	2.57	2.56	2.34	2.19	2.17	2.07	2.04	1.96	1.82	1.72	1.60	1.54
Germany	3.38	3.20	2.93	2.71	2.53	2.38	2.36	2.28	2.26	2.32	2.34	2.31	2.24	2.27
Greece	4.01	3.98	4.04	3.93	3.58	3.43	3.40	3.43	3.44	3.18	2.96	2.69	2.73	2.41
Iceland	1.30	1.95	1.72	1.70	1.75	1.50	1.36	1.34	1.40	1.16	1.32	1.29	1.13	0.96
Ireland	2.93	3.05	2.91	2.66	2.67	2.53	2.50	2.44	2.10	2.06	1.95	1.80	1.80	1.80
Italy	4.39	4.07	4.18	4.01	3.61	3.60	3.47	3.32	3.27	3.08	2.96	2.85	2.70	2.62
Japan	3.07	2.86	2.64	2.32	2.04	1.85	1.98	1.49	1.53	1.42	1.31	1.24	1.17	1.13
Luxembourg	3.15	2.62	3.11	2.86	2.98	2.40	2.68	2.04	1.70	1.75	2.49	2.25	1.40	1.53
Netherlands	1.79	1.70	1.70	1.58	1.48	1.44	1.47	1.34	1.36	1.32	1.27	1.21	1.17	1.15
New Zealand	2.26	2.28	–	–	–	–	–	–	–	–	1.68	–	–	–
Norway	1.89	–	–	–	–	–	–	–	–	–	1.27	–	–	–
Portugal	7.75	8.88	7.86	7.31	6.90	6.49	6.47	5.92	6.11	5.58	5.51	5.19	4.14	4.48
Spain	4.37	4.62	4.16	4.06	3.92	3.78	3.60	3.40	3.24	3.02	2.81	2.81	2.29	2.15
Sweden	1.66	1.58	1.54	1.54	1.42	1.33	1.26	1.29	1.31	1.17	1.10	1.11	1.08	0.99
Switzerland	2.11	2.10	2.12	2.05	1.90	1.78	1.71	1.75	1.61	1.54	1.44	1.33	1.33	1.32
Turkey	–	–	–	18.00	–	15.70	–	–	13.30	–	12.30	–	–	12.00
United Kingdom	2.25	2.21	2.23	2.18	2.06	1.96	1.96	1.88	1.87	1.86	1.85	1.79	1.75	1.72
United States	2.60	–	–	–	–	2.47	–	–	–	–	2.00	–	1.65	1.77

Country	1974	1975	1976	1977	1978	1979	1980	1981	1982	1983	1984	1985	1986	1987
Australia	1.61	1.43	1.38	1.25	1.22	1.14	1.07	1.00	1.03	0.96	0.92	0.99	0.88	0.87
Austria	2.35	2.05	1.82	1.68	1.50	1.47	1.43	1.27	1.28	1.19	1.14	1.12	1.03	0.98
Belgium	1.74	1.61	1.53	1.36	1.33	1.23	1.21	1.15	1.11	1.05	1.00	0.94	0.97	0.97
Canada	1.50	1.43	1.35	1.24	1.20	1.09	1.04	0.96	0.91	0.85	0.81	0.80	0.79	–
Denmark	1.07	1.04	1.02	0.87	0.88	0.88	0.84	0.79	0.82	0.77	0.77	0.78	0.82	0.83
Finland	1.10	1.00	0.92	0.88	0.77	0.76	0.76	0.66	0.61	0.61	0.63	0.63	0.59	0.62
France	1.46	1.36	1.25	1.15	1.06	1.01	1.01	0.96	0.93	0.89	0.83	0.81	0.80	0.76
Germany	2.11	1.97	1.74	1.54	1.47	1.36	1.27	1.16	1.09	1.02	0.96	0.89	0.87	0.83
Greece	2.39	2.40	2.25	2.04	1.93	1.87	1.79	1.63	1.51	1.46	1.43	1.41	1.22	1.17
Iceland	1.17	1.25	0.77	0.95	1.13	0.54	0.77	0.60	0.71	0.62	0.61	0.57	0.54	0.72
Ireland	1.78	1.75	1.55	1.55	1.49	1.24	1.11	1.06	1.05	0.98	1.01	0.89	0.87	0.74
Italy	2.29	2.22	1.95	1.81	1.69	1.57	1.43	1.41	1.29	1.24	1.17	1.09	0.98	0.96
Japan	1.08	1.00	0.93	0.89	0.84	0.79	0.75	0.71	0.66	0.62	0.60	0.55	0.52	0.50
Luxembourg	1.35	1.48	1.79	1.06	1.06	1.30	1.15	1.38	1.21	1.12	1.17	0.90	0.80	0.93
Netherlands	1.13	1.06	1.07	0.95	0.96	0.87	0.86	0.83	0.83	0.84	0.70	0.69	0.64	–
New Zealand	–	–	–	–	–	1.26	1.29	1.17	1.17	1.25	1.16	1.08	1.12	0.98
Norway	–	1.11	1.05	0.92	0.86	0.88	0.81	0.75	0.81	0.79	0.83	0.85	0.78	0.84
Portugal	3.79	3.89	3.34	3.03	2.91	2.60	2.43	2.18	1.98	1.92	1.67	1.78	1.58	1.42
Spain	1.99	1.89	1.71	1.60	1.53	1.43	1.23	1.25	1.13	1.09	0.94	–	0.87	–
Sweden	0.96	0.86	0.83	0.80	0.78	0.75	0.69	0.69	0.68	0.70	0.64	0.68	0.59	0.61
Switzerland	1.25	1.07	1.07	0.98	0.88	0.85	0.91	0.76	0.77	0.76	0.71	0.69	0.68	0.68
Turkey	–	–	–	–	11.00	–	9.00	–	9.50	–	8.30	–	–	–
United Kingdom	1.68	1.60	1.45	1.41	1.32	1.28	1.21	1.12	1.10	1.01	0.96	0.94	0.95	0.91
United States	1.67	1.61	1.52	1.41	1.38	1.31	1.26	1.19	1.12	1.09	1.07	1.06	1.04	1.00

SOURCE: Organization for Economic Cooperation and Development: Health Data File, 1989.

Table 59
Perinatal mortality, by country: 1960-87

Percent of live and still births

Country	1960	1961	1962	1963	1964	1965	1966	1967	1968	1969	1970	1971	1972	1973
Australia	2.90	—	—	—	2.51	2.48	2.52	2.43	2.26	2.26	2.25	2.11	2.34	2.33
Austria	3.50	3.18	3.18	3.19	3.01	2.95	2.95	2.74	2.69	2.70	2.70	2.59	2.59	2.46
Belgium	3.19	3.01	2.99	2.88	3.03	2.73	2.74	2.64	2.47	2.48	2.33	2.29	2.20	2.12
Canada	2.84	2.81	2.86	2.80	2.74	2.60	2.55	2.47	2.37	2.23	2.18	2.01	1.90	1.76
Denmark	2.62	2.69	2.49	2.43	2.31	2.39	2.16	1.95	1.89	1.87	1.79	1.74	1.61	1.45
Finland	2.75	2.75	2.62	2.36	2.37	2.36	2.06	2.03	1.91	1.88	1.70	1.67	1.71	1.48
France	3.13	2.98	2.98	2.94	2.86	2.77	2.72	2.67	2.57	2.50	2.33	2.25	2.13	2.03
Germany	3.58	3.41	3.26	3.07	2.86	2.86	2.76	2.69	2.64	2.66	2.64	2.53	2.39	2.30
Greece	2.64	2.59	2.72	2.86	2.88	2.94	3.02	2.96	2.86	2.91	2.74	2.79	2.73	2.55
Iceland	1.97	2.78	2.16	2.41	2.27	2.40	2.06	2.07	2.36	1.83	1.85	1.78	1.95	1.62
Ireland	3.77	3.61	3.44	3.20	3.18	3.00	2.86	2.85	2.66	2.58	2.42	2.28	2.32	2.29
Italy	4.19	4.03	3.99	3.94	3.73	3.65	3.61	3.41	3.34	3.19	3.12	3.04	2.92	2.83
Japan	3.73	3.68	3.49	3.27	3.02	2.77	2.82	2.44	2.28	2.14	2.03	1.92	1.79	1.70
Luxembourg	3.23	3.02	3.08	2.71	3.01	3.06	2.30	2.37	2.43	2.13	2.47	2.16	1.60	1.77
Netherlands	2.66	2.59	2.57	2.45	2.34	2.31	2.24	2.11	2.02	1.96	1.86	1.76	1.66	1.63
New Zealand	2.70	—	—	—	—	—	—	—	—	—	2.00	—	—	—
Norway	2.40	—	—	—	—	—	—	—	—	—	1.90	—	—	—
Portugal	4.11	4.09	4.26	3.96	3.86	3.86	3.84	3.85	3.87	3.86	3.70	3.82	3.45	3.31
Spain	3.66	—	—	—	—	—	—	—	—	—	2.55	—	—	—
Sweden	2.62	2.42	2.36	2.31	2.16	1.99	1.88	1.88	1.83	1.62	1.64	1.56	1.43	1.40
Switzerland	—	—	—	—	—	—	—	—	—	—	1.81	—	—	—
Turkey	—	—	—	—	—	—	—	—	—	—	—	—	—	—
United Kingdom	3.36	3.27	3.15	3.00	2.88	2.76	2.67	2.58	2.50	2.37	2.38	2.26	2.21	2.13
United States	2.86	—	—	—	—	—	—	—	—	—	2.30	—	—	—

Country	1974	1975	1976	1977	1978	1979	1980	1981	1982	1983	1984	1985	1986	1987
Australia	2.33	2.02	2.02	1.79	1.61	1.50	1.41	1.32	1.34	1.22	1.19	1.18	1.15	1.06
Austria	2.30	2.12	1.82	1.73	1.49	1.41	1.41	1.20	1.13	1.12	1.02	1.01	0.91	0.76
Belgium	2.05	2.01	1.80	—	1.54	1.47	1.41	1.32	1.26	1.22	1.14	—	—	—
Canada	1.67	—	—	1.38	1.28	1.18	1.09	1.07	1.01	0.95	0.87	0.87	0.84	0.88
Denmark	1.31	1.33	1.26	1.06	1.08	0.99	0.90	0.90	0.87	0.90	0.84	0.81	0.84	0.88
Finland	1.46	1.24	1.14	1.12	0.94	0.93	0.84	0.79	0.74	0.74	0.76	0.73	0.64	0.69
France	1.93	1.81	1.67	1.56	1.47	1.38	1.29	1.23	1.19	1.14	1.12	—	—	—
Germany	2.14	1.93	1.71	1.49	1.37	1.26	1.16	1.05	0.96	0.93	0.86	0.79	0.76	0.73
Greece	2.58	2.55	2.51	2.26	2.16	2.13	2.03	1.84	1.68	1.65	1.68	1.58	1.47	1.45
Iceland	1.67	1.56	0.93	1.14	1.31	0.80	0.88	0.76	0.90	0.73	0.61	0.52	0.82	0.86
Ireland	2.20	2.15	1.97	1.92	1.76	1.62	1.48	1.34	1.35	1.37	1.37	1.23	—	—
Italy	2.61	2.41	2.26	2.08	1.99	1.85	1.75	1.70	1.60	1.52	1.45	—	—	—
Japan	1.61	1.52	1.40	1.34	1.24	1.19	1.11	1.03	0.96	0.89	0.83	0.76	0.70	0.66
Luxembourg	1.67	1.60	1.80	1.06	1.20	1.22	0.98	1.11	1.20	0.98	0.88	0.99	0.72	—
Netherlands	1.54	1.39	1.44	1.29	1.24	1.19	1.10	1.07	1.01	1.01	1.00	0.99	0.97	0.92
New Zealand	—	—	—	—	—	1.21	1.22	1.05	1.06	0.99	0.86	0.89	0.87	0.79
Norway	—	—	1.33	1.32	1.11	1.18	1.11	0.96	0.98	0.99	0.89	0.93	0.80	0.74
Portugal	3.22	3.13	2.93	2.89	2.69	2.55	2.39	2.27	2.21	2.11	1.98	1.97	1.82	1.67
Spain	—	2.11	1.98	1.87	1.73	1.65	1.44	1.44	1.29	1.21	1.12	—	—	—
Sweden	1.32	1.13	1.08	1.02	0.95	0.92	0.87	0.77	0.78	0.73	0.73	0.73	0.75	0.71
Switzerland	—	—	—	—	—	1.08	0.95	0.91	0.90	0.91	0.81	0.83	0.76	—
Turkey	—	—	—	—	—	—	—	—	—	—	—	—	—	—
United Kingdom	2.08	1.97	1.80	1.73	1.56	1.46	1.34	1.20	1.13	1.04	1.01	0.96	0.90	0.88
United States	—	1.77	1.67	1.54	1.46	1.38	1.32	1.26	1.23	1.15	1.10	1.07	1.03	1.00

SOURCE: Organization for Economic Cooperation and Development, Health Data File, 1989.

194

Table 80

Crude mortality rates, by country: 1960-87

Deaths per 1,000 population

Country	1960	1961	1962	1963	1964	1965	1966	1967	1968	1969	1970	1971	1972	1973
Australia	8.5	8.4	8.6	8.8	9.0	8.7	9.0	8.6	9.1	8.5	8.9	8.4	8.2	8.2
Austria	12.7	12.1	12.7	12.8	12.3	13.0	12.5	12.9	12.9	13.3	13.2	13.0	12.6	12.2
Belgium	12.3	11.5	12.1	12.4	11.6	12.1	12.1	12.0	12.6	12.4	12.3	12.3	12.0	12.1
Canada	7.8	7.6	7.7	7.7	7.5	7.5	7.4	7.3	7.3	7.3	7.3	7.3	7.4	7.4
Denmark	9.6	9.3	9.6	9.8	9.9	10.0	10.2	9.9	9.6	9.8	9.7	9.8	10.2	10.1
Finland	9.0	9.2	9.5	9.3	9.4	9.6	9.6	9.5	9.7	10.0	9.6	9.9	9.5	9.2
France	11.3	10.7	11.3	11.5	10.6	11.0	10.6	10.9	11.0	11.3	10.6	10.8	10.6	10.7
Germany	11.5	11.1	11.3	11.6	11.0	11.4	11.5	11.5	12.1	12.2	11.9	11.9	11.8	11.8
Greece	7.3	7.6	7.9	7.9	8.1	7.8	7.9	8.2	8.3	8.2	8.4	8.4	8.6	8.7
Iceland	6.6	7.0	6.8	7.2	7.0	6.7	7.1	7.0	6.9	7.2	7.1	7.3	6.9	7.0
Ireland	11.7	12.4	12.0	11.9	11.5	11.5	12.1	10.7	11.3	11.6	11.4	10.3	11.1	10.6
Italy	9.5	9.1	9.9	10.0	9.4	9.9	9.4	9.6	10.0	9.9	9.8	9.5	9.5	9.9
Japan	7.6	7.4	7.5	7.0	6.9	7.1	6.8	6.8	6.8	6.8	6.9	6.6	6.5	6.6
Luxembourg	11.7	11.3	12.4	12.0	11.8	12.3	12.2	12.2	12.2	12.4	12.4	12.8	11.8	11.9
Netherlands	7.5	7.5	7.9	8.0	7.6	7.9	8.1	7.9	8.2	8.3	8.4	8.3	8.5	8.2
New Zealand	8.7	8.9	8.7	8.6	8.8	8.6	8.9	8.4	8.7	8.6	8.8	8.3	8.4	8.3
Norway	9.2	9.1	9.3	10.1	9.4	9.4	9.6	9.5	9.9	9.8	10.0	10.0	9.9	10.1
Portugal	10.5	11.1	10.7	10.8	10.6	10.5	11.0	10.5	10.4	11.1	10.3	11.0	10.0	10.6
Spain	8.6	8.3	8.7	8.7	8.4	8.3	8.3	8.3	8.4	8.8	8.3	8.8	8.1	8.5
Sweden	10.0	9.8	10.2	10.1	10.0	10.1	10.1	10.1	10.4	10.5	10.0	10.2	10.4	10.5
Switzerland	9.6	9.3	9.8	9.9	9.3	9.5	9.4	9.1	9.3	9.4	9.2	9.3	8.9	9.0
Turkey	–	–	–	–	–	–	–	–	–	–	–	–	–	–
United Kingdom	11.5	11.9	11.9	12.2	11.3	11.5	11.8	11.2	11.9	11.9	11.7	11.5	12.0	11.9
United States	9.4	9.2	9.4	9.5	9.3	9.4	9.5	9.3	9.7	9.5	9.3	9.2	9.3	9.3

Country	1974	1975	1976	1977	1978	1979	1980	1981	1982	1983	1984	1985	1986	1987
Australia	8.4	7.8	8.0	7.6	7.5	7.3	7.4	7.2	7.5	7.1	7.2	7.4	7.2	7.2
Austria	12.4	12.7	12.6	12.2	12.5	12.2	12.2	12.3	12.1	12.3	11.7	11.9	11.5	11.2
Belgium	11.9	12.1	12.1	11.4	11.7	11.4	11.6	11.5	11.5	11.7	11.3	11.5	11.4	11.4
Canada	7.4	7.3	7.3	7.2	7.2	7.1	7.2	7.0	7.1	7.0	7.0	7.2	7.3	7.2
Denmark	10.1	10.1	10.6	10.0	10.4	10.7	10.9	10.9	10.8	11.2	11.2	11.3	11.3	11.3
Finland	9.6	9.3	9.5	9.3	9.2	9.2	9.2	9.1	8.9	9.2	9.2	9.8	9.6	9.7
France	10.5	10.6	10.5	10.1	10.2	10.1	10.1	10.2	9.9	10.2	9.9	10.0	9.9	9.5
Germany	11.7	12.2	11.9	11.5	11.8	11.6	11.6	11.7	11.6	11.7	11.4	11.5	11.5	11.2
Greece	8.5	8.8	8.9	9.0	8.6	8.6	9.0	8.8	8.8	9.1	8.9	9.4	9.2	9.5
Iceland	6.9	6.5	6.1	6.5	6.4	6.6	6.7	7.2	6.8	7.0	6.6	6.8	6.6	7.0
Ireland	10.7	10.6	10.1	10.0	10.1	10.0	9.6	9.2	9.4	9.4	9.1	9.3	9.6	8.8
Italy	9.6	10.0	10.0	9.8	9.6	9.6	9.9	9.6	9.5	9.9	9.4	9.6	9.5	9.3
Japan	6.5	6.3	6.3	6.1	6.1	6.0	6.2	6.1	6.0	6.2	6.2	6.3	6.2	6.2
Luxembourg	12.0	12.2	12.5	11.3	11.6	11.0	11.2	11.2	11.5	11.2	11.2	10.9	10.9	10.8
Netherlands	8.0	8.3	8.3	7.9	8.2	8.0	8.0	8.1	8.2	8.2	8.3	8.5	8.6	8.3
New Zealand	8.1	8.0	7.9	8.2	7.9	7.9	8.5	7.8	8.0	8.1	7.6	8.2	8.2	8.1
Norway	9.8	10.0	9.9	9.9	10.1	10.3	10.3	9.8	9.9	10.2	10.4	10.6	10.0	10.0
Portugal	10.5	10.2	10.5	9.8	9.8	9.4	9.9	9.8	9.4	9.6	9.6	9.6	9.4	9.3
Spain	8.3	8.3	8.3	8.0	8.0	7.8	7.7	7.6	7.4	7.7	7.7	8.0	7.9	–
Sweden	10.6	10.8	11.0	10.7	10.8	11.0	11.1	11.1	10.9	10.9	10.8	11.3	11.1	11.1
Switzerland	8.8	8.9	9.1	8.9	9.2	9.0	9.3	9.4	9.3	9.5	9.2	9.3	9.2	9.2
Turkey	–	–	–	–	–	7.0	7.5	7.3	9.1	9.0	8.7	9.0	8.8	8.5
United Kingdom	11.9	11.8	12.1	11.7	11.9	12.0	11.7	11.7	11.8	11.7	11.4	11.9	11.6	11.3
United States	9.0	8.7	8.7	8.6	8.6	8.4	8.7	8.6	8.5	8.6	8.6	8.7	8.7	8.7

SOURCE: Organization for Economic Cooperation and Development: Health Data File, 1989.

Table 61
Population in thousands, by country: 1960-87

Mid-year estimates

Country	1960	1961	1962	1963	1964	1965	1966	1967	1968	1969	1970	1971	1972	1973
Australia	10,547	10,774	10,986	11,196	11,418	11,648	11,865	12,074	12,300	12,553	12,817	13,067	13,304	13,505
Austria	7,048	7,086	7,130	7,176	7,224	7,271	7,322	7,377	7,415	7,441	7,467	7,500	7,544	7,586
Belgium	9,153	9,184	9,221	9,290	9,378	9,464	9,528	9,581	9,619	9,646	9,651	9,673	9,709	9,739
Canada	17,909	18,269	18,615	18,965	19,325	19,678	20,048	20,412	20,729	21,028	21,324	21,595	21,822	22,072
Denmark	4,581	4,612	4,647	4,684	4,720	4,757	4,797	4,839	4,867	4,893	4,929	4,963	4,992	5,022
Finland	4,430	4,461	4,491	4,523	4,549	4,564	4,581	4,606	4,626	4,624	4,606	4,612	4,640	4,666
France	45,684	46,163	46,998	47,816	48,310	48,758	49,164	49,548	49,915	50,315	50,772	51,251	51,701	52,118
Germany	55,585	56,175	56,837	57,389	57,971	58,619	59,148	59,286	59,500	60,067	60,651	61,302	61,672	61,976
Greece	8,327	8,398	8,448	8,480	8,510	8,551	8,614	8,716	8,741	8,773	8,793	8,831	8,889	8,929
Iceland	176	179	182	185	189	192	196	199	201	203	205	206	209	212
Ireland	2,834	2,819	2,830	2,850	2,864	2,876	2,884	2,900	2,913	2,926	2,950	2,978	3,024	3,073
Italy	50,198	50,524	50,844	51,199	51,601	51,988	52,332	52,667	52,987	53,317	53,661	54,005	54,400	54,779
Japan	93,260	94,100	94,980	95,890	96,900	97,950	98,860	99,920	101,070	102,320	103,720	104,750	107,180	108,660
Luxembourg	314	317	321	324	328	332	334	335	336	338	340	342	347	351
Netherlands	11,486	11,639	11,806	11,966	12,127	12,292	12,455	12,597	12,730	12,878	13,039	13,194	13,329	13,439
New Zealand	2,377	2,427	2,485	2,537	2,589	2,635	2,683	2,728	2,754	2,780	2,820	2,864	2,913	2,971
Norway	3,585	3,615	3,639	3,667	3,694	3,723	3,753	3,785	3,819	3,851	3,879	3,903	3,933	3,961
Portugal	9,037	9,032	9,020	9,082	9,123	9,129	9,109	9,103	9,115	9,097	9,044	8,990	8,970	8,976
Spain	30,583	30,904	31,158	31,430	31,741	32,085	32,453	32,850	33,240	33,566	33,876	34,190	34,498	34,810
Sweden	7,480	7,520	7,562	7,604	7,662	7,734	7,807	7,869	7,912	7,968	8,043	8,098	8,122	8,137
Switzerland	5,362	5,512	5,666	5,789	5,887	5,943	5,996	6,063	6,132	6,212	6,267	6,343	6,401	6,441
Turkey	27,755	28,447	29,156	29,883	30,628	31,391	32,192	33,013	33,855	34,719	35,605	36,554	37,502	38,451
United Kingdom	52,373	52,807	53,292	53,625	53,991	54,350	54,643	54,959	55,214	55,461	55,632	55,907	56,079	56,210
United States	180,671	183,691	186,538	189,242	191,889	194,303	196,560	198,712	200,706	202,677	205,052	207,661	209,896	211,909

Country	1974	1975	1976	1977	1978	1979	1980	1981	1982	1983	1984	1985	1986	1987
Australia	13,723	13,893	14,033	14,192	14,358	14,514	14,695	14,923	15,184	15,394	15,579	15,788	16,018	16,263
Austria	7,599	7,579	7,566	7,568	7,562	7,549	7,549	7,565	7,574	7,552	7,553	7,558	7,566	7,576
Belgium	9,768	9,795	9,811	9,822	9,830	9,837	9,847	9,853	9,856	9,855	9,855	9,858	9,862	9,868
Canada	22,395	22,727	23,027	23,295	23,535	23,768	24,070	24,366	24,657	24,905	24,995	25,181	25,374	25,652
Denmark	5,045	5,060	5,073	5,088	5,097	5,117	5,122	5,124	5,119	5,116	5,112	5,114	5,121	5,130
Finland	4,691	4,712	4,726	4,739	4,753	4,765	4,780	4,800	4,827	4,856	4,882	4,902	4,918	4,932
France	52,460	52,699	52,909	53,145	53,376	53,606	53,880	54,182	54,480	54,729	54,946	55,170	55,393	55,627
Germany	62,054	61,829	61,531	61,400	61,327	61,359	61,566	61,682	61,638	61,423	61,175	61,024	61,066	61,077
Greece	8,962	9,046	9,167	9,309	9,430	9,548	9,642	9,730	9,790	9,847	9,900	9,934	9,966	9,998
Iceland	215	218	220	222	223	226	228	231	234	237	239	241	243	246
Ireland	3,124	3,177	3,228	3,272	3,314	3,368	3,401	3,443	3,483	3,505	3,529	3,540	3,541	3,542
Italy	55,130	55,441	55,701	55,929	56,127	56,292	56,434	56,508	56,639	56,836	57,005	57,141	57,246	57,345
Japan	110,158	111,520	112,768	113,880	114,920	115,880	116,800	117,650	118,450	119,260	120,020	120,750	121,490	122,091
Luxembourg	355	359	361	361	362	363	364	366	366	366	366	367	370	372
Netherlands	13,545	13,666	13,774	13,856	13,942	14,038	14,150	14,247	14,313	14,367	14,424	14,491	14,572	14,671
New Zealand	3,032	3,087	3,116	3,128	3,129	3,138	3,144	3,157	3,183	3,226	3,258	3,272	3,279	3,309
Norway	3,985	4,007	4,026	4,043	4,060	4,073	4,087	4,100	4,116	4,128	4,141	4,153	4,169	4,184
Portugal	9,098	9,426	9,666	9,736	9,802	9,857	9,851	9,892	9,969	10,050	10,129	10,185	10,230	10,280
Spain	35,147	35,515	35,937	36,367	36,778	37,108	37,386	37,751	37,961	38,180	38,342	38,505	38,668	38,830
Sweden	8,160	8,192	8,222	8,251	8,275	8,294	8,311	8,324	8,327	8,329	8,337	8,350	8,370	8,399
Switzerland	6,460	6,404	6,333	6,316	6,333	6,351	6,385	6,429	6,467	6,482	6,505	6,533	6,573	6,619
Turkey	39,399	40,348	40,925	41,835	42,774	43,741	44,737	45,757	46,780	47,804	49,420	50,664	51,731	52,893
United Kingdom	56,224	56,215	56,206	56,179	56,167	56,227	56,314	56,379	56,335	56,377	56,488	56,618	56,763	56,930
United States	213,854	215,973	218,035	220,239	222,585	225,055	227,757	230,138	232,520	234,799	237,011	239,279	241,625	243,934

Table 62
Employment in thousands, by country: 1960-87

Mid-year estimates

Country	1973	1972	1971	1970	1969	1968	1967	1966	1965	1964	1963	1962	1961	1960
Australia	5,783	5,610	5,516	5,395	5,183	5,136	5,010	4,891	4,733	4,587	4,347	4,226	4,127	4,115
Austria	3,159	3,115	3,092	3,059	3,052	3,058	3,099	3,150	3,176	3,198	3,203	3,225	3,241	3,223
Belgium	3,774	3,725	3,729	3,691	3,630	3,670	3,573	3,585	3,567	3,561	3,513	3,488	3,433	3,404
Canada	8,860	8,447	8,214	8,034	7,952	7,719	7,583	7,377	6,974	6,728	6,498	6,351	6,176	6,084
Denmark	2,375	2,346	2,298	2,284	2,268	2,248	2,223	2,237	2,226	2,186	2,142	2,116	2,084	2,054
Finland	2,253	2,209	2,188	2,202	2,156	2,124	2,153	2,192	2,188	2,163	2,165	2,155	2,165	2,124
France	21,303	21,037	20,934	20,856	20,596	20,308	20,350	20,298	20,148	20,086	19,867	19,709	19,713	19,715
Germany	26,849	26,661	26,721	26,560	26,228	25,826	25,804	26,673	26,755	26,604	26,581	26,518	26,426	26,063
Greece	3,172	3,157	3,143	3,171	3,138	3,149	3,186	3,225	3,309	3,278	3,320	3,367	3,424	3,386
Iceland	90	88	86	81	78	78	77	77	76	75	72	71	69	68
Ireland	1,057	1,050	1,055	1,053	1,066	1,063	1,060	1,066	1,069	1,071	1,066	1,060	1,053	1,055
Italy	20,243	19,816	19,928	19,949	19,818	19,723	19,732	19,510	19,812	20,161	20,277	20,592	20,812	20,762
Japan	56,348	55,102	54,818	54,434	54,300	53,920	53,120	52,170	51,200	–	–	–	–	48,200
Luxembourg	151	148	–	140	140	137	136	137	137	–	–	–	–	132
Netherlands	4,685	4,683	4,724	4,709	4,641	4,564	4,523	4,537	4,502	4,464	4,387	4,328	4,243	4,182
New Zealand	1,154	1,115	1,103	1,090	1,058	1,035	1,051	1,026	990	957	929	911	895	875
Norway	1,571	1,565	1,558	1,547	1,528	1,519	1,509	1,499	1,497	1,485	1,475	1,460	1,423	1,401
Portugal	3,303	3,331	3,352	3,362	3,188	3,208	3,228	3,248	3,268	3,088	3,107	3,127	3,153	3,173
Spain	12,952	12,642	12,609	12,539	12,410	12,280	12,051	11,944	11,993	11,485	–	–	–	11,641
Sweden	3,932	3,918	3,905	3,912	3,837	3,766	3,727	3,767	3,762	3,736	3,683	3,665	3,645	3,616
Switzerland	3,203	3,189	3,167	3,124	3,082	3,031	3,013	2,997	3,009	3,030	2,983	2,938	2,828	2,701
Turkey	14,015	13,802	13,504	13,283	13,097	13,071	13,013	12,989	12,837	12,719	12,558	12,372	12,394	12,253
United Kingdom	25,057	24,391	24,399	24,753	24,857	24,836	24,987	25,351	25,199	24,946	24,657	24,627	24,452	24,178
United States	93,370	89,786	87,839	87,854	88,060	85,718	83,742	81,823	78,303	76,023	74,532	73,543	72,018	71,906

Country	1987	1986	1985	1984	1983	1982	1981	1980	1979	1978	1977	1976	1975	1974
Australia	7,195	6,994	6,817	6,559	6,369	6,303	6,390	6,315	6,151	6,008	5,982	5,966	5,841	5,854
Austria	3,216	3,219	3,209	3,199	3,195	3,223	3,269	3,277	3,244	3,230	3,219	3,187	3,176	3,200
Belgium	3,216	3,698	3,662	3,635	3,634	3,672	3,722	3,797	3,799	3,753	3,751	3,758	3,782	3,828
Canada	12,033	11,711	11,388	11,075	10,810	10,655	11,014	10,735	10,449	10,053	9,728	9,559	9,364	9,220
Denmark	2,614	2,593	2,532	2,463	2,428	2,421	2,410	2,442	2,453	2,424	2,399	2,379	2,338	2,367
Finland	2,297	2,297	2,308	2,312	2,305	2,296	2,279	2,256	2,192	2,144	2,167	2,210	2,252	2,262
France	21,445	21,434	21,394	21,467	21,680	21,752	21,716	21,847	21,836	21,818	21,730	21,389	21,236	21,461
Germany	25,891	25,702	25,452	25,283	25,262	25,651	26,092	26,278	25,995	25,644	25,490	25,530	25,746	26,497
Greece	3,738	3,776	3,589	3,500	3,509	3,491	3,529	3,356	3,312	3,276	3,262	3,230	3,190	3,190
Iceland	132	125	121	117	115	114	111	106	103	102	99	98	95	93
Ireland	1,088	1,081	1,074	1,104	1,122	1,146	1,146	1,156	1,145	1,110	1,083	1,064	1,073	1,060
Italy	22,924	22,786	22,613	22,413	22,325	22,182	22,060	22,062	21,641	21,315	21,201	20,989	20,698	20,646
Japan	62,432	61,833	61,311	60,899	60,602	59,609	59,116	58,657	58,253	57,665	57,108	56,432	55,973	56,110
Luxembourg	170	165	161	159	158	158	159	158	157	156	157	157	158	155
Netherlands	4,741	4,684	4,589	4,528	4,531	4,619	4,736	4,807	4,773	4,713	4,680	4,669	4,670	4,687
New Zealand	1,554	1,544	1,341	1,293	1,279	1,285	1,272	1,274	1,275	1,257	1,265	1,246	1,225	1,204
Norway	1,873	1,829	1,772	1,725	1,709	1,718	1,722	1,714	1,686	1,675	1,657	1,624	1,596	1,593
Portugal	4,191	4,084	4,076	3,729	3,787	3,850	3,901	3,865	3,879	3,797	3,857	3,279	3,259	3,277
Spain	11,648	11,052	10,808	10,952	11,220	11,272	11,378	11,683	11,953	12,215	12,551	12,654	12,789	13,019
Sweden	4,288	4,277	4,271	4,241	4,195	4,211	4,233	4,234	4,181	4,127	4,104	4,111	4,089	4,010
Switzerland	3,260	3,219	3,171	3,142	3,149	3,033	3,054	3,016	2,962	2,940	2,923	2,918	3,017	3,187
Turkey	16,450	16,092	15,790	15,611	15,412	15,292	15,168	15,032	15,393	15,029	14,881	14,613	14,296	14,190
United Kingdom	25,033	24,544	24,446	24,060	23,610	23,908	24,345	25,327	25,393	25,015	24,865	24,845	25,056	25,148
United States	122,109	118,912	116,914	114,308	109,484	108,339	109,519	108,607	108,081	104,748	100,019	96,515	94,089	95,766

SOURCE: Organization for Economic Cooperation and Development: Health Data File, 1989.

Table 63
Gross domestic product, by country: 1960-87

National currency in millions

Country	1960	1961	1962	1963	1964	1965	1966	1967	1968	1969	1970	1971	1972	1973
Australia	14,841	15,208	16,416	18,238	20,078	21,098	23,259	24,828	28,026	31,041	34,266	38,367	43,717	52,407
Austria	162,890	180,730	192,130	207,080	226,730	246,490	268,530	285,590	306,830	335,000	375,880	419,620	479,540	543,460
Belgium	563,951	600,210	642,669	691,091	773,379	842,133	905,033	969,689	1,037,500	1,151,309	1,280,924	1,402,401	1,568,509	1,782,338
Canada	38,720	40,115	43,433	46,542	50,884	56,040	62,597	67,258	73,325	80,493	86,454	95,365	106,005	124,506
Denmark	41,149	45,659	51,448	54,765	62,601	70,320	77,183	84,813	94,358	107,319	118,626	131,120	150,728	172,859
Finland	16,199	18,362	19,661	21,352	24,083	26,634	28,554	31,321	35,908	40,986	45,743	50,257	58,625	71,364
France	301,733	329,161	367,531	412,017	457,073	492,010	532,643	575,353	625,348	713,039	796,353	887,811	998,409	1,133,839
Germany	302,710	331,710	360,780	382,370	420,180	459,170	488,230	494,350	533,280	596,950	675,300	750,560	823,740	917,270
Greece	105,167	118,637	126,005	140,714	157,999	179,765	199,988	216,097	234,508	266,460	298,917	330,300	377,726	484,151
Iceland	85	98	117	139	178	215	258	261	280	349	438	557	696	972
Ireland	631	680	736	791	901	959	1,010	1,104	1,245	1,438	1,620	1,853	2,238	2,701
Italy	26,749,000	29,747,000	33,423,000	38,283,000	41,907,000	45,095,000	48,860,000	53,820,000	58,337,000	64,403,000	67,178,000	72,994,000	79,810,000	96,738,000
Japan	16,680,000	20,170,800	22,328,800	26,228,600	30,399,700	33,765,300	39,688,900	46,445,400	54,947,000	65,061,400	75,298,500	82,899,300	96,486,300	116,715,000
Luxembourg	26,106	26,116	27,501	29,341	33,495	35,098	36,879	37,117	40,609	47,024	54,966	55,943	63,070	76,666
Netherlands	44,421	46,898	50,486	54,775	64,454	71,986	78,383	85,994	95,352	107,990	121,180	136,530	154,260	176,040
New Zealand	2,813	2,872	3,114	3,397	3,721	4,013	4,190	4,374	4,642	5,132	5,832	6,874	7,901	9,200
Norway	33,058	36,062	38,844	41,682	45,837	50,564	54,568	59,700	63,749	69,417	79,878	89,107	98,403	111,854
Portugal	71,441	76,879	81,804	88,737	96,251	107,484	117,756	131,625	145,706	159,802	177,792	199,094	231,837	282,209
Spain	685,500	780,800	902,300	1,064,800	1,202,200	1,398,900	1,618,300	1,817,800	2,037,500	2,317,000	2,576,200	2,920,000	3,432,300	4,139,700
Sweden	72,128	78,466	85,097	92,106	102,716	113,032	122,952	133,458	141,621	153,798	172,226	186,215	203,758	226,744
Switzerland	37,370	42,040	46,620	51,265	56,825	60,860	65,355	70,350	75,120	81,395	90,665	102,995	116,710	130,060
Turkey	46,977	49,827	57,876	66,910	71,477	76,439	90,775	101,186	112,190	124,472	145,491	187,133	232,115	295,501
United Kingdom	25,744	27,471	28,778	30,593	33,334	35,785	38,174	40,361	43,781	46,764	51,333	57,668	63,856	73,626
United States	513,564	531,980	572,419	604,108	646,682	701,665	768,633	812,723	888,072	958,833	1,009,218	1,095,417	1,203,650	1,344,963

Country	1974	1975	1976	1977	1978	1979	1980	1981	1982	1983	1984	1985	1986	1987
Australia	63,188	74,642	85,270	92,717	105,293	118,818	138,700	155,788	169,921	192,276	214,735	236,236	260,400	291,887
Austria	618,560	656,120	724,750	796,190	842,330	918,540	994,700	1,055,970	1,133,530	1,201,230	1,276,780	1,348,130	1,423,050	1,481,560
Belgium	2,090,875	2,313,136	2,627,049	2,838,323	3,052,341	3,258,821	3,525,670	3,658,471	3,978,528	4,215,334	4,525,400	4,843,019	5,121,000	5,337,800
Canada	148,891	166,751	194,117	213,382	236,596	270,061	307,730	353,454	371,820	402,229	442,180	475,766	502,200	544,900
Denmark	193,629	216,256	251,215	279,311	311,377	346,893	373,786	407,790	464,467	512,540	565,284	619,575	667,141	693,028
Finland	90,055	104,291	117,775	130,001	143,620	166,959	192,825	218,817	246,187	275,230	309,567	336,824	360,300	393,600
France	1,300,834	1,477,919	1,707,549	1,917,603	2,182,588	2,481,097	2,808,295	3,164,804	3,626,021	4,006,498	4,364,893	4,692,476	5,035,000	5,289,000
Germany	984,580	1,026,900	1,121,720	1,197,820	1,285,320	1,392,300	1,478,940	1,540,930	1,597,920	1,674,840	1,755,840	1,830,490	1,931,220	2,009,090
Greece	564,205	672,158	824,932	963,728	1,161,392	1,428,757	1,710,934	2,050,057	2,574,652	3,077,837	3,804,705	4,614,166	5,543,000	6,390,000
Iceland	1,418	2,029	2,871	4,145	6,480	9,630	15,480	24,412	38,231	66,046	87,719	119,175	158,167	207,640
Ireland	2,988	3,792	4,653	5,703	6,757	7,917	9,361	11,359	13,381	14,683	16,320	17,316	18,540	19,780
Italy	122,190,000	138,630,000	174,870,000	214,400,000	253,540,000	309,830,000	387,670,000	464,030,000	545,120,000	633,440,000	727,230,000	812,750,000	896,320,000	979,680,000
Japan	138,451,100	152,361,600	171,293,400	190,084,500	208,602,200	225,288,400	245,349,400	260,135,700	272,243,900	283,654,400	302,434,900	320,078,700	333,236,800	348,911,300
Luxembourg	93,783	86,442	99,715	102,351	111,825	122,003	132,929	141,691	158,786	174,743	196,511	210,910	220,500	223,500
Netherlands	199,780	219,960	251,930	274,930	297,010	315,960	336,740	352,850	368,860	381,020	400,250	416,590	429,900	431,800
New Zealand	10,117	11,668	14,106	14,879	16,856	19,688	22,947	27,746	31,097	34,307	38,838	44,861	53,079	59,257
Norway	129,729	148,702	170,709	191,534	213,080	238,669	285,046	327,674	362,269	402,199	452,512	501,816	514,600	556,900
Portugal	339,283	377,203	468,854	625,835	787,260	993,305	1,256,051	1,501,131	1,850,410	2,301,710	2,805,500	3,526,300	4,403,000	5,169,000
Spain	5,102,000	6,018,300	7,234,200	9,178,400	11,230,700	13,130,500	15,209,100	16,989,000	19,567,300	22,234,700	25,121,300	27,853,500	31,955,000	35,710,000
Sweden	256,127	300,785	340,197	370,016	412,450	462,307	525,099	573,040	627,678	705,365	789,583	860,884	931,784	1,005,226
Switzerland	141,100	140,155	141,960	145,790	151,675	158,545	170,330	184,755	195,980	203,865	213,230	227,950	243,400	255,180
Turkey	409,746	519,173	663,937	862,968	1,274,781	2,155,894	4,327,964	6,413,610	8,620,394	11,532,000	18,212,000	27,509,000	39,290,000	57,770,000
United Kingdom	83,788	105,902	126,340	145,459	167,699	196,360	230,700	254,269	275,631	300,057	319,130	352,600	376,500	409,900
United States	1,456,411	1,583,918	1,764,805	1,967,489	2,218,908	2,464,805	2,688,467	3,009,474	3,121,397	3,353,473	3,722,337	3,959,610	4,191,000	4,473,000

SOURCE: Organization for Economic Cooperation and Development: Health Data File, 1989.

Table 64
Gross domestic product price index (1980 = 100), by country: 1960-87

Country	1960	1961	1962	1963	1964	1965	1966	1967	1968	1969	1970	1971	1972	1973
Australia	26.5	26.9	27.1	27.9	28.8	29.6	30.6	31.4	32.4	33.9	35.3	37.4	40.2	45.0
Austria	37.2	39.2	40.7	42.2	43.5	46.0	47.5	49.0	50.4	51.8	54.2	57.6	62.0	67.0
Belgium	35.9	36.4	37.0	38.1	39.9	41.9	43.7	45.0	46.2	48.1	50.3	53.2	56.5	60.5
Canada	32.9	33.1	33.6	34.3	35.1	36.3	38.1	39.7	41.1	42.9	44.9	46.4	49.0	53.3
Denmark	21.3	22.2	23.7	25.0	26.2	28.1	30.1	31.9	34.2	36.5	39.6	42.6	46.5	51.5
Finland	19.0	20.1	20.9	21.9	23.5	24.7	25.8	27.7	31.1	32.4	33.6	36.2	39.2	44.8
France	25.5	26.3	27.6	29.3	30.6	31.4	32.3	33.3	34.7	37.0	39.1	41.6	44.5	48.3
Germany	41.5	43.5	45.2	46.6	48.0	49.7	51.3	52.1	53.2	55.4	59.6	64.4	67.8	72.1
Greece	20.3	20.6	21.6	21.9	22.7	23.6	24.7	25.3	25.8	26.6	27.7	28.5	30.0	35.8
Iceland	1.6	1.8	2.0	2.2	2.5	2.9	3.2	3.3	3.7	4.5	5.2	5.9	6.9	9.2
Ireland	16.0	16.4	17.2	17.6	19.2	20.1	21.0	21.8	22.7	24.7	26.9	29.8	33.8	39.0
Italy	16.2	16.7	17.7	19.2	20.4	21.3	21.7	22.3	22.7	23.6	25.1	26.8	28.6	32.3
Japan	28.4	30.6	31.9	33.6	35.4	37.2	39.1	41.2	43.2	43.2	45.2	48.1	53.6	60.5
Luxembourg	36.3	34.9	36.3	37.4	39.6	40.7	42.3	42.5	44.7	47.0	54.1	53.6	56.8	63.5
Netherlands	28.8	30.3	30.5	32.0	34.7	36.9	39.1	40.7	42.4	45.2	47.9	51.8	56.7	61.8
New Zealand	21.0	20.6	21.4	21.8	22.7	23.1	22.6	24.5	26.0	26.2	29.7	33.2	36.4	39.7
Norway	27.8	28.5	29.9	30.9	32.3	33.9	35.2	36.3	37.9	39.5	44.5	47.5	49.9	54.4
Portugal	16.9	17.2	17.2	17.6	17.9	18.6	19.6	20.3	20.7	22.2	22.6	23.8	25.6	28.0
Spain	13.1	13.3	14.1	15.3	16.3	17.8	19.6	20.3	20.7	22.7	24.2	26.2	28.4	31.8
Sweden	26.2	27.0	28.1	28.9	30.1	31.9	34.0	35.7	36.6	37.8	39.8	42.6	45.6	48.8
Switzerland	39.4	41.0	43.4	45.5	47.9	49.7	52.1	54.4	56.1	57.5	60.3	65.8	72.2	78.1
Turkey	3.1	3.2	3.5	3.7	3.8	3.9	4.2	4.5	4.7	4.9	5.5	6.4	7.5	9.1
United Kingdom	17.9	18.5	19.1	19.5	20.2	21.3	22.3	23.0	23.9	25.2	27.1	29.7	32.1	34.2
United States	36.5	36.7	37.6	38.0	38.4	39.4	41.0	42.4	44.5	46.7	49.2	51.7	54.1	57.7

Country	1974	1975	1976	1977	1978	1979	1980	1981	1982	1983	1984	1985	1986	1987
Australia	53.2	61.8	70.0	76.3	82.1	90.2	100.0	109.6	121.8	131.9	140.3	148.8	159.3	171.8
Austria	73.3	78.0	82.4	86.8	91.3	95.1	100.0	106.3	112.9	117.1	122.9	126.5	131.7	135.0
Belgium	68.2	76.4	82.2	88.3	92.2	96.4	100.0	105.1	112.6	119.2	125.1	132.4	136.9	139.6
Canada	61.0	67.0	72.8	77.4	82.1	90.4	100.0	110.8	120.4	126.2	130.2	134.0	137.4	143.3
Denmark	58.2	65.5	71.4	78.2	85.9	92.4	100.0	110.1	121.7	131.0	138.4	145.6	151.7	159.3
Finland	54.8	62.8	70.6	77.8	84.1	91.3	100.0	111.7	121.2	131.6	143.4	150.7	157.7	165.9
France	54.0	61.0	67.8	74.0	81.5	89.8	100.0	111.4	124.4	136.6	146.7	155.4	163.2	167.8
Germany	77.2	81.8	84.8	88.0	91.7	95.4	100.0	104.0	108.6	112.1	114.3	116.9	120.5	122.9
Greece	43.3	48.7	56.1	63.4	71.6	85.0	100.0	119.8	149.8	178.4	214.6	252.5	299.5	346.6
Iceland	12.7	17.9	24.0	31.8	46.6	65.7	100.0	151.0	231.5	416.7	537.1	703.0	870.0	1051.0
Ireland	41.3	50.6	61.3	69.4	76.7	87.2	100.0	117.4	135.3	149.8	160.3	168.6	176.4	182.5
Italy	38.7	45.1	53.4	63.3	72.3	83.3	100.0	118.6	138.8	159.5	177.8	193.6	208.2	221.0
Japan	73.1	78.7	84.3	89.2	93.5	96.3	100.0	103.2	105.1	105.9	107.2	108.7	110.8	110.6
Luxembourg	74.3	73.4	82.4	83.2	87.7	93.0	100.0	106.8	117.9	126.0	131.6	136.0	138.1	136.6
Netherlands	67.4	74.3	81.0	86.4	91.1	94.6	100.0	105.5	111.9	114.0	116.1	118.1	118.9	117.9
New Zealand	40.9	46.5	55.2	67.0	75.4	86.4	100.0	115.3	128.5	138.0	148.1	168.3	196.4	219.8
Norway	60.0	66.1	71.0	76.9	81.8	87.3	100.0	114.0	125.6	133.2	141.8	148.8	146.9	157.6
Portugal	33.3	38.8	45.1	57.0	69.4	82.8	100.0	118.0	142.4	177.1	219.8	267.4	320.4	359.2
Spain	37.0	43.2	50.3	62.0	74.8	87.6	100.0	112.0	127.4	142.2	157.8	171.3	190.0	201.2
Sweden	53.4	61.2	68.5	75.7	82.9	89.5	100.0	109.5	118.9	130.5	140.5	150.0	160.6	169.2
Switzerland	83.5	89.5	91.9	92.1	95.5	97.4	100.0	106.9	114.7	118.5	121.8	125.1	129.9	133.1
Turkey	11.7	13.8	16.2	20.2	29.0	49.4	100.0	142.0	181.8	234.5	350.2	504.1	663.6	909.2
United Kingdom	39.4	50.1	57.6	65.6	73.0	83.6	100.0	111.5	119.9	126.1	132.0	139.4	144.4	151.5
United States	62.9	69.1	73.4	78.4	84.1	91.6	100.0	109.5	116.5	120.5	124.8	128.2	131.5	135.5

SOURCE: Organization for Economic Cooperation and Development: Health Data File, 1989.

Table 65
Compensation per employee, by country: 1960-87

In national currency units

Country	1960	1961	1962	1963	1964	1965	1966	1967	1968	1969	1970	1971	1972	1973
Australia	–	–	–	–	2,636	2,760	2,858	3,014	3,242	3,538	3,898	4,248	4,671	5,548
Austria	32,200	35,300	38,300	41,300	45,000	49,200	54,000	59,000	63,200	68,500	74,000	83,400	92,500	104,800
Belgium	99,910	102,710	110,569	119,398	131,011	143,598	155,814	167,253	177,788	192,579	212,916	237,707	271,119	306,113
Canada	3,932	4,044	4,174	4,322	4,515	4,764	5,096	5,480	5,811	6,287	6,899	7,396	8,008	8,721
Denmark	12,658	14,294	15,903	16,516	18,389	20,917	23,049	25,566	28,010	31,204	34,633	38,664	41,744	47,214
Finland	5,197	5,608	6,128	6,791	7,811	8,562	9,255	10,158	11,255	12,088	13,102	15,101	17,289	20,432
France	9,381	10,367	11,580	12,902	14,022	15,006	15,911	17,002	18,906	21,002	23,022	25,680	28,292	31,935
Germany	7,132	7,860	8,573	9,094	9,840	10,773	11,593	11,974	12,777	13,995	16,230	18,115	19,917	22,330
Greece	28,300	30,100	32,200	34,600	39,200	44,100	49,700	54,300	59,500	65,600	71,900	78,400	88,100	103,600
Iceland	–	–	44,538	47,963	55,650	–	–	–	–	–	–	–	–	6,621
Ireland	278	495	–	–	–	676	733	792	875	997	1,165	1,328	1,555	1,860
Italy	809,313	875,690	994,227	1,190,389	1,337,239	1,440,721	1,554,242	1,685,312	1,809,696	1,947,037	2,208,000	2,503,000	2,769,000	3,258,000
Japan	268,692	304,802	347,397	396,632	443,721	494,871	543,788	609,870	701,426	800,003	904,861	1,040,824	1,190,658	1,438,284
Luxembourg	119,362	122,979	128,276	135,584	155,971	162,952	172,726	176,821	186,364	197,917	226,868	244,800	269,967	304,579
Netherlands	6,037	6,485	6,900	7,600	8,800	9,800	10,000	12,000	13,000	14,700	16,600	18,800	21,200	24,400
New Zealand	–	–	–	–	–	–	–	–	–	–	–	–	–	–
Norway	–	–	18,163	19,259	20,575	22,340	24,354	26,752	28,574	30,536	33,100	37,900	42,000	47,200
Portugal	–	–	–	–	–	–	–	–	–	–	–	37,900	44,200	52,100
Spain	40,725	45,706	52,641	63,607	72,334	84,837	99,431	114,579	124,492	139,377	154,570	176,658	207,572	244,882
Sweden	12,790	13,942	15,460	16,836	18,322	20,032	22,085	24,085	25,578	27,168	29,577	32,251	34,980	37,376
Switzerland	7,912	–	–	–	11,135	12,964	13,011	14,058	14,920	15,864	17,597	20,096	22,527	25,420
Turkey	–	–	–	–	–	–	–	–	–	–	–	–	–	–
United Kingdom	–	724	758	795	851	909	967	1,027	1,107	1,187	1,337	1,488	1,682	1,902
United States	4,715	4,841	5,055	5,250	5,499	5,724	6,012	6,287	6,744	7,223	7,739	8,273	8,892	9,538

Country	1974	1975	1976	1977	1978	1979	1980	1981	1982	1983	1984	1985	1986	1987
Australia	7,091	8,201	9,254	10,078	10,887	12,114	13,684	15,627	17,582	18,407	19,777	20,965	22,661	24,452
Austria	119,300	134,400	146,900	159,500	173,200	183,200	195,400	211,100	224,300	235,600	247,000	260,300	274,400	285,800
Belgium	361,706	421,547	488,775	531,277	570,908	602,169	654,389	696,780	754,255	800,238	847,067	884,195	917,680	935,030
Canada	9,978	11,428	12,984	14,166	14,954	16,151	17,629	19,779	21,930	22,862	24,037	25,222	26,039	27,253
Denmark	55,920	63,714	71,145	78,046	85,196	93,240	102,606	112,078	124,973	133,014	140,150	146,650	157,586	170,494
Finland	25,359	31,543	36,839	40,281	42,859	47,870	54,471	62,200	68,507	75,371	83,254	92,112	98,912	107,856
France	37,540	44,527	51,065	57,517	64,650	73,290	83,498	95,495	108,590	120,107	129,687	138,280	143,700	154,224
Germany	24,900	26,694	28,797	30,707	32,430	34,337	36,711	38,620	40,235	41,730	43,171	44,498	46,201	47,550
Greece	123,000	147,300	182,500	230,971	282,954	346,583	402,425	489,340	623,792	757,836	928,238	1,116,196	1,290,900	1,405,602
Iceland	9,650	12,612	16,413	24,089	37,159	54,960	84,965	124,270	189,451	295,668	379,684	538,826	688,824	978,456
Ireland	2,211	2,798	3,355	3,815	4,401	5,186	6,272	7,578	8,579	9,414	11,100	11,900	12,200	12,823
Italy	3,993,000	4,823,000	5,831,000	7,043,000	8,204,000	9,836,000	11,945,000	14,642,000	17,009,000	19,734,000	22,056,000	24,283,000	26,076,000	28,511,000
Japan	1,811,878	2,106,313	2,324,325	2,559,442	2,736,969	2,906,468	3,026,886	3,224,595	3,363,140	3,453,300	3,597,483	3,728,965	3,874,000	3,959,960
Luxembourg	369,405	411,200	465,560	509,256	537,744	569,823	614,447	663,399	712,118	759,398	808,250	842,400	881,500	936,530
Netherlands	28,300	32,000	35,500	37,428	40,061	42,567	47,336	48,977	51,819	53,455	53,582	54,294	55,117	56,048
New Zealand	–	–	–	–	–	10,552	12,481	14,422	15,705	13,505	–	–	20,534	22,193
Norway	53,700	63,500	72,000	79,300	85,800	88,918	97,963	109,606	122,406	133,121	143,430	154,270	169,815	184,210
Portugal	70,600	94,500	114,700	110,784	131,785	156,711	235,866	285,934	341,000	414,400	472,800	596,000	712,900	747,422
Spain	299,531	360,985	448,694	571,181	719,205	861,447	958,277	1,110,540	1,259,070	1,433,085	1,575,601	1,734,300	1,864,400	1,969,649
Sweden	42,211	49,340	58,185	65,297	72,444	78,652	87,062	95,091	101,304	109,771	118,603	126,782	139,833	150,735
Switzerland	28,291	30,443	31,535	33,144	33,449	34,864	36,758	39,543	42,812	45,236	47,213	49,675	52,043	–
Turkey	–	–	–	–	–	–	–	–	–	–	–	–	–	–
United Kingdom	2,261	2,968	3,400	3,757	4,262	4,889	5,896	6,674	7,292	7,954	8,362	8,964	9,556	10,223
United States	10,295	11,152	12,088	12,995	14,019	15,235	16,730	18,317	19,604	20,597	21,538	22,451	23,344	24,341

Table 66
Exchange rates, by country: 1960-87

National currency units per U.S. dollar

Country	1960	1961	1962	1963	1964	1965	1966	1967	1968	1969	1970	1971	1972	1973
Australia	0.89	0.89	0.89	0.89	0.89	0.89	0.89	0.89	0.89	0.89	0.89	0.88	0.84	0.70
Austria	25.96	25.93	25.82	25.83	25.83	25.82	25.83	25.83	25.84	25.86	25.86	24.96	23.12	19.58
Belgium	50.00	50.00	50.00	50.00	50.00	50.00	50.00	50.00	50.00	50.00	50.00	48.87	44.01	38.98
Canada	0.97	1.01	1.07	1.08	1.08	1.08	1.08	1.08	1.08	1.08	1.05	1.01	0.99	1.00
Denmark	6.91	6.91	6.91	6.91	6.91	6.91	6.91	6.96	7.50	7.50	7.50	7.42	6.95	6.05
Finland	3.20	3.20	3.20	3.20	3.20	3.20	3.20	3.45	4.20	4.20	4.20	4.18	4.15	3.82
France	4.94	4.94	4.94	4.94	4.94	4.94	4.94	4.94	4.94	5.19	5.55	5.54	5.04	4.46
Germany	4.20	4.03	4.00	4.00	4.00	4.00	4.00	4.00	4.00	3.94	3.66	3.49	3.19	2.67
Greece	30.00	30.00	30.00	30.00	30.00	30.00	30.00	30.00	30.00	30.00	30.00	30.00	30.00	29.63
Iceland	0.34	0.40	0.43	0.43	0.43	0.43	0.43	0.44	0.62	0.88	0.88	0.88	0.88	0.90
Ireland	0.36	0.36	0.36	0.36	0.36	0.36	0.36	0.36	0.42	0.42	0.42	0.41	0.40	0.41
Italy	623.99	625.00	625.00	625.00	625.00	625.00	625.00	625.00	625.00	625.00	625.00	619.93	583.22	583.00
Japan	360.00	360.00	360.00	360.00	360.00	360.00	360.00	360.00	360.00	360.00	360.00	349.33	303.17	271.70
Luxembourg	50.00	50.00	50.00	50.00	50.00	50.00	50.00	50.00	50.00	50.00	50.00	48.87	44.01	38.98
Netherlands	3.80	3.65	3.62	3.62	3.62	3.62	3.62	3.62	3.62	3.62	3.62	3.50	3.21	2.80
New Zealand	0.71	0.72	0.72	0.72	0.72	0.72	0.72	0.73	0.89	0.89	0.89	0.88	0.84	0.74
Norway	7.14	7.14	7.14	7.14	7.14	7.14	7.14	7.14	7.14	7.14	7.14	7.04	6.59	5.77
Portugal	28.75	28.75	28.75	28.75	28.75	28.75	28.75	28.75	28.75	28.75	28.75	28.31	27.05	24.52
Spain	60.00	60.00	60.00	60.00	60.00	60.00	60.00	61.67	70.00	70.00	70.00	69.47	64.27	58.26
Sweden	5.17	5.17	5.17	5.17	5.17	5.17	5.17	5.17	5.17	5.17	5.17	5.12	4.76	4.37
Switzerland	4.37	4.37	4.37	4.37	4.37	4.37	4.37	4.37	4.37	4.37	4.37	4.13	3.82	3.16
Turkey	4.87	9.00	9.00	9.00	9.00	9.00	9.00	9.00	9.00	9.00	11.50	14.92	14.15	14.15
United Kingdom	0.36	0.36	0.36	0.36	0.36	0.36	0.36	0.36	0.42	0.42	0.42	0.41	0.40	0.41
United States	1.00	1.00	1.00	1.00	1.00	1.00	1.00	1.00	1.00	1.00	1.00	1.00	1.00	1.00

Country	1974	1975	1976	1977	1978	1979	1980	1981	1982	1983	1984	1985	1986	1987
Australia	0.70	0.76	0.82	0.90	0.87	0.89	0.88	0.87	0.99	1.11	1.14	1.43	1.50	1.43
Austria	18.69	17.42	17.94	16.53	14.52	13.37	12.94	15.92	17.06	17.96	20.01	20.69	15.27	12.64
Belgium	38.95	36.78	38.61	35.84	31.49	29.32	29.24	37.13	45.69	51.13	57.78	59.38	44.67	37.34
Canada	0.98	1.02	0.99	1.06	1.14	1.17	1.17	1.20	1.23	1.23	1.30	1.37	1.39	1.33
Denmark	6.09	5.75	6.05	6.00	5.51	5.26	5.64	7.12	8.33	9.15	10.36	10.60	8.09	6.84
Finland	3.77	3.68	3.86	4.03	4.12	3.90	3.73	4.32	4.82	5.57	6.01	6.20	5.07	4.40
France	4.81	4.29	4.78	4.91	4.51	4.25	4.23	5.43	6.57	7.62	8.74	8.99	6.93	6.01
Germany	2.59	2.46	2.52	2.32	2.01	1.83	1.82	2.26	2.43	2.55	2.85	2.94	2.17	1.80
Greece	30.00	32.05	36.52	36.84	36.75	37.04	42.62	55.41	66.80	88.06	112.72	138.12	139.98	166.18
Iceland	1.00	1.54	1.82	1.99	2.71	3.53	4.80	7.22	12.35	24.84	31.69	41.51	41.10	42.07
Ireland	0.43	0.45	0.56	0.57	0.52	0.49	0.49	0.62	0.70	0.80	0.92	0.95	0.74	0.67
Italy	650.34	652.85	832.28	882.39	848.66	830.86	856.45	1136.77	1352.51	1518.85	1756.96	1909.44	1490.81	1297.00
Japan	292.08	296.79	296.55	268.51	210.44	219.14	226.74	220.54	249.03	237.51	237.52	238.54	168.52	144.60
Luxembourg	38.95	36.78	38.61	35.84	31.49	29.32	29.24	37.13	45.69	51.13	57.78	59.39	44.67	37.34
Netherlands	2.69	2.53	2.64	2.45	2.16	2.01	1.99	2.50	2.67	2.85	3.21	3.32	2.45	2.03
New Zealand	0.72	0.83	1.00	1.03	0.96	0.98	1.03	1.15	1.33	1.50	1.76	2.02	1.91	1.70
Norway	5.54	5.23	5.46	5.32	5.24	5.06	4.94	5.74	6.45	7.30	8.16	8.60	7.39	6.74
Portugal	25.41	25.55	30.23	38.28	43.94	48.92	50.06	61.55	79.47	110.78	146.39	170.40	149.59	140.79
Spain	57.69	57.41	66.90	75.96	76.67	67.13	71.70	92.32	109.86	143.43	160.76	170.04	140.05	123.52
Sweden	4.44	4.15	4.36	4.48	4.52	4.29	4.23	5.06	6.28	7.67	8.27	8.60	7.12	6.34
Switzerland	2.98	2.58	2.50	2.40	1.79	1.66	1.68	1.96	2.03	2.10	2.35	2.46	1.80	1.49
Turkey	13.93	14.44	16.05	18.00	24.28	31.08	76.04	111.22	162.55	225.46	366.68	521.98	674.51	854.60
United Kingdom	0.43	0.45	0.56	0.57	0.52	0.47	0.43	0.50	0.57	0.66	0.75	0.78	0.68	0.61
United States	1.00	1.00	1.00	1.00	1.00	1.00	1.00	1.00	1.00	1.00	1.00	1.00	1.00	1.00

SOURCE: Organization for Economic Cooperation and Development: Health Data File, 1989.

Table 67

Purchasing power parities for gross domestic product, by country: 1960-87

Country	1960	1961	1962	1963	1964	1965	1966	1967	1968	1969	1970	1971	1972	1973
	National currency units per U.S. dollar													
Australia	0.75	0.76	0.75	0.76	0.78	0.78	0.77	0.77	0.75	0.75	0.74	0.75	0.77	0.81
Austria	17.14	17.91	18.20	18.62	19.01	19.62	19.41	19.38	19.00	18.60	18.50	18.69	19.24	19.50
Belgium	41.99	42.25	42.01	42.75	44.20	45.34	45.37	45.24	44.29	44.28	43.55	43.81	44.52	44.76
Canada	1.02	1.03	1.02	1.03	1.04	1.05	1.06	1.07	1.06	1.05	1.04	1.02	1.04	1.06
Denmark	5.15	5.34	5.57	5.82	6.01	6.31	6.17	6.34	6.47	6.60	6.79	6.95	7.27	7.54
Finland	2.61	2.73	2.77	2.88	3.05	3.13	3.15	3.27	3.49	3.46	3.42	3.50	3.63	3.88
France	4.22	4.34	4.44	4.67	4.81	4.82	4.76	4.75	4.72	4.79	4.81	4.84	4.91	4.97
Germany	3.05	3.17	3.22	3.28	3.34	3.37	3.35	3.28	3.20	3.18	3.25	3.34	3.36	3.36
Greece	21.54	21.71	22.21	22.24	22.78	23.11	23.27	23.05	22.43	22.03	21.74	21.35	21.46	24.04
Iceland	0.29	0.32	0.35	0.38	0.44	0.49	0.52	0.51	0.56	0.64	0.71	0.76	0.85	1.07
Ireland	0.24	0.24	0.25	0.25	0.27	0.28	0.28	0.28	0.28	0.29	0.30	0.32	0.35	0.37
Italy	384.83	392.38	406.11	435.10	457.75	465.79	456.64	454.54	440.78	437.07	443.42	452.18	459.63	480.84
Japan	199.37	213.27	216.23	223.28	230.56	236.54	238.57	244.92	245.99	246.01	251.49	252.62	255.32	270.28
Luxembourg	38.87	37.21	37.74	38.47	40.21	40.38	40.28	39.15	39.22	39.34	42.82	40.33	40.81	42.83
Netherlands	2.13	2.16	2.19	2.27	2.44	2.52	2.57	2.59	2.57	2.60	2.62	2.70	2.83	2.89
New Zealand	0.59	0.57	0.58	0.59	0.61	0.62	0.60	0.60	0.60	0.59	0.62	0.66	0.70	0.71
Norway	5.54	5.64	5.79	5.91	6.12	6.26	6.25	6.22	6.19	6.15	6.58	6.68	6.71	6.88
Portugal	14.46	14.65	14.34	14.50	14.57	14.80	14.91	15.01	14.57	14.88	14.42	14.38	14.87	15.31
Spain	25.17	25.44	26.27	28.11	29.92	32.00	33.16	34.58	34.58	34.41	34.92	35.88	37.32	39.12
Sweden	4.95	5.05	5.14	5.22	5.39	5.58	5.70	5.79	5.66	5.57	5.56	5.67	5.80	5.83
Switzerland	2.64	2.73	2.83	2.93	3.05	3.09	3.11	3.14	3.08	3.01	3.00	3.11	3.27	3.32
Turkey	3.47	3.59	3.85	4.02	4.08	4.15	4.23	4.36	4.32	4.34	4.59	5.15	5.73	6.69
United Kingdom	0.25	0.26	0.26	0.27	0.27	0.28	0.28	0.28	0.28	0.28	0.28	0.29	0.30	0.31
United States	1.00	1.00	1.00	1.00	1.00	1.00	1.00	1.00	1.00	1.00	1.00	1.00	1.00	1.00

Country	1974	1975	1976	1977	1978	1979	1980	1981	1982	1983	1984	1985	1986	1987
Australia	0.88	0.92	0.99	1.01	1.01	1.02	1.04	1.06	1.11	1.16	1.20	1.24	1.30	1.35
Austria	19.58	18.97	18.87	18.61	18.27	17.47	16.63	16.38	16.35	16.42	16.63	16.60	16.83	16.80
Belgium	46.18	47.12	47.88	48.20	46.83	45.02	42.92	41.73	42.02	43.09	43.63	44.63	45.07	44.50
Canada	1.11	1.11	1.13	1.13	1.12	1.13	1.15	1.18	1.20	1.22	1.22	1.22	1.22	1.23
Denmark	7.81	8.00	8.22	8.43	8.62	8.54	8.52	8.69	9.03	9.41	9.60	9.80	10.01	10.20
Finland	4.36	4.54	4.82	4.97	4.99	4.96	5.02	5.20	5.31	5.58	5.86	5.97	6.02	6.21
France	5.07	5.22	5.42	5.55	5.64	5.72	5.94	6.13	6.44	6.85	7.09	7.27	7.41	7.43
Germany	3.29	3.18	3.10	3.01	2.93	2.80	2.70	2.60	2.56	2.56	2.51	2.48	2.49	2.47
Greece	26.65	27.22	29.68	31.42	33.00	35.98	38.81	43.06	50.66	58.41	67.73	77.34	89.68	100.00
Iceland	1.35	1.73	2.19	2.72	3.71	4.80	6.78	9.49	13.68	23.85	29.63	37.80	46.05	54.20
Ireland	0.36	0.40	0.45	0.48	0.49	0.52	0.54	0.59	0.64	0.68	0.71	0.72	0.74	0.74
Italy	522.67	558.60	621.86	694.21	735.35	783.79	866.97	952.15	1040.31	1161.63	1234.22	1302.00	1370.28	1399.00
Japan	299.31	293.45	296.10	293.69	286.92	271.54	258.51	247.12	236.74	231.01	225.44	221.90	220.01	213.00
Luxembourg	45.86	40.91	43.46	41.06	40.25	39.09	39.76	39.35	40.84	42.26	43.02	43.13	43.10	41.00
Netherlands	2.89	2.90	2.98	2.98	2.93	2.79	2.73	2.67	2.67	2.63	2.58	2.55	2.50	2.40
New Zealand	0.67	0.69	0.77	0.84	0.91	0.97	1.00	1.09	1.14	1.16	1.21	1.35	1.54	1.69
Norway	6.95	6.96	7.04	7.15	7.10	6.95	7.33	7.74	8.02	8.24	8.46	8.63	8.28	8.64
Portugal	16.65	18.56	17.67	20.67	26.99	27.33	31.43	34.37	38.91	47.01	56.14	66.22	76.07	84.10
Spain	41.78	44.35	48.85	56.17	62.85	67.49	70.55	73.20	78.33	84.67	90.52	95.34	103.23	106.00
Sweden	5.85	6.10	6.42	6.65	6.80	6.74	6.89	6.99	7.14	7.58	7.87	8.15	8.51	8.69
Switzerland	3.25	3.17	3.07	2.88	2.78	2.61	2.44	2.42	2.44	2.44	2.42	2.42	2.44	2.43
Turkey	7.59	7.95	8.64	10.01	13.39	21.13	38.57	50.75	61.10	76.32	109.88	153.30	196.10	262.00
United Kingdom	.032	0.37	0.40	0.43	0.45	0.47	0.52	0.53	0.54	0.55	0.55	0.57	0.57	0.58
United States	1.00	1.00	1.00	1.00	1.00	1.00	1.00	1.00	1.00	1.00	1.00	1.00	1.00	1.00

Contributors

Morris L. Barer, Ph.D., M.B.A., is Director, Division of Health Services Research and Development, and Associate Professor, Department of Health Care and Epidemiology, at the University of British Columbia. He received his doctorate degree in health economics in 1977 and a masters degree in business administration in 1988 from the University of British Columbia. He is the senior editor for health economics with *Social Science and Medicine*.

A. J. Culyer has been a Professor of economics at the University of York, England since 1979. He has also taught or held visiting positions at the University of California, Los Angeles, Exeter, Otago, Queen's Kingston, Trent, and Australian National University. He is the co-editor of the *Journal of Health Economics* and a member of an English District Health Authority.

Karen Davis, Ph.D., is Chairman of the Department of Health Policy and Management in the School of Hygiene and Public Health and has a joint appointment as Professor of economics at Johns Hopkins University. She received her doctorate degree in economics from Rice University in Houston, Texas. She serves as regional editor USA/Canada for the journal *Health Policy* and as a consultant for the World Health Organization, European Regional Office.

Alain C. Enthoven, Ph.D., is Marriner S. Eccles Professor of public and private management at the Graduate School of Business, and Professor of health care economics at the School of Medicine, Stanford University. He has written extensively on reforming the incentives in the health care financing and delivery system.

Robert G. Evans, Ph.D., is Professor of the Department of Economics, at the University of British Columbia. He is a Fellow and Director of the Program in Population Health, Canadian Institute for Advanced Research, and a National Health Research Scientist. He received his doctorate degree in economics from Harvard University in 1970.

Klaus-Dirk Henke, Ph.D., is Professor of economics at the University of Hannover, in Hannover, Federal Republic of Germany. He received his doctorate degree in economics from the University of Cologne in 1970. Previously, he was Assistant Professor at the Universities of Cologne and Marburg, Associate Professor at the University of Marburg, and Guest Scholar at the Brookings Institution in Washington, D.C.

Jeremy Hurst, M.Sc., is a senior economic adviser in the Department of Health in England. He has a particular interest in international comparisons of the financing and organization of health services.

Bengt Jönsson, Ph.D., is Professor of health economics at the Department of Health and Society, Linköping University and Director of the Center for Medical Technology Assessment. He received his doctorate degree in economics from Lund University in 1976. He was Director for the Swedish Institute for Health Economics for 1980-82. He is a member of the Scientific Advisory Board to the National Board of Health and Welfare, Sweden and he has acted as adviser to the World Health Organization.

Björn Lindgren, Ph.D., is Professor of health economics at the University of Lund, and director of the Swedish Institute for Health Economics, Lund, Sweden. His current work includes research on productivity and efficiency measurement in hospital care, organization and financing of health care, and methods for economic evaluation in health care.

Klim McPherson, Ph.D., is a university lecturer in medical statistics in the Department of Community Medicine at Oxford University. He was affiliated with the Medical Research Council and Harvard Medical School before going to Oxford in 1976. His research focuses on organizational aspects of health care delivery and chronic disease epidemiology.

Jack A. Meyer, Ph.D., is President of New Directions for Policy, Inc., a research organization based in Washington, D.C. Current areas of interest include health care for the uninsured, long-term care, and labor markets and demographic change. An economist by training, he is principal author of *The Common Good: Social Welfare and the American Future*, recently published by the Ford Foundation.

Jean-Pierre Poullier has been an economist with the Organization for Economic Cooperation and Development in Paris since 1972. He was with the Brookings Institution in Washington, D.C. from 1963 to 1967, and then worked as an economic consultant until 1972. He was educated at the University of Geneva and received a masters degree in economics from Yale University in 1962. He has published several books and articles on health issues.

Uwe E. Reinhardt, Ph.D., received his doctorate degree in economics from Yale University in 1970. He has taught at Princeton University since September 1968 and is the James Madison Professor of Political Economy. His research interests have centered primarily on topics in health economics. In 1988, he was elected President of the American Association of Health Services Research.

Simone Sandier is Director of Research at CREDES (Centre de Recherche, d'Etude et de Documentation en Economic de la Santé) in Paris and has degrees in mathematics and statistics from the University of Paris. She specializes in the macroeconomic aspects of the health sector, including National Health Accounts, forecasting and planning, regional studies, and international comparisons. She is an expert adviser for various French and International Commissions.

George Schieber, Ph.D., is Director of the Office of Research, Health Care Financing Administration. He served as Administrator in the Directorate for Social Affairs, Manpower, and Education at the Organization for Economic Cooperation and Development in Paris for 1985-87. Prior to that, he was the Director of the Office of Policy Analysis, Office of Legislation and Policy, Health Care Financing Administration.

WHERE TO OBTAIN OECD PUBLICATIONS
OÙ OBTENIR LES PUBLICATIONS DE L'OCDE

Argentina – Argentine
Carlos Hirsch S.R.L.
Galeria Güemes, Florida 165, 4° Piso
1333 Buenos Aires
          Tel. 30.7122, 331.1787 y 331.2391
Telegram: Hirsch-Baires
Telex: 21112 UAPE-AR. Ref. s/2901
Telefax:(1)331-1787

Australia – Australie
D.A. Book (Aust.) Pty. Ltd.
648 Whitehorse Road, P.O.B 163
Mitcham, Victoria 3132   Tel. (03)873.4411
Telex: AA37911 DA BOOK
Telefax: (03)873.5679

Austria – Autriche
OECD Publications and Information Centre
4 Simrockstrasse
5300 Bonn (Germany)   Tel. (0228)21.60.45
Telex: 8 86300 Bonn
Telefax: (0228)26.11.04

Gerold & Co.
Graben 31
Wien I   Tel. (0222)533.50.14

Belgium – Belgique
Jean De Lannoy
Avenue du Roi 202
B-1060 Bruxelles
          Tel. (02)538.51.69/538.08.41
Telex: 63220   Telefax: (02) 538.08.41

Canada
Renouf Publishing Company Ltd.
1294 Algoma Road
Ottawa, ON K1B 3W8   Tel. (613)741.4333
Telex: 053-4783   Telefax: (613)741.5439
Stores:
61 Sparks Street
Ottawa, ON K1P 5R1   Tel. (613)238.8985
211 Yonge Street
Toronto, ON M5B 1M4   Tel. (416)363.3171

Federal Publications
165 University Avenue
Toronto, ON M5H 3B9   Tel. (416)581.1552
Telefax: (416)581.1743

Les Publications Fédérales
1185 rue de l'Université
Montréal, PQ H3B 3A7   Tel.(514)954-1633

Les Éditions La Liberté Inc.
3020 Chemin Sainte-Foy
Sainte-Foy, PQ G1X 3V6
          Tel. (418)658.3763
          Telefax: (418)658.3763

Denmark – Danemark
Munksgaard Export and Subscription Service
35, Norre Sogade, P.O. Box 2148
DK-1016 Kobenhavn K
          Tel. (45 33)12.85.70
Telex: 19431 MUNKS DK
          Telefax: (45 33)12.93.87

Finland – Finlande
Akateeminen Kirjakauppa
Keskuskatu 1, P.O. Box 128
00100 Helsinki   Tel. (358 0)12141
Telex: 125080   Telefax: (358 0)121.4441

France
OECD/OCDE
Mail Orders/Commandes par correspon-
dance:
2 rue André-Pascal
75775 Paris Cedex 16   Tel. (1)45.24.82.00
Bookshop/Librairie:
33, rue Octave-Feuillet
75016 Paris   Tel. (1)45.24.81.67
                     (1)45.24.81.81
Telex: 620 160 OCDE
Telefax: (33-1)45.24.85.00

Librairie de l'Université
12a, rue Nazareth
13602 Aix-en-Provence   Tel. 42.26.18.08

Germany – Allemagne
OECD Publications and Information Centre
4 Simrockstrasse
5300 Bonn   Tel. (0228)21.60.45
Telex: 8 86300 Bonn
          Telefax: (0228)26.11.04

Greece – Grèce
Librairie Kauffmann
28 rue du Stade
105 64 Athens   Tel. 322.21.60
Telex: 218187 LIKA Gr

Hong Kong
Swindon Book Co. Ltd.
13 - 15 Lock Road
Kowloon, Hongkong   Tel. 366 80 31
Telex: 50 441 SWIN HX
Telefax: 739 49 75

Iceland – Islande
Mal Mog Menning
Laugavegi 18, Postholf 392
121 Reykjavik   Tel. 15199/24240

India – Inde
Oxford Book and Stationery Co.
Scindia House
New Delhi 110001   Tel. 331.5896/5308
Telex: 31 61990 AM IN
Telefax: (11)332.5993
17 Park Street
Calcutta 700016   Tel. 240832

Indonesia – Indonésie
Pdii-Lipi
P.O. Box 269/JKSMG/88
Jakarta 12790   Tel. 583467
Telex: 62 875

Ireland – Irlande
TDC Publishers - Library Suppliers
12 North Frederick Street
Dublin 1   Tel. 744835/749677
Telex: 33530 TDCP EI Telefax : 748416

Italy – Italie
Libreria Commissionaria Sansoni
Via Benedetto Fortini, 120/10
Casella Post. 552
50125 Firenze   Tel. (055)645415
Telex: 570466   Telefax: (39.55)641257
Via Bartolini 29
20155 Milano   Tel. 365083
La diffusione delle pubblicazioni OCSE viene
assicurata dalle principali librerie ed anche
da:
Editrice e Libreria Herder
Piazza Montecitorio 120
00186 Roma   Tel. 679.4628
Telex: NATEL I 621427

Libreria Hoepli
Via Hoepli 5
20121 Milano   Tel. 865446
Telex: 31.33.95 Telefax: (39.2)805.2886

Libreria Scientifica
Dott. Lucio de Biasio "Aeiou"
Via Meravigli 16
20123 Milano   Tel. 807679
Telefax: 800175

Japan– Japon
OECD Publications and Information Centre
Landic Akasaka Building
2-3-4 Akasaka, Minato-ku
Tokyo 107   Tel. 586.2016
Telefax: (81.3)584.7929

Korea – Corée
Kyobo Book Centre Co. Ltd.
P.O. Box 1658, Kwang Hwa Moon
Seoul   Tel. (REP)730.78.91
Telefax: 735.0030

**Malaysia/Singapore –
Malaisie/Singapour**
University of Malaya Co-operative Bookshop
Ltd.
P.O. Box 1127, Jalan Pantai Baru 59100
Kuala Lumpur
Malaysia   Tel. 756.5000/756.5425
Telefax: 757.3661

Information Publications Pte. Ltd.
Pei-Fu Industrial Building
24 New Industrial Road No. 02-06
Singapore 1953   Tel. 283.1786/283.1798
Telefax: 284.8875

Netherlands – Pays-Bas
SDU Uitgeverij
Christoffel Plantijnstraat 2
Postbus 20014
2500 EA's-Gravenhage   Tel. (070)78.99.11
Voor bestellingen: Tel. (070)78.98.80
Telex: 32486 stdru   Telefax: (070)47.63.51

New Zealand – Nouvelle-Zélande
Government Printing Office
Customer Services
P.O. Box 12-411
Freepost 10-050
Thorndon, Wellington
Tel. 0800 733-406   Telefax: 04 499-1733

Norway – Norvège
Narvesen Info Center – NIC
Bertrand Narvesens vei 2
P.O. Box 6125 Etterstad
0602 Oslo 6
                Tel. (02)57.33.00
Telex: 79668 NIC N   Telefax: (02)68.19.01

Pakistan
Mirza Book Agency
65 Shahrah Quaid-E-Azam
Lahore 3   Tel. 66839
Telex: 44886 UBL PK. Attn: MIRZA BK

Portugal
Livraria Portugal
Rua do Carmo 70-74
Apart. 2681
1117 Lisboa Codex   Tel. 347.49.82/3/4/5

**Singapore/Malaysia
Singapour/Malaisie**
See "Malaysia/Singapore"
Voir "Malaisie/Singapour"

Spain – Espagne
Mundi-Prensa Libros S.A.
Castello 37, Apartado 1223
Madrid 28001   Tel. (91) 431.33.99
Telex: 49370 MPLI   Telefax: 275 39 98
Libreria Internacional AEDOS
Consejo de Ciento 391
08009 –Barcelona   Tel. (93) 301-86-15
Telefax: (93) 317-01-41

Sweden – Suède
Fritzes Fackboksföretaget
Box 16356, S 103 27 STH
Regeringsgatan 12
DS Stockholm   Tel. (08)23.89.00
Telex: 12387   Telefax: (08)20.50.21
Subscription Agency/Abonnements:
Wennergren-Williams AB
Box 30004
104 25 Stockholm   Tel. (08)54.12.00
Telex: 19937 Telefax: (08)50.82.86

Switzerland – Suisse
OECD Publications and Information Centre
4 Simrockstrasse
5300 Bonn (Germany)   Tel. (0228)21.60.45
Telex: 8 86300 Bonn
Telefax: (0228)26.11.04

Librairie Payot
6 rue Grenus
1211 Genève 11   Tel. (022)731.89.50
Telex: 28356

Maditec S.A.
Ch. des Palettes 4
1020 Renens/Lausanne Tel. (021)635.08.65
Telefax: (021)635.07.80
United Nations Bookshop/Librairie des Na-
tions-Unies
Palais des Nations
1211 Genève 10
          Tel. (022)734.60.11 (ext. 48.72)
Telex: 289696 (Attn: Sales)
Telefax: (022)733.98.79

Taiwan – Formose
Good Faith Worldwide Int'l. Co. Ltd.
9th Floor, No. 118, Sec. 2
Chung Hsiao E. Road
Taipei   Tel. 391.7396/391.7397
Telefax: (02) 394.9176

Thailand – Thaïlande
Suksit Siam Co. Ltd.
1715 Rama IV Road, Samyan
Bangkok 5   Tel. 251.1630

Turkey – Turquie
Kültur Yayinlari Is-Türk Ltd. Sti.
Atatürk Bulvari No. 191/Kat. 21
Kavaklidere/Ankara   Tel. 25.07.60
Dolmabahce Cad. No. 29
Besiktas/Istanbul   Tel. 160.71.88
Telex: 43482B

United Kingdom – Royaume-Uni
HMSO
Gen. enquiries   Tel. (071) 873 0011
Postal orders only:
P.O. Box 276, London SW8 5DT
Personal Callers HMSO Bookshop
49 High Holborn, London WC1V 6HB
Telex: 297138 Telefax: 071 873 8463
Branches at: Belfast, Birmingham, Bristol,
Edinburgh, Manchester

United States – États-Unis
OECD Publications and Information Centre
2001 L Street N.W., Suite 700
Washington, D.C. 20036-4095
                Tel. (202)785.6323
Telefax: (202)785.0350

Venezuela
Libreria del Este
Avda F. Miranda 52, Aptdo. 60337
Edificio Galipan
Caracas 106
          Tel. 951.1705/951.2307/951.1297
Telegram: Libreste Caracas

Yugoslavia – Yougoslavie
Jugoslovenska Knjiga
Knez Mihajlova 2, P.O. Box 36
Beograd   Tel. 621.992
Telex: 12466 jk bgd

Orders and inquiries from countries where
Distributors have not yet been appointed
should be sent to: OECD Publications
Service, 2 rue André-Pascal, 75775 Paris
Cedex 16, France.
Les commandes provenant de pays où
l'OCDE n'a pas encore désigné de dis-
tributeur devraient être adressées à : OCDE,
Service des Publications, 2, rue André-
Pascal, 75775 Paris Cedex 16, France.

6/90

OECD PUBLICATIONS, 2 rue André-Pascal, 75775 PARIS CEDEX 16
PRINTED IN FRANCE
(81 89 05 1) ISBN 92-64-13310-0 - No. 44985 1990